ST ANDREW'S HOSPITAL NORTHAMPTON

THE FIRST 150 YEARS

(1838–1988)

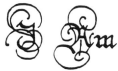

I Am

I am: yet what I am none cares nor knows,
My friends forsake me like a memory lost;
I am the self-consumer of my woes,
They rise and vanish an oblivious host,
Shadows of life whose very soul is lost;
And yet I am, I live tho', I am tossed
Into the nothingness of scorn and noise,
Into the living sea of waking dream,
Where there is neither sense of life nor joys,
But the huge shipwreck of my own esteem
And all that's dear — even those I loved the best
Are strange — nay, they are rather stranger
than the rest.

I long for scenes where man has never trod,
Scenes where woman never smiled nor wept,
And there to abide with my creator — God,
And to sleep as I in childhood sweetly slept;
Full of high thoughts unborn, so let me lie;
The grass below — above the vaulted sky.

John Clare

ST ANDREW'S HOSPITAL NORTHAMPTON

THE FIRST 150 YEARS
(1838–1988)

ARTHUR FOSS AND KERITH TRICK

GRANTA EDITIONS

GRANTA EDITIONS

© St Andrew's Hospital 1989
ISBN 0 906782 44 9

Published by Granta Editions
47 Norfolk Street, Cambridge CB1 2LE

Design by Jim Reader
Jacket design by Alan Moore
Design and production in association with
Book Production Consultants, Cambridge
Printed in Great Britain at The Bath Press, Avon

CONTENTS

ILLUSTRATIONS

PREFACE

*C*urrent policy in the management of mental illness is directed to treating the patient in the community. Most of the large mental hospitals which began their life as county asylums in the 1850s are scheduled to close. As this movement develops momentum, predictable problems are becoming apparent and a number of institutions designed to contain the more disturbed and disturbing patients are being opened. It is in this period of change and uncertainty that St Andrew's celebrates its 150th anniversary, and this seems an appropriate time to review its history.

St Andrew's foundation, prior to the statutory requirement that counties built asylums, reflected the philanthropic views of some of the country's leading families and the willingness of the public at large to contribute sums of money to its establishment and maintenance.

The development of the hospital reflected the views of its Medical Superintendents, supported by successive generations of Governors, who have given unstintingly of their time and energy. The Medical Superintendents in turn reflected the views and attitudes of their professional peers and the constraints of knowledge and available techniques.

A hospital, however, is not merely a setting for medical treatments; it is also a complex social structure, influencing and being influenced by the society in which it exists. This volume attempts to record some of the attitudes and activities of those charged with the treatment of the mentally disordered from 1838 to 1988.

INTRODUCTION

*T*his is a history of the first 150 years of St Andrew's Hospital, Northampton, which was opened in 1838 under the name of the Northampton General Lunatic Asylum; it was renamed after St Andrew forty years later. Its foundation was the result of the united efforts of the nobility, gentry, clergy and the professional and commercial classes of county and town. Its establishment reflects both the regeneration of Christian values and sentiments aroused by the horrors of the Industrial Revolution, and the slow change in climate, starting in the mid eighteenth century, from indifference to caring, marked by the gradual ending of restraint in asylums and the promotion of 'moral treatment', first introduced by the Quakers at their York Retreat during the Regency.

Several hospitals for lunatics were opened during the second half of the eighteenth century, but it was the 2nd Earl Spencer of Althorp who, as Home Secretary, 1806–7, initiated an inquiry into the situation of 'the Criminal and Pauper Lunatics in England'. The resulting County Asylum Act of 1808 recommended but did not make it obligatory for each county to establish an asylum for lunatics to be financed from the local rates; it was not until 1845, that a comprehensive Bill making it compulsory for each county to set up its own asylum for pauper lunatics received the royal assent. The legal regulations, which have moulded the way in which the mentally sick have been increasingly caringly treated, are here covered in sufficient detail to explain why the Hospital has developed in the way it has, for St Andrew's was erected, not through the rates, but by public subscription and has been a charity from its inception. At first it took both private paying patients and a percentage of pauper lunatics from the parishes. The fees from the private patients made possible the development of the Hospital's facilities and gave support to many in Northamptonshire who had successfully maintained themselves while able to work but who, if inflicted with insanity, would otherwise except for St Andrew's have suffered the undeserved indignities of pauper status.

The Governors, among whom the local clergy were strongly represented, were interested in character as well as charity. John Stuart Mill wrote: 'The worth of a State in the long run is the worth of the individuals composing it'. According to Samuel Smiles, who quoted Mill's aphorism at the head of his first chapter of *Self-Help*, first drafted soon after the opening of St Andrew's, 'the spirit of self-help is the root of all genuine growth in the individual . . . . Help from without is often enfeebling in its effects, but help from within invariably invigorates'. These sentiments were probably shared by the majority of those who contributed to and served the Hospital so well in its formative years. The support of the deserving poor was a corner-stone of their philosophy.

As a result of the 1845 Bill, the Commissioners in Lunacy exerted increasing pressure first to convert St Andrew's into the county asylum for paupers and then, when the Governors refused to abandon their charitable intentions, to force the local magistrates to build a separate county asylum. By 1876, the latter course had been achieved and the paupers withdrawn from St Andrew's.

From then onwards, the Governors have concentrated on the pursuit of excellence; not only have they continued to give charitable support to deserving cases but they have sought out, both in Britain and overseas, the latest developments in psychiatric medicine. Their membership has come from a wide cross-section of the local community and their names and achievements are an essential part of this history. In particular, there is pride in those families who in successive generations have taken a keen and continuing interest in the Hospital's work. Among the present Governors are descendants of those who helped found St Andrew's. Many, who have served the Institution, have been well-known in other fields.

Of outstanding importance has been the role played by the Superintendents. Each of them has introduced new vigour and new ideas and the Hospital's success reflects their strength of character, enterprise and dedication. Care was consistently taken to adopt new ideas as soon as they had been thoroughly tested and much of this has been reflected in the living conditions of the patients. Attention has also been paid to staff at all levels and their working conditions. Also recorded are the legal, social and economic problems which have had to be surmounted: the differences which occasionally emerged in the Victorian era between county land-owners and the Northampton town community and between the established Church and Nonconformism are also part of this history.

The authors have been given full access to the Hospital's archives and acknowledge their debt to the writings of Kathleen Jones, Denis Leigh and Andrew T. Scull. They are grateful to the staff of the Northampton Public Library for their help.

The letters of John Clare quoted in Chapter 7 are copyright © Eric Robinson 1985. 'I AM' by John Clare is copyright © Eric Robinson 1967; these are all reproduced by kind permission of Curtis Brown Ltd. We gratefully acknowledge permission from Northamptonshire Libraries to publish material from manuscripts in their possession.

Chapter One

THE ORIGINS OF THE GENERAL LUNATIC ASYLUM, LATER ST ANDREW'S HOSPITAL, NORTHAMPTON

T he first mention of providing 'accommodation for lunatics' in Northampton was in 1789. The occasion was a meeting of the Governors of the Northampton General Infirmary to give serious consideration to erecting a new, purpose-built hospital, as the original Infirmary, opened in George Row in 1744, was no longer large enough to cope with the demand for room. The Infirmary had first been raised by the leading citizens of the county and town in 1743 and was supported entirely by voluntary donations; it was governed by the subscribers who were responsible for drawing up and, when necessary, amending its rules and statutes. It was open to all poor persons who could produce tickets provided by subscribers, a pattern which was to be largely followed by the Northampton General Lunatic Asylum when it became established some fifty years later.

The Governors of the Infirmary acquired eight acres on the Billing Road for their new building, the site of the present Northampton General Hospital. They decided, however, against including room for lunatics because it was thought that mentally disturbed patients would prove too noisy for the physically ill.

Then in March 1804, some fifteen years later, an unusual bequest was received by the Committee of the Infirmary, whose president was the 2nd Earl Spencer, later to play a highly important role in legislation regarding the insane when he was Home Secretary in 1806–7. This was the gift of £100 from an anonymous donor on condition that 'the interest of the money be applied to the annual purpose of the charity, and if it meets with the approbation of the Governors that the principal be reserved towards their design of making a provision for persons of disordered mind, when a suitable opportunity shall offer itself'.

In September 1806, the Treasurer of the Infirmary reported that he had received a letter from the Rev. J. Wye, recently appointed to the living of Wootton, asking 'Whether there be already established a ward for the reception of lunatics, if not, whether such a plan be in contemplation', and offering one hundred guineas 'whenever there is a probability that such a plan may be carried into execution'.

These two offers illustrated how at the beginning of the nineteenth century the established, educated classes were becoming slowly but increasingly aware of the plight of the poor, especially those afflicted with insanity. At this time both the Agricultural and the Industrial Revolutions were in full swing. The population had begun to grow steadily as medical knowledge increased and the death-rate reduced. This in turn led to improved food production on the great estates to meet increased demand. The need for more food led to enclosures of common land and the eviction of the small tenant farmers and independent yeomen who had depended on it for their livelihood. By the time Queen Victoria came to the throne, over half of Northamptonshire had been enclosed.

The now landless labourers who, until they lost their rights, had been able to cope with their sick, were now forced to search for work in the new, ramshackle towns of the Industrial Revolution where conditions made it increasingly difficult to maintain such family obligations. Their plight became even worse with the collapse of the labour market at the end of the Napoleonic Wars. Whereas the lives of the rural poor had in many areas been cushioned by the paternal benevolence of the traditional landowning hierarchy, those in the new industrial areas were at the mercy of the factory owners, intent only on uncontrolled profits.

The machinery to deal with the insane paupers was still that laid down by the Elizabethan Poor Law Acts of 1597 and 1601. These had been introduced as a result both of the enclosures in the late Tudor period and of the dissolution of the monasteries. Before the reign of Henry VIII, those insane who had not been looked after by their families were often given succour by the religious houses. When these no longer existed, the sick and elderly of families displaced by the enclosures, became a financial burden on their local community. These two Acts imposed on each parish the obligation to raise a rate for its needy and worthy poor. These funds were used for household relief or for care in almshouses, often established as private charities. For the more rebellious, including those who refused to work and the more dangerous lunatics, there was the county Bridewell (house of correction) or the common jail.

These Acts were later confirmed by Charles II's Act of Settlement in 1662. The system became the responsibility of the unpaid Justices of the Peace, who were nominally appointed by the Crown, but in practice by the Lord-Lieutenant of the County. The Justices understandably reflected the thinking of the local gentry who were usually anxious that the poor rate be kept as low as possible, an attitude still evident during the early years of the Northampton General Lunatic Asylum.

The situation of the insane was at its bleakest in the first half of the eighteenth century. Emphasis was on confinement, not cure. What treatment there was, consisted of blood-letting, purging and emetics. Medical practice was based on the theories of classical authors, rarely on clinical experiment and observation. Expense was held to a minimum, especially in the private madhouses. Because the staff, kept as small as possible, were usually of the lowest calibre and ill-paid accordingly, restraint on inmates was often savage, sometimes achieved through a poor diet which, combined with bleeding and purging, left them too weak to become a nuisance. There was, in any case, no distinction between paupers afflicted with insanity and other vagrants until this was established by the 1744 Vagrancy Act.

During the second half of the eighteenth century came the first signs of a change of attitude towards the insane. Several new mental hospitals were founded in which attempts were made to restrict restraints and to effect cures. Attention was also paid to the horrors of the private madhouses, as a result of a scandal, publicised by an article in the *Gentleman's Magazine* in January 1763, which revealed how quite sane people were unlawfully confined in them with the connivance of their relatives. The Act for Regulating Private Madhouses of 1774 established five important principles:

1. Private institutions run for profit must be licensed by a public authority.
2. The reception by a madhouse of a person alleged to be insane must be recorded.
3. Madhouses must be visited by Commissioners who were to be appointed by procedures laid down by Parliament.
4. There must be inspection to ensure that those wrongfully detained were released and those rightfully detained were treated humanely.
5. There must be supervision by the medical profession.

A further impetus to the public interest in, and concern about the treatment of, the insane was given by the madness of George III. His sovereignty did not protect him from the bullying, the restraints, the cauterising irons and the vomiting and purging medicines which the more enlightened practitioners were beginning to eschew.

Perhaps the most influential institution for the care and treatment of the insane was The Retreat, founded at York in 1792 by the Society of Friends. Its name was chosen to suggest 'a quiet haven in which the shattered bark might find the means of reparation or of safety'. William Tuke, the first Superintendent, evolved with Dr Thomas Fowles a therapeutic approach, which became known as 'moral treatment', 'moral' at that time being roughly equivalent in this context to what would now be called 'psychological'. Having found the standard treatments then advocated ineffective, they instituted a humanitarian regime. Patients were never punished for failure to restrain themselves but there were extra amenities for those who showed improved self-control. Patients were encouraged to dress well, attend tea parties given by the female Superintendent, to garden, read, sew and take an interest in domestic animals. Medical treatment took second place to good food, exercise and occupation. The Retreat being a Quaker organisation, the staff was of a much higher calibre than those usually associated with mental asylums. As a result, The Retreat became renowned not only in Britain but in Europe as well.

So it was that by the beginning of the nineteenth century, there was coming into being a far more Christian and caring attitude, together with a growing feeling of responsibility, towards the insane, especially towards the deserving, hard-working poor. A leading Benthamite, interested in lunacy reform – and there were now several groups working in this field – was Sir George Onesiphorus Paul, Bt, High Sheriff of Gloucestershire. In 1806, he wrote to the Home Secretary, the 2nd Earl Spencer, proposing that the government should establish tax-supported district asylums for pauper and criminal lunatics: 'I believe there is hardly a parish of any considerable extent in which there may not be found some unfortunate creature of this descripton who, if his ill-treatment has made him phrenetic, is chained in the cellar or garret of a workhouse, fastened to the leg of a table, tied to a post in an outhouse, or perhaps shut up in an uninhabited ruin; or, if his lunacy is inoffensive, left to ramble half-naked and half-starved through the streets and highways, teased by the scoff and jest of all that is vulgar, ignorant and unfeeling'.

It was a timely letter and Lord Spencer acted at once. In January 1807, he appointed a Select Committee 'to enquire into the State of Criminal and Pauper Lunatics in England, and the laws relating thereto'. A leading figure was Charles Williams-Wynn, then Under-Secretary of State for the Home Department; others included Samuel Romilly, William Whitbread and William Wilberforce, all three of them well-known reformers. The Select Committee's report was published that year, but the County Asylum Act of 1808, 'for the better Care and Maintenance of Lunatics, being Paupers or Criminals in England', was passed after Lord Spencer had left office. Known as Wynn's Law, it implemented the main recommendations of the Committee, which was that each county should establish an asylum to which pauper and criminal lunatics might be sent.

These asylums were to be financed out of the local rates and governed by a committee of local Justices of the Peace, who were to be responsible for their erection and for periodical inspection. The Justices, who were not to derive personal advantage from any asylum contract, were empowered to raise a county rate for this purpose and to invite voluntary subscriptions. Detailed guidance was given on the choice of site, the separation of male from female patients, the need for separate wards for convalescents and incurables, 'and also separate and distinct Day Rooms and Airing Grounds for the Male and Female Convalescents and dry and airy Cells for Lunatics of every Description'. Dangerous or criminal lunatics were to be admitted on a warrant from two Justices.

Here, potentially, was a great step forward. The importance of the Act was its conclusion that, not only was there a need to deal with the problem of insanity itself, but also that this should be a public responsibility. The Act did not place a statutory duty upon the county authorities to erect asylums and its effectiveness was therefore limited; only nine were built during the next twenty years, partly because of the reluctance of local magistrates to raise the necessary funds. The first to be established was at Nottingham in 1810. Built to accommodate some eighty patients, it became badly overcrowded within a year. An amendment to the 1808 Act was therefore passed in 1811, giving discretionary powers to the magistrates to grant or withhold warrants for the admission of patients, depending upon the availability of accommodation.

Meanwhile, the Court of Governors of the Northampton Infirmary, encouraged by the passing of the County Asylum Act of 1808, decided in July 1809 to hold a special Court in the following September 'for the purpose', according to an announcement in the local Press, 'of taking into Consideration the Expediency and Propriety of joining with the County of Northampton in the Erection and Establishment of a LUNATIC ASYLUM under the provisions of an Act of Parliament lately passed for that Purpose'. The notice was signed by Edward Bouverie of Delapré Abbey, whose uncle was created Earl of Radnor. Bouverie, who was for a time MP for Northampton, was to play a major role throughout the early history of the General Lunatic Asylum almost up to his death in 1858. The Special Court, however, resolved unanimously 'that it does not seem expedient to them to do so'. The reason for this was probably fear that subscriptions and donations to the Infirmary might be adversely affected.

Notwithstanding, further gifts were received, including £50 from the 'Parish of Hardington (guaranteed by Edw. Bouverie) . . . to be advanced whenever the Building was decided upon'. By 1814, the fund for the Lunatic Asylum had reached £522.16s.10½d., reported in the local Press as a result of the decision of the Governors of the Infirmary to publish regularly a list of contributions 'in the hope of exciting the Sympathy of the Charitable towards promoting the Erection and Establishment of a GENERAL ASYLUM FOR LUNATICS in some eligible situation at a convenient Distance from the Site of the present Infirmary'. A book for recording subscriptions was also opened at the Infirmary. The notice, dated 22 October 1814, was signed by H. Harday, Secretary of the General Infirmary, who later became Secretary of the Asylum.

1814 also saw the establishment of a Sub-Committee to investigate the way in which the sums already donated had been invested and the interest used. It was found that the wishes of the donors had not always been followed and in due course £261.4s.10d. was used to purchase Government Securities. Lord Althorp, W. R. Cartwright, Lord Compton and William Hanbury, then the Parliamentary Representatives for the County and Town, were appointed Trustees of this fund. It was also agreed that subsequent gifts should be similarly invested.

Further donations included an anonymous one of £2.10s., 'being an Ebenezer Gift on completing fifty years', and £8.0s. found in Northampton with the request that this sum be advertised and, if not claimed, added to the fund. Much later, in 1826, the Treasurer was sent a letter anonymously from London, containing the halves of five £100 notes with the instruction to advertise their receipt in the *Northampton Mercury*. The donor promised to send the remaining halves when he saw that this had been done.

Throughout the second and third decades of the nineteenth century, increasing publicity was given to the ill-treatment of the mentally sick. In 1815, a Parliamentary Select Committee was instructed to examine the situation and produced a number of reports. One revealed the dreadful conditions at the Bethlem Hospital, the oldest asylum in England, originally founded in 1247, where visitors could up to 1770 watch the antics of the inmates for a few pence. Here patients were found to be confined in rooms with only shutters to exclude the winter. The more troublesome were chained to their beds or the wall and many were virtually naked except for a blanket over their shoulders.

A further report in 1816 revealed even worse conditions in the private madhouses. Bills were drafted by supporters of reform in the House of Commons in 1816, 1817 and 1819 with the aim of setting up an efficient inspectorate to cover both madhouses and single lunatics but the House of Lords rejected every attempt. Their Lordships' attitude was clearly expressed by Lord Chancellor Eldon when he said: 'There could be no

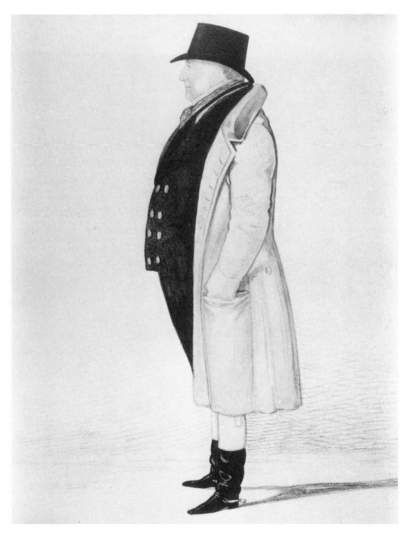

Sir William Wake, 9th Bt. (1768–1846), from the portrait by Richard Deighton.

more false humanity than an over-humanity with regard to persons afflicted with insanity'.

In 1827, another Select Committee investigated the appalling conditions still prevalent in the private madhouses. Its membership included young Lord Ashley, later the 7th Earl of Shaftesbury, who carried through the 1845 Lunatics Act, and Lord Althorp, who was Chancellor of the Exchequer from 1830 to 1834, the year he succeeded his father as 3rd Earl Spencer and became greatly involved in the formation and administration of St Andrew's until his death in 1845. Two Bills emerged in 1828 from their deliberations. The County Asylums Act instructed visiting Justices to make annual returns of admissions, discharges and deaths to the Home Secretary, who was empowered to have asylums inspected as considered necessary; this was the first move towards bringing all institutions for the insane under central control. The Madhouses Act introduced regular inspections by visiting Justices of both private madhouses and subscription hospitals with the power to grant and to recommend withdrawal of licenses. Each institution had to provide regular medical attention, keep detailed records for inspection by the visiting Justices and apply restraint only on the instructions of a qualified medical attendant.

It was in the same year, 1828, that the Governors of the Northampton Infirmary were informed at a public meeting at the George Inn by Sir William Wake, 9th Bt., of Courteenhall, that the subscribers to the Northamptonshire Yeomanry, formed during the Napoleonic Wars and now disbanded, had decided that the surplus fund of £6,000 should be given to the Asylum fund.

By February 1833, the total sum raised to build the Asylum had reached £12,038.18s.9d. The Governors accordingly resolved to recommend to the Grand Jury at the next Lent Assizes that a public meeting be called 'to consider the expediency of commencing the erection of a Lunatic Asylum by voluntary subscription'. It was obviously intended that this establishment should be independent of the county authorities. The Grand Jury's reaction was that 'such an application would be at present premature' and they were 'very fearful that the General Infirmary might suffer from such an undertaking at the present time'. This was not, however, the end of the project, but merely the end of the beginning.

Chapter Two

THE ESTABLISHMENT OF THE GENERAL

LUNATIC ASYLUM

*I*n spite of the reaction of the Grand Jury in 1833, the Governors of the Northampton Infirmary set up a Sub-Committee to plan the Asylum. On 14 July 1834, they decided to acquire at auction the freehold of 21½ acres of the estate of the late Robert Harding, situated off the Billing Road in an area once occupied by the St Andrew Priory, a Cluniac foundation of 1100, from which the Hospital's present name is taken. The site cost £2,900 and, finally, the decision to erect the Asylum was taken at a public meeting on 17 October of that year.

That some thirty years elapsed from the receipt of the first donation until this decision was taken, is symptomatic of those troubled years: first the Napoleonic Wars, followed by the Luddite Riots, the Chartist Movement and, in 1832, the passing of the first Reform Bill. The advance of humanitarianism was slow. In 1816, a law was introduced whereby a starving cottager could be transported for life if caught at night with nets for snaring hares and rabbits. It was legal until 1827 to protect pheasant reserves with hidden mantraps and firing guns which could kill or maim the innocent as well as those guilty of poaching.

By the 1830s, compassion for the state, both physical and spiritual, of the oppressed and incapable was widespread as exemplified by the many charitable organisations mentioned in the local press. There were, among others, the 'Institute for the Deaf and the Blind', a charity to help the 'Distressed Highlanders and Islanders of Scotland', the 'Peterborough Diocesan Association for Promoting the Enlargement and the Building of Churches and Chapels' and the 'National Society for Educating the Poor in the Principles of the Established Church of

England', the lead usually taken by the landowning magnates of the county. It was thus the 3rd Baron Lilford who took the chair at the meeting of 17 October 1834, when the 10th Earl of Westmorland, KG, Lord-Lieutenant of the County, was elected Perpetual President of the proposed Institution; from then onwards it has been the Hospital's tradition that the Lord-Lieutenant down to the present incumbent of that office, John Lowther of Guilsborough Court, should be its President. The following were then elected Vice-Presidents:

The 5th Duke of Buccleuch and Queensberry
The 4th Duke of Grafton
The 2nd Marquess of Northampton
The 2nd Earl Spencer
The 5th Earl Fitzwilliam
Viscount Althorp, MP, later the 3rd Earl Spencer
Viscount Brudenell, MP
Viscount Milton, MP
The Bishop of Peterborough
The 3rd Baron Southampton
The 3rd Baron Lilford
W. R. Cartwright, Esq., MP

The principal advocate in favour of establishing the Asylum was the Rev. Dr George Butler, later Dean of Peterborough. He explained that £13,226 had by then been received, including the Yeomanry donation which had now increased to £7,000. Out of this total, £2,900 had been spent in purchasing the land. The cost of fitting out a hospital for about one hundred patients would be £20,000 so that a further £10,000 would be needed. As for objections about timing, these could always be said to apply in some degree. The building of the Infirmary had taken place at an even more unfavourable time, but it was now flourishing. The motion was carried in spite of one or two objections, after Edward Bouverie had moved that books be opened for receiving subscriptions. A further £800 was immediately raised or promised. It was also agreed that the Asylum should be completely independent of the Infirmary.

In its editorial of the following week, the *Northampton Mercury*, which supported the Liberal cause, warmly favoured the enterprise and showed considerable understanding of the problem of the pauper lunatic.

Of all benevolent institutions [it declared], a Lunatic Asylum seems most free from the objection which has occasionally been urged against charities for the relief of the poor – that the direct good they produce is counterbalanced by indirect and injurious consequences – that the prospect that they hold out of gratuitous assistance tends to foster those habits of improvidence to which the lower classes are without doubt peculiarly tempted. Against a calamity of so overwhelming a nature as insanity no degree of forethought, no previous economy, however rigid, on the part of the poor man, can enable him to make provision . . .

The expense of procuring a proper keeper, added to the difficulty of providing any place where the insane person can be safely secured, makes it in general impossible to retain him among his connexions. Unless, therefore, the very objectionable practice is resorted to of placing him in a workhouse, he is generally sent to one of those larger establishments, which exist in various parts of the country for the reception of lunatics of the poorer classes. Many of our readers will recollect the disclosures which took place some years ago, of the wretched treatment to which the inmates of some of these madhouses were subjected. The regulations which have been subsequently enforced by the Legislature for the licensing and inspection of all houses for the reception of the insane, afford, we are willing to believe, an effectual check against the recurrence of cruelty and neglect such as were then brought to light. But no precautions, which mere law can create, will completely remove the objections to this mode of disposing of the pauper lunatic. The proprietors of such houses are doubtless persons of not less natural humanity than others. But their feelings unavoidably become blunted by the constant sight of human nature in its most degraded form, and their interests are strongly at variance with their duties. They in general receive a fixed weekly or quarterly sum for boarding and clothing the patient and providing medical assistance and of course their profits directly depend upon the smallness of the cost at which they can comply with these conditions. They are therefore, strongly tempted to feed and clothe scantily the unfortunate beings committed to their charge, to provide an inadequate supply of medical and other attendance, and to crowd into their houses the utmost number of patients permitted by law. On the other hand, the distance of the connexions of the lunatics in the vast majority of cases renders it impossible that they should exercise any control over the conduct of the proprietor and his agents . . . it can hardly be doubted that instances, if not of positive cruelty, at least of culpable negligence and penurious treatment, will frequently occur. It must be borne in mind that lunacy is a disease eminently dependent for its relief upon the moral no less than the purely medical discipline to which the patient is subjected.

The *Mercury* ended by hoping that, in the unlikely circumstances of serious difficulties preventing the raising of the necessary money, the magistrates of the county would supply the extra sum required out of the county rates.

> Undoubtedly it is undesirable to increase without urgent necessity the burdens which already press heavily upon the occupiers of land. But even as a question of economy, we doubt whether the cost of maintaining an Asylum, added to the interest of the money sunk in the erection, would much exceed the aggregate of the expenses at this moment incurred by various parishes of the country in the support of the pauper lunatics. And when an indisputable good is to be effected, and a large amount of human suffering alleviated, by the expenditure of a few thousands of public money, economy itself ceases to be a duty.

At another public meeting on 9 April 1835, held again at the George with the 3rd Lord Spencer in the chair, it was again agreed to set about erecting an asylum without further delay, 'upon a plan which will admit of enlargement when necessary'. The meeting had been encouraged by Lord Fitzwilliam, who said that the York Asylum was able to support itself, and by Mr William Collins who reported that the Hanwell Asylum, Middlesex, had a surplus of £7,000 at the end of its first two years, in spite of the fact that this asylum was for paupers only, at a rate of 9s. per week; this was 20 per cent lower than the parishes had been accustomed to pay to private institutions. A Special Committee was appointed to procure plans and estimates for a building eventually to accommodate a hundred patients; its members were:

The Earl Fitzwilliam
The Earl of Euston (later the 5th Duke of Grafton)
Sir William Wake, 9th Bt.
The Rev. Sir George Robinson, 7th Bt.
W. R. Cartwright, MP
Edward Bouverie
The Rev. Dr Butler
Dr Robertson
Dr Kerr
C. R. Thornton
Langham Christie
L. H. Forbes
A. A. Young

William Collins
John and Samuel Percival

Details about these plans were circulated to 'different persons of property connected with the county'.

It was forthwith decided to advertise in the local and the London Press for architects to submit plans for the proposed Asylum. Later that month, the following notice was published:

To Architects
It being in contemplation to erect a Lunatic Asylum near Northampton for the accommodation of fifty pauper patients and twenty class patients. Such Architects as are desirous of engaging in the undertaking are invited to send or produce plans and specifications on or before Tuesday, the 19th of May next. The class patients for whom it is wished to provide, are persons of indigent circumstances, but above the need of parochial assistance.

Meanwhile, the land was rented out for a year only and Mr Milne, the borough surveyor, was asked to examine it 'to ascertain the nature of the subsoil as to the probability of its producing material for the building'. Milne, in addition to being borough surveyor, practised as an architect and among his buildings are the old gaol at Brackley (1837), the Hanging Houghton Lodge Farm (1837), which he designed for Sir Justinian Isham, Bt., and the Lodges and Boardroom for the General Infirmary (1844).

Milne did not, however, draw up the original plans for the Asylum. The Minutes of the 11 June 1835 state:

(1)   'that Mr Wallet's plan, providing for the accommodation of 122 patients, be adopted according to the recommendations of the Special Commitee, provided the expense does not exceed £14,500,
(2)   that Mr Milne be directed to prepare specifications according to Mr Wallet's plan,
(3)   that such specifications be laid before the Special Committee by Mr Milne as soon as prepared,
(4)   that Mr Milne be employed to superintend the execution of the work when commenced.

Little else seems to be known of Mr Wallett other than that he had been an apothecary at Bethlem Hospital and left there under a cloud. A note in the Minutes for 8 April 1837 reads:

That Mr George Wallett be appointed the Medical Superintendent and Mrs Wallett the Matron at a salary of two hundred pounds to take effect from Michaelmas.

That one hundred pounds be given to Mr Wallett for the use of his models and for his service previous to the regular commencement of his duties.

The next entry in the Minutes in this connection, accompanied by no explanation, is that of 19 May 1838 which reads:

Resolved that Mr and Mrs Thomas Prichard be appointed Medical Superintendent and Matron.

Thus Mr and Mrs Wallett vanish from the history of St Andrew's.

Not everyone was enthusiastic about building the Asylum immediately. W. R. Cartwright, the Conservative Member of Parliament for Northampton, declared at a public meeting of the subscribers, as reported in the *Northampton Mercury* of 24 October 1835, that in his opinion it would have been advisable to postpone its erection for two or three years until more funds had become available. In any case, all private madhouses were now under the strict control of magistrates at Quarter Sessions so that the possibility of serious misconduct had been materially reduced. Paupers could now be sent to a private asylum for 10s. 6d. a week and, unless the public asylum could offer a lower rate, he did not think that there was much to be gained. However, in view of what had happened, he would give the project his full support.

Lord Spencer in reply believed, according to the *Mercury*, that as soon as it became evident that they were in earnest, there would be many fresh subscriptions. He thought they were running no hazard by proceeding to build directly. It might be true that they might get pauper-patients into other lunatic asylums at nearly the same rate, but he had reason to believe that, because of distance and other objections, parishes were not disposed to resort to them, although they would readily send them to a county asylum. And although, as far as money was concerned, the charity might not be very great yet, in a far more important aspect – in ascertaining the best means of alleviating and preventing so melancholy a calamity – it was a charity of the highest order. He thought, too, that it was a duty which they owed to many subscribers who had come forward on the express understanding that they should begin immediately. Many years had elapsed since the scheme was first proposed, and he hoped that they should all now agree to go actively to work.

A new Committee was elected to deal with the erection of the Asylum; its members were: Lord Northampton, Lord Spencer, the Rev. Sir George Robinson, Edward Bouverie, Dr Robertson, Dr Kerr, The Rev. Dr Butler, and Messrs Samuel Percival, William Collins, William Strong and George Baker, any three of whom could form a quorum. John and Samuel Percival were appointed Treasurers to the Asylum and Mr Harday of the Northampton Infirmary its Secretary. The work was put out to tender and on 9 January 1836, the estimate submitted by John Elliott of Rolls Buildings, Fetter Lane, London, was accepted, subject to satisfactory references.

In the meanwhile, fund-raising activities increased. Of particular interest was the annual morning concert organised for some years at the end of each August on the second day of the races by Mr M'Corkell, a local music teacher. The first took place in 1835 when, according to the *Mercury*, 'the greater number of the most distinguished families in the county were present', and £96.10s.0d. was raised; the whole amount was donated to the Asylum, Mr M'Corkell refusing to accept half, as suggested by Lord Spencer at a public meeting, 'for the risk and trouble which he had incurred in his undertaking'. In 1836 a full list of patrons and stewards for the August concert, over 120 names in all, was published in the local Press. The musical director was Mr Charles M'Corkell of the Royal Academy of Music, son of the organiser; he also arranged the overture to Handel's *Semiramide* for five harps, played by himself and his four sisters. On this occasion, the organisers shared the profits of the concert equally with the Asylum, which gained £35, making a total of over £120 for the two years.

On the afternoon of the 26 May 1836, the foundation stone was laid by Lord Spencer in front of a multitude which, according to the *Mercury*, could 'scarcely have been less than from eight to ten thousand persons on the ground at one time'. In the morning, the Mayor, Corporation and the Pomfret Lodge of Free and Accepted Masons, with deputations from the Leamington, Leicester and other Lodges present at the request of Lord Spencer, himself a prominent Mason, went in procession to All Saints Church, where the sermon, preached by the Hon. and Rev. Henry Watson of Rockingham Castle, lasted nearly an hour. The collecting plates were held by Lord Spencer, Lady Isham, the Rev. Sir George Robinson, Miss Wake, the Hon T. Trevor and Mr T. Bruton, Provincial Grand Treasurer for Staffordshire, when £80 was collected.

According to the Tory *Northampton Herald*,

> The gentry and others then proceeded to the George Hotel to partake of a splendid cold collation . . . Three o'clock had now arrived, and the day being fine thousands were assembled to witness the reforming of the

procession – This shortly took place, and moved slowly up St Giles Street to the scite [sic] of the building in the following order.

Two Trumpeters on horseback
Band of Music
Special Constables   Charity Children   Special Constables
The Mayor and Corporation
The Secretary
The Treasurers
The Under Sheriff
The High Sheriff
Lord Spencer
Masonic Band
Masonic Lodges, in the following order:-
A Band of Music
Tyler with drawn sword
Banner
Visitors not belonging to any Lodge – Two and two
Visiting Lodges
The Pomfret Lodge in the following order:-
Tyler with drawn sword
Entered apprentice Masons – Two and two
Rough Ashlar – carried by a Master Mason
Second Light
Third Light
Master Masons– Two and two
Past Masons – Two and two
Glass Vase
Brass Plate

Silver trowel on Crimson   Mallet carried by an
Velvet cushion   Operative Mason

Architect carrying a Plan of the Intended Building
Two Deacons each carrying a Silver Ewer
Director of Ceremonies, with Cornucopia
Terrestrial globe   Celestial globe
Secretary with the Book of Constitutions carried on
a crimson velvet cushion
Treasurer with the Coins
Junior Warden with Plumb
Banner of the Pomfret Lodge, Steward with Ward on each side

Senior Warden with level

Chaplain

Bible Square and Compass
on a crimson velvet cushion

Steward with Wand		Steward with Wand

The Worshipful Master with Square

Two Stewards with Wands

Inner Guard with drawn Sword

Steward with Wand		Steward with Wand

'On arriving at the ground', reported the *Mercury*, 'the rush of persons anxious to secure a favourable situation for viewing the ceremony was so tremendous, that the order of the procession was entirely broken.' It had originally been intended that admission should be by ticket at one shilling each, but in the event the public were, on the insistence of Lord Spencer, allowed free entry. The *Herald* regretted that 'the arrangements for viewing the ceremony were not of the best description, there being very few of the many thousands present, who were able to obtain a knowledge of what was going on'.

When order had eventually been restored, the start of the ceremony was heralded by a flourish of trumpets. Coins were put into a glass vase which was placed in a cavity under the foundation stone and covered by a brass plate, bearing the inscription:

> The first stone of this building was laid by the Rt. Honourable John
> Charles, Earl Spencer, attended by the Pomfret Lodge of Free and
> Accepted Masons and the Mayor and Corporation of Northampton,
> May 26, 1836.

According to the *Mercury*, 'the silver trowel was then handed to Earl Spencer, who applied the cement; after which the upper stone was lowered by three distinct stops – a flourish of trumpets sounded between each stop'. The plumb-rule, level and square were in succession handed to Lord Spencer by the Master and Wardens of the Pomfret Lodge and the stone properly adjusted. There followed this proclamation by James Marshall, the Worshipful Master:

> In the name of the Great Architect of the Universe, on behalf of the
> Pomfret Lodge of Ancient, Free and Accepted Masons, and by the desire
> of the Right Honourable Earl Spencer, I declare the stone to be properly
> laid.

23

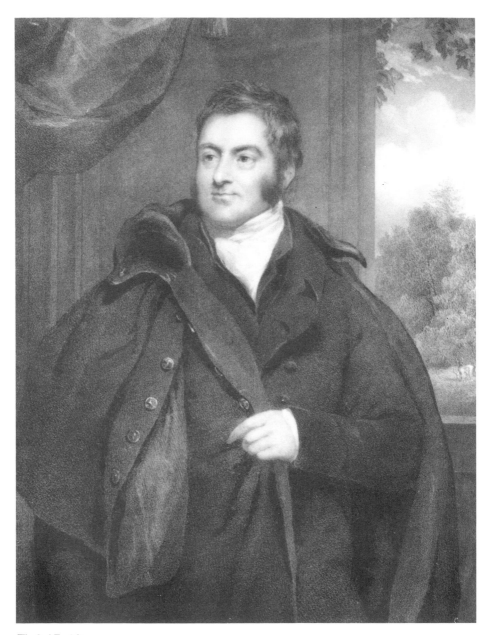

The 3rd Earl Spencer.

The splendour of the stone-laying ceremony was in marked contrast to the opening two years later which went unreported.

By early April 1837, Lord Spencer was able to announce that the external walls and one of the principal staircases had been completed and the roof and most of the doors and windows fixed in position. A considerable sum over and above what had been subscribed was, however, required to complete and furnish the building. It was therefore decided to appeal at once, in the words of the Minutes, 'to those of the Nobility, Gentry, Clergy and others resident in or connected with the County who have not already subscribed and to the public for further contributions in aid of the humane object of the Institute'. It was also agreed that benefactors of £20 and upwards at one time should be Governors for life. In the meanwhile, the Committee was empowered to acquire fixtures and furniture as considered necessary. Statutes and rules for the Asylum were to be drawn up and circulated to subscribers by mid June.

By February 1838, notices inviting tenders for the supply of blankets, sheets and other materials for the Northampton General Lunatic Asylum (this now being its agreed title) appeared in the local Press, details being available by application to Mrs Wallett. It was very soon after this that the Walletts departed as, on 7 April, the local Press advertised vacancies for a Medical Superintendent and a Matron. Candidates 'must have been previously connected with some similar establishment; and with the aim of uniting the two offices, a married Gentleman would be preferred'. These two posts were again advertised on 2 May when the Committee's wish to appoint a Chaplain was also announced. A Special Court was to meet on 19 May to reach a decision. At this meeting, Mr and Mrs Thomas Prichard were chosen, and their joint salary fixed at £200 per annum. The appointment of a Chaplain was deferred.

On Saturday, 26 May, the local Press carried a notice addressed to the Governors of the Northampton General Lunatic Asylum, which read:

My Lords, Ladies and Gentlemen, the flattering result of the Election which took place last Saturday, imposes upon Mrs Prichard and myself the grateful duty of returning our sincerest thanks for the patronage with which we have been honoured; as well as to assure you, that a remembrance of the uniform kindness I experienced during the progress of my canvass, will act as an ever present stimulus to merit its continuance – [signed Thomas Prichard].

On the same day, the Bishop of Chester preached at a service in All Saints Church on behalf of the Asylum which, according to the *Herald*, 'drew together a very numerous and intelligent congregation comprising, in addition to the usual attendance at the church, a large number of the gentry and clergy of the district. The Town Council, the majority of whom are Dissenters, for once laid aside their prejudices, and joined in promoting

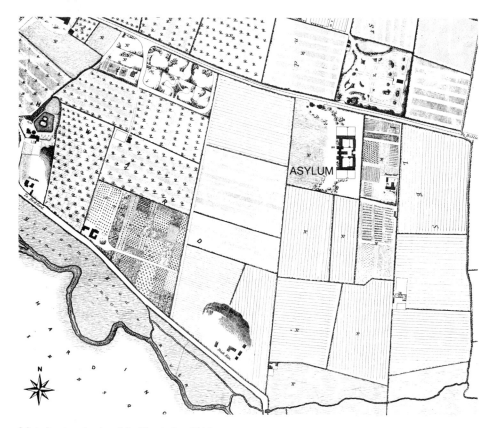

Map showing the site of the Hospital, c.1845.

the object for which the service was designed . . . The discourse of his lordship occupied more than an hour and was listened to with the most profound attention'. The collection raised the large sum of £129.9s.3d.

The Asylum was advertised as being open on the 8 August 1838:

> Strangers will be allowed to visit the Asylum upon being introduced either personally or in writing by a Director . . . And in thus giving an opportunity to persons who feel an interest in the welfare of the Institution, and may wish to inspect its arrangements, it is ultimately to be understoood that they cannot be carried further than is consistent with the personal comfort and privacy of the patients, which must always be preserved.

There was to be no admittance for curiosity or amusement.

Chapter Three

THE ACHIEVEMENTS OF

DR THOMAS PRICHARD

(1838–1844)

T here is no doubt that Thomas Octavius Prichard (1808–47), a Member of the Royal College of Physicians, had unusual intelligence, drive and ambition. He was nominated the first Superintendent of the Asylum in 1838 when only thirty, having already held a similar position at the Glasgow Royal Asylum for two years. Over the next seven he was to establish the reputation of this new Institution in the forefront of its field. He seems to have possessed great gifts of persuasion and, from the notice which he published in the local Press, his 'canvass' of the Governors successfully contributed towards his appointment. He was essentially kind and commanded considerable loyalty from staff and patients. He was however of a somewhat excitable nature, was not always compliant to his employers and on occasion indiscreet in his habits. These were to lay him open to charges of drunkenness which, although probable, were never definitively proved. He also made powerful enemies through his criticism of those parishes which placed their pauper lunatics in the local workhouse for purely economic reasons, only sending them to the Asylum when they were virtually beyond recovery. He was described by G. J. De Wilde, then editor of the *Northampton Mercury*, in a letter printed posthumously in the *The Times Literary Supplement*, 30 June 1921, as a man 'not mad, but just on the other side of that thin partition by which madness is said to be bounded. A tall athletic handsome man, impulsive, energetic, daring, he possessed a peculiar faculty of influencing his patients, even when they were far from his presence'.

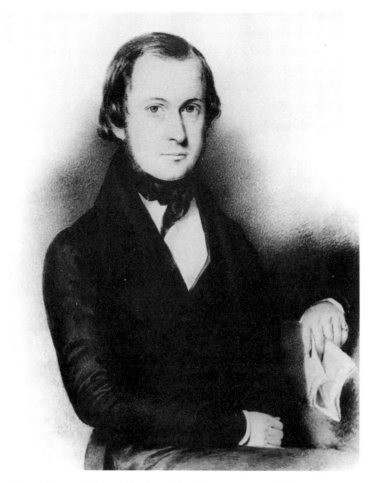

Thomas Octavius Prichard, the first Medical Superintendent, 1838–45.

When Prichard assumed office in 1838, the Asylum was intended to accommodate 70 patients. By January 1844, just before he was first attacked for the apparent neglect of his patients and later for inebriation and accepting outside fees, the number had grown to 261. Throughout the intervening years, he received nothing but praise. The Minutes of 9 July 1840 record: 'it is impossible not to advert to the assiduous care and persevering good management of the Superintendent and Matron and through whose apposite management the finances appear so prosperous'. Both in January and July 1840, the local Press was asked to publish the Directors' satisfaction with them: Mrs Prichard, it should be noted, was, in addition to her duties as Matron, also responsible for bringing up a young family of five. They started with a joint salary of £200 per annum. In 1841, they were voted an increase of £100 per annum which was followed by a similar increment in August 1843 because of their increased duties and 'their continued zeal and ability'. This brought their salary to £400 per annum; in addition they were provided with accommodation, food and service, amounting in all to what was then a handsome income.

The Directors took a close interest in their new Institution. A detailed set of statutes and rules was drawn up, to be adjusted as required. They held Quarterly Courts, and the Annual General Meeting took place at the end of August until 1855, subsequently in February, when a Committee of Management was elected for the following year. This Committee met monthly or more frequently as necessary and appointed Sub-Committees to deal with special projects or problems. It was agreed in September 1839 that no serving member of the Management Committee should supply goods or receive any emolument.

Members appear to have given generously of their time. In addition, a rota of members, whose names were published, undertook to visit the Asylum regularly over specific periods and to report on conditions. This was a measure warmly welcomed by Prichard. In his second Annual Report, 1839–40, he wrote that: 'an infallible remedy for these evils [i.e. the ill-treatment of patients] and an efficient source of further improvement, are alike to be found in the constant inspection of "insane establishments" by the *intelligent visitor* . . . opportunity has thus been afforded for enquiry, the rectification of erroneous impressions, and the rescue of commonsense from the thraldom of misrepresentation, too frequently promoted for the basest purposes. This increase of public intelligence has reacted most favourably; and institutions, once esteemed merely lunatic prisons, have in proportion to their exposure to this salutary influence, assumed characteristics more suitable to their position as *instruments of care*'.

The Superintendent had overall medical and administrative responsibility for the Asylum. The growth in the number of patients must have made it increasingly difficult for him to give detailed medical attention regularly to each individual. This situation appears to have been recognised to some extent by the Directors. In October 1838, he was given permission to call in a physician or a surgeon when considered necessary. In January 1839, having pointed out that his domestic duties, added to the medical and moral treatment of his patients, were more than he could handle with credit to himself and to the Institution, he was allowed to take on as Medical Assistant, but without pay, his cousin, Thomas Prichard, MD, who had then completed his training; the excellence of his work was soon recognised and rewarded accordingly. The family presence was further augmented in July 1841 when William Prichard, a brother of Thomas, was admitted as a trainee pupil. There were other additions to the qualified medical staff: in November 1842, for example, Prichard was authorised to engage a Mr Peter Titley as Medical Assistant at an annual salary of £35. He was allowed to arrange regular visits to the Asylum by medical students for a small fee to gain experience. He was also expected to liaise with other asylums through correspondence and by visits: he was away for a week in April 1840 for this purpose and was allowed £5 towards his expenses.

In July 1841, the Committee expressed thanks to Samuel Tuke of the York Retreat for the gift of 'a valuable work on the Construction and Management of Lunatic Asylums with introductory observations by himself', presumably his *Description of The Retreat, York*, 1813. In November of the following year, Dr Powell, Medical Superintendent of the Nottingham Asylum, was thanked for sending a model of its padded cell. No doubt Prichard was the contact responsible for these communications.

Prichard's outstanding contribution to the history of St Andrew's and to the development of psychiatry was his abolition of all mechanical restraint. A reduction in restraint, whenever possible, had already been practised to a growing extent at The Retreat, York, at the Hanwell Asylum in Middlesex and at the much smaller Lincoln Hospital, the last under Dr Robert Gardiner Hill, who had also in 1838 abolished the use of chains, handcuffs, strait-waistcoats and other mechanical devices. It was Gardiner Hill who wrote in 1857 that 'the first person who adopted the [non-restraint] system in its full extent was the late Dr T. O. Prichard of the Northampton Asylum'. He added: 'I had the pleasure of his acquaintance, and had many opportunities of observing the satisfactory way in which he and Mrs Prichard conducted the Institution.'

Prichard described non-restraint as Dr R. G. Hill's system. Several years later, reporting on events in 1838, he stated that:

Many difficulties and apparent dangers interposed to check our adoption of Mr R. G. Hill's system; an unfinished building, numerous workmen employed in every direction, the inexperience and timidity of the attendants – few in number, in consequence of a prevalent disinclination to enter into our service – all contributed, during the first year, to add to the anxieties of direction and thwart my intentions, as well as to excite occasional doubts of their practicability. These impediments have long been surmounted, for they but stimulated repeated exertion and more extended enquiry; and we have the gratification of knowing that similar results have rewarded the labours of the majority of the superintendents of the largest and most celebrated hospitals in the kingdom; and that unanimity of opinion on this vital question is rapidly pervading not only our own country, but also the great continents of Europe and America.

Once more, in his second Annual Report, Prichard explained in some detail the reasoning leading to this decision. He did not believe that 'moral depravity is the *essential* cause of madness' nor 'guilt and sin its real causes'. He was of the opinion that 'the same physical conditions which constitute diseases acknowledged to be corporeal become, when modified by the specific influences of predisposition and excitement, equally the sources of those mis-termed mental. The brain differs widely as regards its functions from less important or grosser organs, yet when it is diseased, it announces the changes which are taking place in its condition or structure by aberration or suspension of them, in the manner precisely similar to that which obtains in every other instance of organic lesion. The immaterial principle remains intact. But its *agent* being impaired, it does not receive correct data'. It followed that insanity always had a physical cause and the derangement of the intellectual faculties were but the effect. Insanity was thus firmly brought into the field of medicine.

Because people often regarded insanity as a punishment, they accepted confinement or imprisonment in a madhouse together with the use of mechanical restraints, scourging and starvation. Those who were conscious of their mental deterioration were often pushed into madness through fear of the treatment they would be likely to receive in such establishments. Prichard was convinced that the condition of the mentally afflicted was made worse by the use of restraints. Again in his second Annual Report, he wrote that: 'nervous excitability owes its origins to irritation, either morally or physically induced . . . No one can deny that personal coercion must be a source of irritation, especially as the necessity for its appliance so far from being understood will be entirely misconstrued and give rise to terror'. Even the sane might become violent if they were chained up. From his experience the insane were not insensible of the impression they made on others, and were grateful for kindness shown to them. 'Too long have they sustained the weight of an affliction, rendered doubly burdensome by the unskilful; the mind, highly excitable from morbid action, may have sometimes been destroyed by the violence of emotions, excited by the ignorant and injudicious; but the fury which renders them dangerous has been more frequently aroused by the coarse and unsympathising, if not by the deliberately cruel.'

He appreciated that the total abolition of restraint was an experiment that required 'on the part of Superintendents of Asylums the most unceasing watchfulness, on the part of attendants perfect self-command, forbearance, gentleness and a spirit of mildness, moderation and forgiveness, directed by a merciful and intelligent understanding . . . it is not shewn that the employment of instrumental restraint confers these requisites'. Restraints merely encouraged the cowardly and indolent attendant. 'By interdicting the employment of *coercion*, we hope to afford freer scope to the operation of *moral influences*, – stimulate the subordinate, to their constant and prominent cultivation, by rendering his own comfort contingent on success, – and decrease the temptations which allure him from the conscientious discharge of his duty'.

Those who had experience of the orderly, quiet and apparently contented demeanour of patients who had full personal liberty and who were protected as much as possible from external causes of excitement by kindly, gentle and intelligent supervision, appreciated how groundless were the arguments of those who favoured restraints. Prichard quoted the case of two patients who arrived at the Asylum, their legs 'confined by heavy irons, which barely allowed one foot to be shuffled a few inches before its fellow; and their wrists by "figure of eight" handcuffs'. Once these restraints were removed, they became peaceful and helpful. Under systems of restraint, suicides were known to be numerous, 'but open dormitories and constant employment with supervision, deprived of its offensive character by a participation in their various duties and amusements, have hitherto prevented the occurrence of any attempt at self-destruction in this Institution'. He considered that the patient's admission to a new establishment provided an excellent opportunity for a fresh start and a chance for 'the creation of new impressions, favourable to general improvement'. The setting at liberty of every patient immediately on admission 'was attended with some few outbreaks, evidently springing from the remembrance of past grievances and a consequent distrust of unaccustomed professions; but these soon subsided, placing the advantages obtained in so conspicuous a position, that the *attendants* became no less anxious than their superiors to extend its operation'.

Prichard firmly believed that the sooner patients were admitted to the Asylum and the sooner 'moral treatment', as this caring attitude was then called, was started, the better the prospect for their recovery. He showed from an analysis of the fate of private and pauper patients admitted to the Asylum that the private patients had a higher recovery-rate and a lower death-rate; he was later to be attacked by his enemies on the grounds that this was due to private patients being treated better than the paupers. In

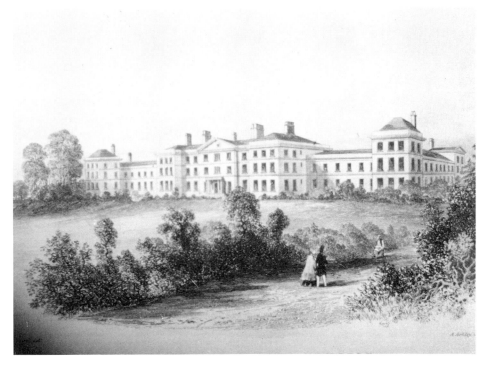

The Lunatic Asylum, Northampton, from an engraving by A. Ashley and J. F. Burrell, c.1845.

reply to this cynical suggestion, he deplored the way many parishes improperly kept their pauper lunatics in the local workhouse on purely economic grounds, only sending them to the Asylum when 'incurable and so dirty in their habits as to become an insupportable nuisance, in which case, not earlier, they are considered "dangerous" and certified as fit and proper objects of a Lunatic Asylum'. This was often too late for their stay in the Asylum to be effective. He also pointed out that a high proportion of the pauper lunatics sent to the Northampton Asylum were 'confirmed and incurable idiots, or involving combinations of epilepsy and palsy', as well as those 'fatuous from old age, and the deplorable, helpless and degraded victims of intemperance, to whom the workhouse or the madhouse too frequently afford but a temporary resting place before sinking into the grave'. In the first two years, nearly 200 paupers were sent to the Asylum not only from Northamptonshire but also from Buckinghamshire, Lincolnshire, Cambridgeshire, Huntingdonshire and Warwickshire, encouraged by 'the low rate of our terms at the opening of the Institution and the liberality of its Directors in rendering it available to the exigencies of the adjoining counties.' Inevitably, death-rates were high among such patients but the number of recoveries was greater than might have been expected.

At first in 1838, county pauper patients were charged 7s. per week and those from other counties 12s. Rates were altered that October; pauper patients from Northamptonshire were charged 9s. per week and those from outside the county 10s. 6d., plus six weeks' deposit. Then in September 1839, it was agreed that all pauper patients should pay at the same rate of 9s. There were higher charges for non-pauper patients of 12s., 15s., £1.1s.0d. and £1.11s.6d., according to circumstances. Applications for the entry of non-pauper patients had to be accompanied by a certificate signed by 'the officiating Minister of the parish and two respectable householders' together with answers to such specific questions as 'What are the Patient's general circumstances?', 'Has he or she any independent property?', 'What trade or occupation did the Patient follow up to the period of the present attack of insanity?', 'Has the Patient ever been at any other Asylum public or private – and at what charge?' Details were also required about any near relative.

Prichard considered it important that the patients led an ordered and disciplined life. 'By the operation of the same wholesome discipline, the patient on quitting the Asylum is restored to his friends and family, endowed with those habits of industry which may secure him against being a burden to them or, through the effects of idleness, relapsing into his recent malady.'

As might be expected, religion was considered an important element in helping the mentally ill. It was hoped that the Rev. William Wales, who at the early age of twenty-nine became Vicar of All Souls (Church of England) Northampton, would accept the chaplaincy to the Asylum, but because of many other church commitments he felt unable to accept. Instead, the Rev. John Little, curate at St Sepulchre, was appointed Chaplain at the annual salary of £45. His duties were to hold a service, including a sermon, at the Asylum every Sunday afternoon, to administer the Sacrament quarterly to those wishing to participate as approved by the Superintendent, to visit the Asylum occasionally during the week in order to consult with the Superintendent about the moral and religious condition of the patients and, at the Superintendent's request, to give religious consolation and instruction to specified patients. A deputy was only acceptable under exceptional circumstances, and absence of leave was to be given only by the Committee. The committee room was supplied with suitable furniture so that it could be used as a chapel. Through the Rev. Dr Butler, the Directors agreed that the Christian Knowledge Society should supply books and tracts.

Little resigned in January 1841 on moving from the district. In March, the Rev. Sir George Robinson proposed that the Bishop of Peterborough, in whose diocese the Asylum was situated, be asked to nominate a Chaplain who would be paid £50 per annum and 'that such a chaplain shall not be engaged in any other duties with parochial care of souls'. His work was to consist of one service with a sermon each Sunday and two weekly services; until this position was filled, a clergyman was to be appointed to take the Sunday service for a guinea on each occasion.

The choice of Chaplain fell on the Rev. John Thornton, who did much to extend his responsibilities. At the Annual Court, held in August 1843, his salary was increased to £100 per annum and Dr Prichard 'requested to observe' that the Chaplain's whole time should be at his disposal for the benefit of the patients. He was further to keep a book 'in which he shall enter the times he visits the House and such observations as he may think fit to make'. According to his Annual Report in 1844, he held services daily, attended on average by about eighty patients. He also undertook regular pastoral visiting and provided books from two local libraries, the most popular subjects being history, biography, travel and poetry. His work was warmly commended.

In addition to Prichard's overall medical and 'moral' responsibilities, he had evergrowing administrative duties. These included the purchasing of food supplies, the employment and payment of staff, who amounted to 161 persons by January 1844, the initiation and supervision of alterations and additions to the buildings, the examination of new methods of heating, drainage, cleaning and a host of other details. When he told the Committee in 1843 that his correspondence was very large, he was authorised to employ a patient competent to help him in return for a gratuity. In the following month, he was allowed fifty guineas a year to take on a fit person to keep the accounts of the Asylum and to take charge of the stores. The pressures of the administration, when added to his medical responsibilities, must have been enormous in the days before the advent of the telephone, typewriter, and trained secretarial assistance.

The Minutes during Prichard's superintendency give a clear picture of the Institution's development. The Directors, Committees and staff were active on a wide front. In August 1838, £28.13s.10d. was authorised to be paid to John Perkins for eight weeks' wages for his foreman, for the use of sixty-five and a half days of his horse and cart and for seeds for the garden which Perkins had undertaken to lay out and for which he was later congratulated. In the following month, Messrs Elliott and Barwell were authorised to provide a pair of entrance gates, a handgate and a sham gate for the grounds for not more than £31; much of the early building work appears to have been carried out by them. In April 1839, the Court resolved that Mr Barwell was not entitled to vote as a Director, in spite of the fact that he had paid £20 in 1835 into the funds, but this was before the decision in 1837 that donors of £20 upwards should become Directors for life had been taken. Later that month, the *Mercury* reported that Mr Barwell had given £20 to the Institution; from October 1839 onwards he appears to have been an active member of the Committee. A further announcement was published in January 1840, that: 'Benefactors of twenty pounds in one or two payments shall be Directors for Life'; the reason for this was that while 'the Establishment is just able to maintain itself from debt . . . it has not the smallest available surplus fund to meet any incidental or unlooked for expenses'.

Unexpected problems inevitably arose from time to time. In October 1838, the Superintendent reported that there had been several escapes over the wall of the men's airing court; these courts, where the open air could be enjoyed, were provided for both male and female patients. It was therefore decided to raise the height of the walls with stones from the farm buildings on the estate. Again at the Annual Court in September, the auditors were of the opinion that certain expenses were unwarranted because caused by poor workmanship, 'particularly the great expense of the Yorkshire paving stones in the yards, making cess pools, laying down pipes etc. for the purpose of carrying the water away from and preserving the back part of the Building, none of which would have been required had the Building been properly set out in the first instance, independent of the advantage not only to the building itself, but to its healthy effect and general appearance'. The language of the Minutes is occasionally obscure but the meaning is plain.

In spring 1840, it was decided that the valuable building material in the grounds, such as stone from the old farm and sand dug up by patients, presumably of the pauper class, should be sold on the best terms obtainable. It was also agreed to inform the clergy of the Established Church and the Ministers of Dissenting Congregations that extra funds were still needed. Accordingly, the Bishop of Peterborough that April preached at All Souls Church on behalf of the Asylum. The *Northampton Herald* of 2 May 1840, reported:

> After describing the distressful circumstances attendant upon a state of lunacy, adverting to the judicious choice of the site of the building, the excellent rules by which the Institute was managed, the care which had been taken for the spiritual as well as the bodily comforts of the patients, and touching slightly upon the inestimable benefits of religion to society

at large, his Lordship stated, that notwithstanding the liberality which had already been manifested, the funds were not sufficiently ample for the purposes of the Institution. There existed a great necessity for adding to the building – a necessity for a separation, a classification of the patients. It must be obvious to every one that the different shades of characters of the patients rendered it requisite that they should be kept out of sight, even out of hearing of each other. [The report ended]: There was not a very numerous congregation, but the collections amounted to £102.8s.5d.

The collecting plates were held by, among others, Lord Spencer, the Rev. Sir George Robinson, Sir William Wake and Miss Wake.

Because of the increasing demand for places, a Special Court decided on 6 August 1840, to provide accommodation for sixty more patients, thirty of each sex, and Sub-Committees were appointed to deal with this. Mr Milne, the surveyor, was able to state in January 1841, that the new wings for seventy patients 'of the lowest rank' would be ready before the end of March. It was therefore decided to publicise this information to counties without asylums and to make it known that out-county patients of this rank would pay the same as in-county patients.

In April 1841, Prichard was begging for the installation of an improved hot-water system. In December 1841, a Special Court decided to build a new laundry and washing house and, during the course of 1842, Mr Perkins's system for 'heating the laundry with hot water and for boiling by steam in the Washing House, the Brewhouse and the Cooking Kitchen' was approved and completed in six weeks during the summer. Mr Milne's plan for enlarging the kitchen was also accepted. At the Annual General Court that August, the auditors were able to announce that income had exceeded expenditure by £1,013.15s.9d. At the same Court it was agreed that a charge of one shilling per week should be made on all patients sent in by the parishes to cover the expense of clothing, wine and spirits and all other extras except for removals and burials.

In April 1843, Dr Prichard considered that a further enlargement of the Asylum was necessary, a view supported by a Special Court held in the following month. Accordingly, an appeal over the signature of Lord Northampton, then Chairman of the Asylum, was published in the local Press on 8 August. At the Annual General Court, held later that month, the auditors reported:

From this continued favourable statement of the financial operations of the Institution we are induced to hope that, when the whole of the

Buildings and alterations now in course of erection shall be completed, a continuance of the preference shewn to our Institution by those who from their situation in life can afford to reimburse the Institution in a more liberal manner than many of the unfortunate beings who through their friends are compelled to seek a residence in this or similar Institutions will be the means in a few years of enabling the Directors to reduce the rates at which they at present receive the poorer classes of patients into the Asylum.

The fundraising campaign continued throughout the year. On the 12 September, the *Mercury* published a letter, signed A.B., which contained the following passage:

To every friend of suffering humanity, our Lunatic Asylum commends itself by its benevolent design; to every Northamptonshire man, and especially to those who are in the habit of frequenting Northampton, it presents itself with a beauty of structure and commanding dignity of position that must needs be felt as adding greatly to the respectability and importance both of the town and county . . . That such a noble edifice should have been erected at an expense of £23,578.6s.2d. is really surprising. But when we further learn from the appeal that this sum includes £3,019.18s.6d., the cost of the site, and the furnishings and internal fitting-up of the numerous apartments, so that (within little more than two years from the laying of the first stone) the Asylum was opened on August 1st, 1838, for the reception of patients – verily, Mr Editor, we are compelled to acknowledge they were faithful stewards who so profitably employed the finances entrusted to their management.

The writer went on to express hopes that the clergy of the Established Church and the ministers of other denominations would continue to raise funds from their congregations.

On 3 October, a leader appeared in the *Mercury* stating that: 'We trust that congregational collections from a much larger proportion of the parishes within this county will appear in our next advertisement, and that the Wesleyan Methodists, and dissenters of every denomination, in proportion to their means, will vie with the Established Church in the promotion of so excellent an Institution. It is in the confident anticipation of this liberality, that the committee of the Lunatic Asylum have actually commenced the erection of the two additional wings . . . ' The *Herald* of the same date described the Asylum to be 'by the beauty of its structure, the chief ornament of the town of Northampton' and went on to say, 'there are upward of 300 parishes in the county of Northampton, of which so few appear as yet to have been addressed from the pulpit, we trust that much more will be speedily coming in through the Clergy of our Establishment, and that their efforts will be seconded by collections from Protestant Dissenters of every denomination'.

At the Annual Court in August 1844, expenses were seen to have grown on account of the new building work, but as the auditors reported, 'this can scarcely be said to produce a feeling of regret in as much as the Establishment is so much the more useful and efficient for carrying out the benevolent intentions of the Founders, by the increased accommodation afforded to a continually increasing number of applicants for admission'. The accounts again showed a surplus in favour of the hospital of close on £1,200, 'a surplus which, even allowing a certain sum annually for necessary repairs, will fully justify a well-grounded belief that, as the future outlay for building purposes will be but trifling, the Institution will, in a very few years, be entirely clear of debt, and consequently in a situation of such prosperity, as to make a considerable reduction in the charges for board of those patients whose pecuniary means shall be inadequate to the present rate of charges'. From this it would appear that the results of the appeal were satisfactory. On this occasion, however, there was no mention for the first time of Dr Prichard who was by then under the shadow to be described in detail in the next chapter.

Throughout this period, the Management Committee took a keen interest in all tenders and payments, queried accounts and on occasion delayed payment until they were satisfied that the charges were fair. In June 1840, for example, the Committee resolved to inform the magistrates at the next Quarter Sessions that the bread and flour supplies from the baking department of the jail had recently been of inferior quality. In February 1839, the Superintendent was instructed not to have work done without an order.

If the Superintendent had to be absent from the Asylum for any reason without first obtaining formal permission, a full explanation was deman-ded, although the Committee's attitude was in general very understanding, at least up until the events of 1844. The Minutes for 25 January 1843 record that:

> Dr Prichard having stated that he was a fortnight ago under the necessity of being absent from the House upon business over which he had no control. The explanation of Dr Prichard is deemed perfectly satisfactory to the Committee.

The Committee was also appreciative. Dr Prichard was authorised from time to time to pay a specified amount in gratuities to deserving staff. On 26 December 1839, it thanked Mr Atkins, a nurseryman, whose land adjoined that of the Asylum, for allowing a ditch bordering their lands to be filled in and expressly declared that the hedge and four foot of land on the Asylum side of the hedge was to be his. It also investigated complaints. Mr Bouverie and Mr Stone personally enquired into one that a woman, who had been discharged from the Asylum as restored to health, proved to be pregnant. It emerged that the woman had been visited by her husband in the Asylum, and that they had been left alone for sometime: 'this', according to the Minutes, 'occurred at such a period previous to her delivery as to account completely for her having been pregnant'.

Chapter Four

EVENTS LEADING TO DR PRICHARD'S

RESIGNATION (1844–1845)

*D*uring Dr Prichard's superintendency, continued progress was made towards a national system whereby all asylums and madhouses were to be inspected regularly. As a result of moves by Lord Granville Somerset, supported by Lord Ashley, a Bill to this effect became law in August 1842. This Act (5 and 6 Vict., *c.* 87), empowered the Metropolitan Commissioners in Lunacy, whose increased numbers were to include four legal Commissioners and six or seven physicians or surgeons, to visit all houses licensed by Justices of the Peace for the reception of insane persons; their inspection of every aspect was to be rigorous and recorded. These visits were to be made twice a year unless the Lord Chancellor, under whose jurisdiction the Commissioners now came, saw fit to reduce the number.

In 1844 the Commissioners produced a report. Their recommendations were aimed at unifying the forms of statutory control exercised over asylums and madhouses and to ensure that all houses containing lunatics should be subject to the Lunacy Laws. The Lunatics Act of 1845 (8 and 9 Vict., *c.* 100) followed together with a subsidiary Bill (8 and 9 Vict., *c.* 126) which dealt with the erection and management of county asylums. How the Northampton Asylum was to be affected by these two Acts will be discussed in Chapter Five. Thus, as a result of this intense activity, there was an increasing interest by the public in the treatment of the insane, which no doubt contributed to the local concern aroused by reports of mismanagement of the Northampton Asylum.

The first indication of trouble appeared in the local Press. According to the *Mercury*, an inquest was held at the Asylum on 17 April 1844, on the body of one John Bannard.

> The coroner in charging the jury stated that the inquiry was made at the request of Mr Bouverie, Dr Prichard and other gentlemen interested in the welfare of the Institution. Remarks had been made upon the number of deaths in the Asylum, and the answer was that it was unduly swelled by the number of persons brought from the Unions in a state of disease so advanced that their recovery was impossible. Under these circumstances it was thought advisable to instigate this inquiry.

It appears that Dr Prichard spoke forcibly and at length against the delay in sending pauper lunatics to the Asylum, perhaps because he feared that these deaths might be adversely affecting both the good name of the Asylum and his own but equally likely because of his own sense of compassion.

He was not alone in this protest. The report, issued a few months later that year by the Metropolitan Commissioners in Lunacy, largely drafted by Lord Ashley, stated that the county asylum Superintendents were virtually unanimous 'that pauper lunatics are sent there at so late a period of their disease as to impede or prevent their ultimate recovery'.

According to the *Mercury*, Mr Lever, surgeon of No. 3 district of the Brackley Union, described Bannard as a farm worker of weak intellect who had previously been insane for five weeks in 1836. At the beginning of that April 1844, after treating him for indigestion, Lever thought him somewhat off-balance but harmless; nevertheless he had him watched. On Monday, 8 April, 'the witness then finding that the person who had charge of him allowed people to come to the house and annoy him – and that he was in fact made a complete puppet-show of – wrote to the relieving officer, advising him that he should be removed to the workhouse where if he was kept quiet, he thought it likely that he might soon recover'. The next day, however, he was so violent that restraint became necessary. On Wednesday, 10 April, the Local Board sanctioned the sending of Bannard, who had refused all nourishment for several days, to the Asylum but this did not take place until Saturday. On arriving there, between 2 p.m. and 3 p.m., he was placed in a cleansing bath and reported by the House Surgeon, Mr W. G. Marshall, who saw him about five minutes after his arrival, to be in a 'moribund or dying condition'. He died the following morning. It was noted that the patient had been attended only by Marshall and not seen at all by Prichard.

The *Herald* gave a very similar account of the inquest. Both newspapers reported Dr Prichard's enquiries about the food and parish allowances granted to the deceased and his wife, which was 3s.6d. and three 4lb loaves a week. The reason for these enquiries was that he and his brother medical officers in similar institutions often found that deaths such as Bannard's arose, in the words of the *Mercury*, from 'maniacal excitement supervening upon dementia arising from insufficient nourishment'. Cases of this character, reported the *Herald*, formed one-fifth of the Asylum's deaths.

There had also been some confusion about the forms which were required to be completed before a patient from a parish could be admitted. Dr Pritchard, according to the *Herald*, drew attention to a printed notice which explained that, in cases where a lunatic could not be conveniently brought to the Asylum, 'a careful and humane conductor will be supplied by the Asylum and his travelling expenses only charged'. That clause, however, was omitted in the form transmitted to the Brackley Board. The verdict returned was:

> That the deceased died for want of the common necessities of life, which he had refused to take; and the jurors consider that there was neglect on the part of the Relieving Officer of the Brackley Union in not conveying the deceased earlier to the Asylum at Northampton, and that the blame also was imputable to the Board of Guardians of the said Union for not immediately enforcing their order of removal, pursuant to the recommendation and report of the surgeon.

The greatest exception to this verdict, however, was taken by the *Herald*, the Tory rival to the Liberal *Mercury*, in its next edition on Saturday, 27 April. The *Herald* was controlled by the Rev. Francis Litchfield, rector of Farthinghoe, a village close to Brackley, who was closely associated with the Brackley Union. The time of the arrival of Bannard at the Asylum was now said to have been at about noon; he was therefore seen, according to the paper, not within five minutes but only some three hours after being admitted. Dr Prichard had attacked the relieving officer and the Brackley Guardians at length, continued the editorial, but no blame whatsoever could fairly be laid upon the former, who had not the slightest suspicion that the man's life was in danger. It was not the relieving officer and the Guardians who were at fault, but Dr Prichard who should be examined by the Asylum Governors not only about the case of Bannard but on the death of every pauper sent in by the Guardians. The leader ended: 'Judging from the published evidence, he, and he only, seems to have been neglectful. We hope the Board of Guardians will initiate a further enquiry into this affair.'

Litchfield, the driving force throughout what became a long sustained attack on Prichard, was prepared to use any weapon that came to hand. Perhaps he was alienated by the strength or abrasiveness of Prichard's attack upon the Brackley Union. He may even have considered himself deeply insulted in some way by Prichard for reasons which may never be known. Whatever the motive, Litchfield's antagonism was extreme and unrelenting.

In its edition of 4 May, the *Herald* reported that the Brackley Board of Guardians had requested the Poor Law Commissioners to send down a Deputy Commissioner for the purpose of getting to the bottom of the Bannard case. It also reported that Dr Prichard had explained to reporters why he had not seen Bannard immediately after his admission. 'As was customary with him, he waited till the man was put into a warm bath. Twice during the afternoon and evening he [Dr Prichard] went to see him, but the man had been put to bed and was asleep on both occasions. He did not disturb him, being of the opinion that sleep would be more beneficial to him than anything he could do for him.' As Bannard had already been seen by Marshall, the House-Surgeon, it would be difficult to fault this approach.

On 25 May, the *Herald* reverted at length to the inquest on Bannard, emphasising that 'not only was the medical chief at the Asylum not examined as to his own care of the deceased pauper, but he was allowed to take so prominent a part in turning the enquiry not towards but away from his own conduct, as a wild accuser of *others*, as actually to have made speeches *ten* times to the jury without being sworn once!' The real purpose of this leader was to announce that the Poor Law Commissioners were reopening the inquest.

On the 8 June, the *Herald* reported the results of that enquiry, stating that 'the inquest on the body had been called and contrived for a private purpose of Dr Prichard, that it was most irregularly conducted, that the witnesses produced were only partially questioned, that he who might have been the most material witness of all was not sworn, yet was permitted to influence the jury by statements irrelevant, partial and inaccurate, and that, in consequence of all this, a most improper and unjust verdict was returned'. Perhaps, it added, the doctor attendant upon Bannard might have given a more detailed report, perhaps the Guardians might have acted more promptly but there was no blame on the relieving officer. The *Herald* went on to 'charge Dr Prichard with incompetency for the post he occupies – with neglect of medical duties such as, if not without precedent in the worst days of madhouse abominations, is at all events unknown at Asylums under modern management; and lastly, with a reckless indifference to accuracy, justice and truth, though perfectly alive to every selfish prompting, such as we have never before witnessed in the case of an educated individual placed as the chief responsible officer at a large medical establishment'.

The *Herald's* leader went on to castigate Prichard and his Medical Assistant, Marshall, because neither knew how to use a thermometer when testing the temperature of the bath water in which Bannard had been placed, implying that the deceased's death might have been hastened by a warm bath. Prichard acknowledged 'that he did not use any other test of heat in a bath than that of his own hands, a test so notoriously fallacious that one hand will often report differently from another to the extent of so many degrees'.

The *Mercury* replied to this attack by the *Herald* upon Prichard in its main editorial of 15 June. From this it appeared that Prichard, having read the *Herald's* recommendation that an appeal should be made to the Poor Law Commissioners to examine the case, had himself written to them before the Brackley Union. Prichard 'was thus, at the enquiry before Mr Austin (the deputy commissioner), made to appear in the light of the accuser of the Brackley Board, while in point of fact his object was to simply defend himself. Dr Prichard's error was in acting upon information derived from the *Northampton Herald*'. The *Mercury* stated that it had 'no intention to defend Dr Prichard against the charge of neglect. But we *do* mean to protest against the endeavour to make Dr Prichard the scape-goat for the misconduct of others . . . We *do* mean to protest against the unfair attempt to insinuate that to Dr Prichard's neglect Bannard's death was owing; when it is as clear as the sun at noon-day that if it was owing to neglect at all it was the neglect of those in whose custody the poor man was kept, harassed and excited from harmless incoherency into intractable madness'.

The *Herald* that same week, 15 June, continued its attack. It had managed to lay hands on a part or all of the private report made by Prichard to the Poor Law Commissioners and proceeded at length to point out petty discrepancies between that report and his evidence given under oath. 'The Doctor,' wrote the *Herald*, 'says the man [Bannard] travelled thirty miles, whereas he travelled five and twenty. The Doctor says the journey must have abridged the man's existence, yet, in his evidence on oath, he says: "five or six miles would have made very little difference . . ." Dr Prichard said the man was nearly seventy years of age. He was only sixty-six . . .'. The *Herald* was anxious to know where Prichard had graduated 'for we have never heard the name of his Alma Mater'.

Litchfield, who was present at the enquiry held by Mr Austin, wrote immediately afterwards to the Secretary of the Asylum; his letter, published in the *Mercury* of 29 June, continued the same line of attack and added that paupers die at Northampton Lunatic Asylum in a far greater proportion than lunatics of better-paying classes.

This letter, as reported by the *Mercury*, was read out on 28 June at a Special Court of the Governors to which Lord Spencer, who took the chair, had replied in a letter dated 11 June. In it he indicated that the Directors admitted that Dr Prichard did not see Bannard before his death 'and that they feel great regret that such should have been the case and they hope that a similar circumstance will never take place again'. However he went on:

> That with respect to your statement of the ignorance and incapacity of Dr Prichard, the Committee have had such experience of his conduct in this Institution that they cannot in any degree admit the justice of such a statement. They cannot believe that in a Lunatic Asylum in which no personal restraint is adopted even in the cases of patients who had long previously been under the severest confinements and where the good order and comfort of the patients is apparent to every one who visits the house, that the Medical Superintendent is incompetent to the performance of his duties. On the contrary, they are satisfied that the reputation which this Institution has obtained, as they believe deservedly, of being one of the best Lunatic Asylums in the Kingdom is entirely owing to the superintendence of Dr Prichard.

In the discussion which followed, as reported by the *Mercury*, there was general agreement that Prichard was at fault in not seeing Bannard but that the patient's life could not have been saved because of his condition. Mr L. H. Forbes agreed that the Poor Law Guardians were in the habit of sending paupers much too late, but the Asylum also needed extra medical help. The Superintendent had managed very well when there were only fifty patients, but now there were 250. He was a good deal absent on the business of the Institution and there ought to be someone who could stand in for him. They had a bye-law allowing their Superintendent to attend private consultations for which he presumed he had his fee, but which certainly took him from the Institution. Lord Spencer agreed as to the need for extra help but considered that they must show their complete confidence in Prichard by making him responsible for such an appointment.

Accordingly the Special Court of 28 June resolved:

1.
That while the Committee had every reason to express their satisfaction at the general good management of the Asylum under the

superintendence of Dr Prichard and at the success which has attended it, they feel called upon to express their great regret that in the case of John Bannard he did not see him before his death, no excuse having been alleged which does in any wise account for such neglect.

2.

That in future Dr Prichard be required to see every patient within one hour of his or her admission into the House, that the case be immediately entered into an entry book and should Dr Prichard be absent that the House Surgeon do perform that duty.

3.

That at every meeting of the Committee a casebook be laid before the Committee in which shall be entered a report containing a classification of all cases within the House together with a specification of any individual case which may require it. The time and proximate cause of death of any of the patients shall be entered in the same book.

4.

That an additional House Surgeon be appointed on the recommendation of Dr Prichard, subject to the approval of the Committee, and that the testimonials of such House Surgeon and of any other who may be engaged in the Asylum be entered in a book.

5.

That it would be advantageous that there should be a coroner's inquest held upon every pauper patient who dies in the House and that in the present state of the funds the Institution can afford to pay for this expense without throwing any burden upon the town of Northampton.

It might have been supposed that this was the end of the matter – but not so. On the 6 July the *Herald* continued its attack on Prichard and those who supported him, including Lord Spencer, who was described as going into a 'towering rage' on receiving Litchfield's letter at Althorp after the enquiry under Mr Austin. Prichard, it was now claimed, was 'a mere licentiate without a diploma'. There are also the first insinuations about drunkenness. Far worse, there was also the first report of the death at the Asylum of a Mrs Elizabeth Lindsey who had been there two nights and one day from the 24 June without having been seen by the Superintendent. 'Dr Prichard told the husband that her confinement was the cause of her death, and *persuaded him not to have an inquest*, as she had been attended by a medical man previous to coming to the Asylum, and as he [the husband] would not like to see her name exposed in the papers.' The coffin was later moved to Whittlesea in the Isle of Ely near her home.

The Lindsey story was expanded further by the *Herald* of 13 July. Her death had been concealed from Lord Spencer while he was presiding at the meeting on 28 June, referred to above. The first he had heard of this case was apparently from the *Herald*'s report: 'Accordingly, we hear that Lord Spencer has expressed himself with something like proper indignation at the trickery practised upon him, and with something like a suitable determination never again to be made a tool by political companions in a similar way,' a reference to the fact that the majority who had supported Prichard at the meeting on 28 June were dissenters. Then there was the question of the post-mortem. 'The body of Mrs Lindsey,' continued the *Herald*, 'has been *cut open* by Dr Prichard – cut open without the husband's authority or even knowledge – cut open without a coroner's warrant – cut open without a jury to decide upon the cause of death – cut open without witnesses being allowed to learn the secret of so sudden – so mysterious – a dissolution . . . Had he meant honestly, with no sinister end in view, he would surely have invited not one or even two but some half dozen professional gentlemen to be present, who might have observed and could testify to the reality of morbid appearances . . . The answer is plain. It would have defeated his purpose of concealment. And, after all this, to have no *inquest* and to hurry off the deceased beyond the power of a Northampton coroner previously so well aware of Dr Prichard's neglect.' Moreover, on the evening that Mrs Lindsey had been brought to the Asylum, he had been at Boughton Fair which was why he did not see her.

Accordingly, the Management Committee met on 22 July 1844 with Sir George Robinson as Chairman and resolved 'that two specific charges against Dr Prichard having been brought under the notice of the Committee, one of disobedience, by neglecting to visit a patient on arrival and another of intoxication, and Dr Prichard having been called in, and asked for an explanation, it is the opinion of the Committee, that by his own confession, he is guilty of the charge of disobedience of the rules of the Institution and that the explanation he had offered on the other charge is not satisfactory.'

As the coroner of the Isle of Ely had decided to carry out a post-mortem on Mrs Lindsey's body without inviting any of the medical officers of the Asylum to attend, the Secretary was instructed to protest against any verdict being reached without hearing evidence from its staff.

The General Court, held on 31 July, decided to adjourn consideration of the charges against Prichard until a Special Court on 14 August. Reporters were to be admitted to all General and Special Courts unless extraordinary objections were raised. At a well-attended Special Court held on 3 August, Prichard, Marshall and Elizabeth Frisby, the nurse who had been responsible for looking after Mrs Lindsey, were instructed to attend the

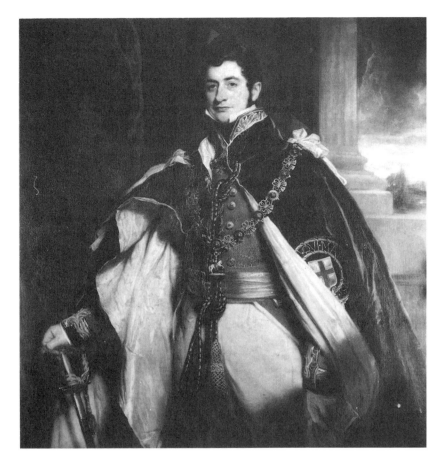

The 2nd Marquess of Exeter, KG, President 1842–66, portrait by Sir Martin Archer Shee (from the Burghley House Collection: photograph: Courtauld Institute of Art).

adjourned inquest on 7 August in the Isle of Ely; the coroner, who agreed, was also asked to provide at the Asylum's expense a full account of the proceedings in time for the Special Court.

The inquest at Whittlesea lasted three days, not finishing until about midnight on the third, and was reported at length in the *Herald*. It appeared that Marshall, the House Surgeon, saw Mrs Lindsey immediately after she had been put to bed on Monday, 24 June. Elizabeth Frisby, the nurse, did not think it necessary to sit with her all night. On the following morning she was very much better and the improvement was maintained throughout the day. Marshall, who visited her on four occasions, was evidently pleased with her. Although he did not know why Dr Prichard had not visited her during Tuesday, he did not consider that this was necessary as he had reported fully on her condition and treatment, nor did he bother the Superintendent about her that evening as she was so much better. Yet on the following morning, Wednesday, 26 June, she was found to have died peacefully in her sleep.

Prichard, during his examination by the coroner, explained that he had returned to the Hospital late on the night of 24 June and was told by Marshall of Mrs Lindsey's arrival. He had a general knowledge of her health from Mr Birdsall, a surgeon who had attended her; he did not visit her as Marshall confirmed Birdsall's statement. He did not visit the patient on the following day but enquired after Mrs Lindsey from Marshall, who told him that there was no need for him to bother. When asked about the rules for visiting patients, Prichard explained, according to the *Herald*, that: 'There is a proposition – not a rule – that I should see every patient within a certain time after admission. No resolution has been passed requiring me to see every patient within an hour. A proposition requires to be confirmed by a subsequent meeting before it becomes a rule.' In fact, the proposition only became a rule on 28 June, two days after Mrs Lindsey's death.

The *Herald* had made great play in its edition of 13 July with the fact that the Superintendent had carried out a private post-mortem without the presence of witnesses in an attempt to conceal that Mrs Lindsey had died from neglect. At the inquest it became clear that Prichard had not performed the autopsy himself but had instructed Marshall to do this. Marshall had explained that he did not like having to make the examination – which the coroner thought a very proper hesitation in the absence of an inquest – but explained that he was implicitly under the direction of Dr Prichard who was responsible, he understood, for all the medical staff.

Prichard in his evidence said that he had discussed Mrs Lindsey's death with two members of the Committee, Mr Sharp and Mr Collins, on that Wednesday morning, 26 June. Prichard had thought there must have been a ruptured blood vessel but could not tell for certain as he had not carried out a post-mortem. They thought he should make one, to which he agreed. He did not report the death formally to the Committee. When Mr Bouverie asked if he was not going to have a coroner's inquest, Prichard reminded him that the Directors had decided to hold inquests on pauper patients, but not on private patients, of which Mrs Lindsey was one; the friends of private patients were at liberty to demand one if they wished but they usually did not like the circumstances of such deaths being published. When the situation was explained to him, Mr Lindsey said that he did not wish for one.

The *Herald* thus reported the conclusion to the inquest:

Elizabeth Frisby's evidence (according to the Coroner) was given in a very satisfactory manner and everything as far as related to her duty and Mr Marshall's appeared to have been properly done. That was not the case with Dr Prichard. It did not appear that he ever saw the patient until after her death. It was a fact that he did not think proper to be present at the post-mortem examination, not did he select a disinterested person to be present. It did not appear that Dr Prichard knew at what time he returned home on Monday night. It was also clear that Mr Marshall was not present when Dr Prichard first saw the body. Such conduct, he must say, was not what it ought to have been . . . The Jury occupied about half an hour in their consultation during which the Propriety of attaching to their verdict censure for Dr Prichard's neglect was discussed. It was ultimately, however, determined to express no opinion on the subject, the jury perceiving it to be a matter strictly and solely in the province of the Directors – The following is the verdict:– 'That the deceased was found dead in bed in the morning of the 26th June, that she died from rupture of the smaller intestine but how such rupture was occasioned there is no evidence in the knowledge of the jurors.'

Because of this situation, the Management Committee on 12 August questioned Mr Fitzhugh, who was described in the Asylum Minute Book as Master of the Union Workhouse, about a statement said to have been made by him that he had twice brought Dr Prichard home to the Asylum in a state of intoxication. Mr Fitzhugh denied ever having said this; he added that he had seen Dr Prichard intoxicated on one occasion six years previously before the opening of the Institution but not since. The Minute continued somewhat enigmatically: 'Mr Tomalin was also present and said that Mr Fitzhugh had never applied to him to know whether he could prudently give evidence of the fact that he had brought Dr Prichard home intoxicated.' Mr Tomalin was Clerk to the Magistrates.

On the 14 August, a Special Court under the chairmanship of Lord Spencer met to consider Dr Prichard's 'disobedience to the Rules of the Institution'. The meeting was on this occasion large, long, heated and confused, to judge from the reports in the local Press. Among those present was Mr Austin, the Deputy Poor Law Commissioner. Unfortunately, contrary to his promise, the Isle of Ely coroner had not had time to prepare a detailed report for the Special Court; instead, a report made by a journalist from the *Mercury* was made available to the meeting by Prichard, much to the indignation of Litchfield and the *Herald*. However, it was decided not to postpone the meeting further as the jury's verdict, that death had been from natural causes, was known.

Lord Spencer said that the points at issue were: whether Mrs Lindsey had been neglected, whether she died in consequence of that neglect and whether Dr Prichard was justified in ordering the post-mortem examination. Mr Litchfield thought that a book had to be kept of each patient's daily treatment but Sir George Robinson considered that, with the present number of patients, this rule, made when their numbers were small, could no longer be complied with. He considered that Mrs Lindsey had not died through any neglect but that Prichard was at fault in not seeing her and for not being present at the post-mortem.

That much of the animosity against Prichard harked back to his supposed attack upon the Brackley Union for their neglect of Bannard became clear when the Hon. P. S. Pierrepont of Evenley Hall, Northampton, the youngest son of the 1st Earl Manvers, said that he regretted intervening but the case had in some measure originated in an attack upon himself as Chairman of a Board of Guardians. An inquiry had taken place and it appeared that the assertion was entirely groundless. He had no feeling against Dr Prichard on that account. Still less was he influenced by party or political prejudice. The sacred stream of charity ought not to be polluted by the poison of politics. He did however wonder whether the resolution regarding Mrs Lindsey should not be coupled with that of Bannard. He was not prepared, however, to press for this but merely wished to explain his feelings on the subject.

Mr Litchfield indicated that Prichard's failure to see Mrs Lindsey on her arrival at the Asylum could be accounted for if he had indeed visited Boughton Fair that same evening, 'when', to quote the *Mercury*, 'all sober people had quitted places of this sort', and if he had taken with him two patients from the Asylum. After a long discussion in which the unreliability of 'hearsay' evidence was admitted, as shown in the case of Mr Fitzhugh's denial, it was suggested that Mr Marshall, the House Surgeon, be asked directly about the Superintendent's drinking habits. However, Mr Charles Markham, the Hospital Auditor, thought that there was some impropriety in examining a servant about his master's behaviour.

Prichard was then questioned directly about his visit to the Boughton Fair, which he did not deny, but refused to give the names of his companions, only one of whom was a patient. Litchfield thought this refusal showed that the relatives of the patient in question would not approve of him being taken to such a place. Prichard replied that Litchfield was talking without the slightest comprehension of his work. It was as much his duty to afford his patients recreation and amusement as it was to prescribe a dose of medicine for them. They were not brought to the

Asylum to be locked up and hidden from society. In spite of Prichard's protests, Marshall was later called into the meeting and questioned in front of him. Marshall declared that Prichard had been sober on his return from Boughton Fair and that he had never seen him incapable of managing the Institution but left a slight shadow of doubt 'when pressed to answer', according to the *Mercury*, 'in a more extended sense', by declining to do so. He hinted that Prichard had been unwell for some weeks.

After Prichard and Marshall had left, Cook, a former House Surgeon, and Thornton, the Chaplain, were then questioned. Both declared that they had never seen the Superintendent drunk or incapable of carrying out his duties but both added that he was very excitable by nature. The meeting was obviously not completely convinced.

At this stage Lord Spencer said, according to the *Mercury*, that he had voted against Prichard's election:

> his hopes as to the prosperity of the Institute were anything but sanguine. But certainly he had seen it go on steadily advancing in prosperity under his management for six years, far beyond their expectations. He was ready to join in the censure of the Bannard case – it was bad: that of Mrs Lindsey was a great deal worse, as coming immediately after the censure arising out of the former. But looking on the other hand at the way in which he had managed the house, he could not consistently declare that Prichard was unfit to continue as superintendent. On the contrary he was sure he was very fit as to the general management. He admitted that he had been guilty of great indiscretion; that he was not a pleasant man to act with. But he thought they would find it very difficult to get another person in whom equal confidence could be placed. Therefore his advice would be to censure Dr Prichard as severely as they pleased, and to continue him in office.

Litchfield pressed hard for Prichard's dismissal which was eventually seconded by Pierrepont, but this proposal received only four votes. The following resolutions, inscribed in the Minute Book, were approved by a large majority:

> That it is the opinion of the meeting that considerable blame attaches to their Superintendent, Dr Prichard, for not having visited Mrs Lindsey from the time of her admission until the time of her death, being two nights and one day, and also for having ordered the House Surgeon to institute a post mortem examination of her body without the knowledge of her husband, and at which examination, neither he himself nor any

other medical authority was present.

That for the time to come there be appointed some medical visitor or visitors, who shall have authority, independent of the Superintendent of the Asylum, to inquire into the practice of the said Superintendent and the general treatment of the patients, and report from time to time thereupon to the Committee of Management.

That the Superintendent be called in and informed of the previous resolutions and that the Directors will forthwith take into their consideration the alterations that will therefore be necessary to the Statutes, and in the salaries of the Officers as at present regulated, if any such alterations in the Salaries should be necessary.

These resolutions were read to Dr Prichard who replied that he had nothing to say but to bow to the decision of the Court as a matter of course.

Whereas the *Mercury* of 17 August gave what would appear to be a comparatively objective report, the *Herald* of the same date continued to attack those it regarded as its enemies. The general theme of its editorial was that Prichard was dishonoured but retained, 'simply, and for no other reason, because of pounds, shillings and pence considerations'. Those who supported Prichard were not forgotten. Mr Collins was described as 'Quaker Collins, the ex-draper' and Thomas Sharp as 'ex-barber'. A final brick: 'It turns out that the Asylum Reports, professedly drawn up by Dr Prichard, have not been drawn up by him, but that his exercise has been done by another hand. We had always suspected as much, because, when Dr Prichard has written letters in the newspapers, and affixed his name to them, they have generally been of the most illiterate, and even ungrammatical description.'

The reverberations in the local Press went on into early September. The *Herald* of 24 August continued its intemperate attack on Prichard and on those Directors of the Asylum, a large majority, who had voted to censure but not dismiss him. The *Mercury*, by contrast, protested that 'Nothing can justify, as nothing can render necessary, the exclusion of every word of the defence, while the amplest scope is given to the accusation. But the sins of our contemporary [the *Herald*] are not those of omission only, but of perversion and commission . . . Let the reader turn to the letter of the Dean of Peterborough, given in an adjoining column, and he will see an instance.' The letter in question had been addressed to the *Herald*, but reproduced in the *Mercury* at Dr Butler's request; it protested in gentle but clear terms at the way both he and Prichard had been misrepresented by the *Herald* with regard to the Asylum's Annual Reports of which they were jointly the authors.

The Annual General Court of 28 August 1844 emphasised the continuing progress of the Asylum, but made no mention of the Superintendent's contribution to this fortunate state of affairs. The only member of the staff to receive the Director's thanks was the Chaplain, the Rev. John Thornton, 'for zealous and successful discharge of his duties during the past year', because, according to the *Herald* of 7 September, 'the present Chaplain did all that a conscientious man could, and perhaps a little more that a scrupulous clergyman would have done, in order to bolster up the character of an intemperate Superintendent'. What else could have induced 'Messrs Collins and Sharp, two bigoted Dissenters, to join in thanking a Chaplain of the Established Church for his religious performances?'.

Unhappily for Prichard, the *Mercury's* report of the meeting of 28 August in its issue of 31 August showed the Superintendent once more under fire. After the conclusion of the Chaplain's report, although there is no reference to this in the Minutes, Sir George Robinson wished to know from Dr Prichard whether he had received any fees under the 13th rule, i.e., 'the Medical Superintendent shall on no account receive money, presents or gratuities of any kind from the patients or their friends, etc.', and, if so, whether they had been cashed to the account of the Institution in compliance with that rule. Prichard replied that he had been called into consultation with other medical men in three cases, but he did not consider that these came within the scope of that rule. When Sir George asked with some warmth how as an honest man he could justify taking a fee under that rule, the Superintendent explained that the question on which he had been called in was legal rather than medical, a question in which deposition of property depended upon the probable recovery of the patient. In one case he had received one hundred guineas, in another ten and in the third one guinea. It was very common in cases of *De Lunatico Inquirendo* for persons in his position to be sent for. Dr Conolly acted in precisely the same way. He always understood that the object of the rule in question was to prevent him from taking charge of patients outside the Asylum, and thus interfering with the regulations and profits of the House; he did not consider these cases came within that rule.

The taking of fees by Dr Prichard is mentioned in the Minutes of the Asylum for the first time at a meeting of the Management Committee on Monday, 28 October, under the chairmanship of Captain the Hon. Frederick Spencer, RN, who was to succeed his brother as the 4th Earl Spencer in the following year. The matter was referred to the General Court, held again under the chairmanship of Captain Spencer two days later. The Court's main task was to consider and adopt the Statutes and

Rules of the Asylum as revised by the Committee of Management in the light of what had happened that year. First, however, at the suggestion of Sir George Robinson, the Court decided to inquire further into the charges that Prichard had received fees, contrary to the rules.

Prichard in explanation said that he had been approached to take on patients in a private capacity. He had himself suggested in 1841 that the rule in question should allow him to 'take charge' of such patients in the neighbourhood and pay the fee into the Asylum. He did not consider that this rule applied to the three quasi-legal consultation cases to which he had referred at the Annual General Court, none of which involved him 'taking charge' of a patient. A heated discussion followed. Asked whether he had received permission to go to the Isle of Wight for one consultation, he was reported to have said that he had told Lord Spencer himself that he was going at the request of a friend of Lord Spencer who was also a Governor. Asked whether he had received a letter on the subject, Prichard said that he had, he thought, shown it to Mr Sharp. He added: 'Everybody who knows anything of me knows that I have been very poor, and am not without ambition. It was a proud day for me, who had stood behind a counter for sixteen hours a day and taken but eight-pence, when by the exercise of my own abilities I received a fee of a hundred guineas. It was not likely I should conceal such a circumstance. I did not conceal it. I spoke of it to different directors; I included it in my income-tax return, and I am assessed for it.'

Eventually after further argument in which Prichard enjoyed support as well as condemnation, it was resolved, according to the Minute Book:

> That in the opinion of this Court Dr Prichard ought not to have received any fee without consulting the Court of Directors, but as there appears to be much doubt in the interpretation of the Rule 13, Page 18, and the Resolution of the Directors passed in connexion with that rule on the 15 July, 1841, this Court does not deem it expedient to make any further notice of the charges against Dr Prichard.

In spite of suggestions of reducing the joint salary of Dr and Mrs Prichard, it remained at £400 per annum by a vote of eleven to five. According to the *Mercury*, a rule prohibiting the Superintendent from receiving any fee under any circumstances was passed unanimously. Moreover, it was agreed to appoint a non-resident physician at a salary of £125 per annum 'to prevent', according to the ever-vindictive *Herald* of 2 November, 'a recurrence of the dreadful deaths which the incompetence, the inattention and absences of the resident superintendent have produced aforetime'. This appointment, as decided by the Court of the 14 August, was to be independent of the Superintendent. Reference was also made to the detailed records the Superintendent would now have to keep according to the amended regulations and to the fact that he was no longer to have access to the spirits and other drinks in the stores.

On 29 January 1845, the General Court confirmed the Statute and Rules as adopted by the previous General Court. Only one rule, rule 14, relating to the votes of Directors and the question of proxies, appears to have been discussed in detail, and threw an interesting light on the relationship between the town and country directors. Mr Young moved an addition to this rule; that 'all Directors residing at any distance beyond ten miles from the town of Northampton shall be entitled to vote at all meetings, except those of the committees, by proxy, given to some director who may be present'. Many directors living at a distance felt it impossible to attend on all occasions; although they had often subscribed ten to fifteen times more than those living in the town, their interests were often unrepresented. Again there were a number of other institutions in Northampton to be attended. Many country gentlemen refused to subscribe because of this situation.

Others considered that this measure would be likely to reduce further the attendance of those living at a distance and might result in too many proxies being exercised by one director which would give him too much influence. The Rev. J. P. Lightfoot introduced a slightly acrimonious tone when, according to the *Mercury* of 1 February, he said that 'it really seemed to be supposed that the gentlemen of Northampton had nothing whatever to do but to attend those meetings, while in point of fact they left their business frequently to their great inconvenience. Many gentlemen living at a distance were comparatively idle and could better afford the time for journey and all'. This proposal was rejected by a large majority.

Another point of interest at this Court was raised by Mr Charles Markham who pointed out that, according to the rules, no medical qualifications were required for the post of Superintendent, although the physician needed to be a Doctor of Medicine and the House Surgeon a member of the Royal College of Surgeons. Mr Lightfoot considered however that this omission was intentional and his view was supported by the meeting.

At a committee meeting held on 28 March, Dr Prichard was asked by Sir George Robinson 'whether', in the words of the *Mercury* of 29 March, 'the rumour was well founded that he had said it was his intention to resign. Dr Prichard replied that it was; that however serious he must feel such a step to be, in reference to its possible consequence to his wife and family, he was driven to it by the recent rules enacted by the Directors. The actual resignation must be made at a quarterly meeting. It is stated to be Dr Prichard's intention to establish a private asylum at his own risk, and it is further stated that he has received promises of extensive support'.

The next Quarterly Court met on 30 April. According to the *Herald* of 3 May, 'so large a number of noblemen and gentlemen has scarcely ever, we believe, been collected within the walls of that Institution, a circumstance, together with the restored good temper and good manners of the meeting, that promises well and, we trust, faithfully, for the future character and welfare of the Charity'. Prichard was asked whether it was his intention to resign. In reply he said, according to the *Mercury* of 3 May, 'I stated at your last meeting it was my intention to give notice at the present court of my resignation of 30 June. I made that statement because although I was not required to do so, and could not then give a legal notice, I considered it due, as an act of courtesy to the governors, such as I feel they would exercise towards myself, to give them the earliest intimation of my intention.' However, as he now found he could not take over his new home until 30 September, he would be happy to remain at the Asylum until then, if it did not in any way inconvenience the Court. He then formally put forward his resignation as Medical Superintendent as from that date and this was accepted.

After Prichard's withdrawal, the Court discussed whether the Asylum should be run according to the new rules or whether these should be held in abeyance until a new Superintendent took over. The new rules were accepted but the Court declined to appoint a visiting physician or a House Surgeon immediately: this latter position was becoming vacant as Marshall was a candidate for a similar appointment at Bethlem which he was thought likely to obtain, being one of three short-listed from 200 applicants. It was, however, decided to proceed with the nomination of a House Steward and Mr Knight, then acting in that capacity, was elected on the strong recommendation of Dr Prichard. The *Herald*, however, was not happy with this decision. It was concerned that the Chaplain had not been consulted as to his knowledge of Knight's religious principles and practices. 'What if he should be a Unitarian?' Knight was required to give security for £200 and a Mr Charles Davies of Kingsthorpe was prepared to stand surety for him. A bond was drawn up accordingly.

The method of finding a new Superintendent was then considered. Both Lord Spencer and Sir George Robinson were against relying upon testimonials, the latter adding that this system would enable any man with a good horse to ride about the county and carry the day, a reference to Prichard's success in gaining the nomination in 1837; he, like Lord Spencer, had not then voted in favour of Prichard. Instead it was agreed on 14 May 'to refer the election to three Medical Gentlemen eminent for their treatment of the insane'. The only restriction was that the successful candidate should be a member of the Church of England.

In spite of the unfortunate misunderstandings and the occasional irresponsible incidents of 1844, Prichard's superintendence of the Asylum must be regarded as a great success. Because, until 1844, he was constantly being told this by the Directors, he may have become conceited and have begun to feel that he was not being allowed sufficient freedom in the management of his patients or in organising his own work. He must, to have achieved so great a responsibility at so young an age in a fairly new and largely uncharted field, have been exposed to immense pressures. Perhaps he began to rely too much upon alcohol as a source of relief. Certainly, when he died on 1 September 1847, barely two years after leaving the Northampton Asylum, the cause of death on his death certificate was given as 'Hepatic disease', of which alcohol is sometimes the cause. Perhaps it was to this that Marshall, the House Surgeon, had been referring during his interrogation by the Court on 14 August 1844, when he said that Prichard had been ill for some weeks before the evening of the Superintendent's visit to Boughton Fair, and had declined to be questioned 'in the more extended sense' on the latter's taking too much wine.

That he was known to drink excessively on occasions may be considered further borne out by the brutal and relentless attacks made by the *Herald*. After one, published on 19 April 1845, in which it declared that the revised rules of the Institution were an attempt to force Prichard to resign, the Superintendent instructed Charles Britten, a local solicitor, to obtain a retraction of the charges made in that article, especially those regarding his professional reputation, or initiate legal action. The *Herald*, nevertheless, in its issue of 3 May swept away Britten's approach by stating 'we cannot retract opinions founded on facts and on events known to all the world, which have so often and so strongly been noticed in this journal'. Prichard made no further move.

The remaining months of Prichard's life can be briefly covered. He established his own private mental hospital at Abington Manor which he leased from Mr Lewis Lloyd of Overstone Park. This hospital was registered as the Abington Abbey Retreat, in November 1845.

> The institution is under the supervision of a Committee; and house visitors [according to a well-worded brochure], being subscribers to a Benevolent Fund, through which invalids of respectability and

education, but of limited incomes, – a class of patients who suffer most severely in mind and body from inappropriate treatment and classification – are enabled to enjoy the benefits which this Establishment confers, at lower rates of payment than they could otherwise be admitted for. By its constitution, then, the *Abington Abbey Retreat* possesses all the advantages that attach to a public Institution, while it is free from the numerous and obvious objections which unavoidably exist in hospitals admitting indiscriminately *criminal, pauper* and private insane patients under the same roof.

Rates were from one guinea a week upwards. Prichard himself earned a salary; the Matron was his wife.

His transformation from being Superintendent of the Asylum to Director of his own institution had not gone completely smoothly. At the Quarterly Court, held on Wednesday, 30 July 1845, Mr Young raised the point that Dr and Mrs Prichard had been canvassing the first-class patients, those paying the most, to transfer to Abington. Both Captain Spencer and Lord Northampton, according to the *Mercury* of 2 August, pointed out that:

> Dr Prichard was no longer their servant, and by accepting his resignation they had virtually given up their right even to enquire into the imputation against him. Because he was going to leave them, they would not be justified in trying to injure his character. The world was wide enough for them all . . . Every institution must expect to receive some such injury from temporary circumstances like these; but that was no reason why they should despair . . . Whatever might be said about Dr Prichard in other respects, no doubt the asylum had derived great advantages from his character for humanity in the treatment of the insane.

Prichard was then questioned on this matter. He made it plain, again according to the *Mercury*, that 'if the patients came from the neighbourhood, and not through his own connexion, he should consider them belonging to the Asylum and he should certainly not interfere with them. But with respect to patients recommended by his own father, or by his wife's connexions, he considered himself as much justified in expecting them to follow him, as Dr Robertson would expect to retain his patients, if he left his present residence . . . shortly before he went to Abington, he meant to send circulars to everyone of them. He considered himself perfectly justified in doing so'. After Prichard had left the meeting, Lord Northampton confessed that he thought there was a great deal of reason in what Prichard had said.

When in July 1846 the Commissioners in Lunacy reported favourably on the Abington Abbey Retreat the inmates numbered twenty-six, including twelve who had followed Prichard from the Asylum. They were provided with books, newspapers and bagatelle. Twelve to fourteen of the patients attended divine service regularly; the men played cricket occasionally and 'the ladies work at their needle and play on the piano'.

On Prichard's death, his cousin, Thomas Prichard, who had joined him at the Asylum, having studied medicine at Glasgow University and later succeeding as Superintendent of the Glasgow Royal Asylum, took charge of the Retreat. He also married his predecessor's widow, who was to die in 1852 at the age of forty-four. This Prichard was also a remarkable man. His humanity and concern for others can be appreciated by his insistence on regularly publishing reports of the work carried out at the Retreat. He was convinced that all who ran private establishments for the insane had a duty to do so. He died in 1878, to be succeeded as Superintendent by his brother, Henry Shutt Prichard, until his death in 1892 when the lease expired. Ownership of Abington Manor then passed to Lord Wantage who in 1897 gave the house and grounds to Northampton Corporation for use as a museum and a park; both are still used as such.

Chapter Five

DR P. R. NESBITT (1845–1860)

*A*t a Special Court, held on 26 July 1845, it was resolved, according to the Minute Book:

1. That Dr Nesbitt, at present one of the resident Medical Officers of Hanwell Asylum be, and is hereby, appointed Medical Superintendent of this Institution.

2. That Mrs Nesbitt be, and is also, elected Matron of this Institution, and that their joint salary be £300 per annum and that they enter upon their respective offices in this House on the first of October next.

Such was the satisfaction that they gave during their fourteen years at the Asylum that their joint salary was raised to £500, a handsome sum when taking into account that board, lodging and service were included. Dr Conolly, when Superintendent at Hanwell with its 1,000 patients, earned no more than £300 per annum. The Special Court also resolved that William Gurslave Marshall, who had failed to gain election to the vacancy at Bethlem, be appointed House Surgeon at an annual salary of £80.

Lord Spencer had not been present at the Special Court of 14 May, over which Lord Southampton had presided, when it was decided to approach three medical authorities, eminent for their treatment of the insane, for their recommendation, rather than rely upon testimonials as in the election of Dr Prichard. The last meeting he chaired or, indeed, attended had been on 30 April, when Prichard had formally resigned. Nevertheless, he acted immediately. He first approached Lord Ashley and Mr Robert Gordon, a Commissioner in Lunacy, and, on their advice, wrote to Dr Conolly of Hanwell, with whom he was well-acquainted, Dr Hitch of Gloucester and Dr Sutherland of Bethlem. He made it clear in his letter that the Asylum was not a county lunatic asylum,

> nor are there any funds subscribed annually for its use; it was built by private subscription and is now entirely self-supporting. It is, therefore, not only essential to its prosperity, but even to its continued existence, that the gentleman who has the care of it should have the confidence of the public. It is not probable that any gentleman already possessing this confidence will come forward as a candidate for the office of Superintendent of our Asylum, and therefore the only mode by which this essential object can be obtained is by placing the election in the hands of those whose names will be a guarantee to the public that the gentleman selected is well qualified in every respect to perform the duties of the office. The directors have consequently resolved to refer the election to three medical gentlemen answering this description, leaving it to me to decide to whom I should apply. I have decided that I cannot do better than apply to yourself [as one of the three].

The recommendation of Dr Nesbitt was made in a letter of 27 June, signed by Messrs Conolly, Hitch and Sutherland. They explained that, in addition to being a member of the Church of England, the successful candidate should, in their judgement, also have had practical experience of managing an asylum and that his wife should be capable of acting as Matron.

> Our selection [they wrote], eventually rested on two gentlemen; namely on Dr Nesbitt, one of the house surgeons of the Hanwell Asylum, and who in a late election of a resident medical officer at Bethlem was one of three candidates retained out of 160; and on Dr Huxley, who was lately elected medical superintendent of the Asylum at Gloucester, having been chosen to that office out of thirty-seven candidates.
>
> The claims of these gentlemen were so nearly equal that it was only after full consideration of all the circumstances in which the application had been made to us, and in consequence of the possession by Dr Nesbitt of a longer professional experience and of his being twelve years the senior of Dr Huxley, that we came to the unanimous determination to recommend Dr Nesbitt.

Dr Conolly wrote Lord Spencer a covering letter:

> Dr Nesbitt is a well-educated Physician. He took his degree at
> Edinburgh, and is practically and perfectly acquainted with his
> profession both as a Physician and Surgeon. His age is 38, and he is a
> man of very quiet and domestic habits; scrupulously attentive to his
> duties in the Asylum and punctual and laborious in the performance of
> them. He is also generally informed and unquestionably a man of talent.
> He further possesses the advantage of a good temper; and I cannot but
> hope that his appointment will be a fortunate thing for the patients, very
> satisfactory to the Directors, and particularly so to your Lordship and
> those who have always taken so great an interest in the welfare of the
> Asylum.
>
> Mrs Nesbitt is a very amiable and lady-like person, of a most kind
> disposition, devoted to the care of her young family, but feeling that kind
> of interest in the patients which is the best security for not neglecting
> them in the capacity of matron.

The Nesbitts at this time had six children with a seventh on the way. The
whole correspondence was entered in the Minute Book.

When Dr Nesbitt took over as Superintendent, there was much uncertainty about the Asylum's reputation as shown by the fluctuations in the
number of its patients. In the first quarter of 1844, before Prichard's much
publicised troubles, their number had been 230. By January 1845 they had
risen to 261 and in March of that year were 264. After the announcement of
Prichard's resignation, numbers began to fall off: in June there were 238
patients and by the end of September, when Prichard left, only 209. At the
end of Nesbitt's first month as Superintendent the figure sank to 191 but
afterwards there was a slow recovery. By January 1846, there were 217
patients, by April 235 and by the end of September, a year after Prichard's
departure, their number had risen to 258.

By 1859, Nesbitt's last complete year, the average number of patients in
the Institution had risen to 317, of which some 28 per cent were private
patients in two classes, first and second; the remainder were paupers from
the parish unions. It is therefore obvious that Dr Nesbitt quickly established public confidence in himself. This is reflected in his address to the
Quarterly Court in April 1846 when, according to the *Mercury* of 6 June
1846, he said:

> I do not propose presenting to the Court anything deserving the name of
> a report, because that I conceive may more appropriately be submitted

at the usual annual period. But any allusion that arrests the public interest cannot but operate beneficially on the establishment and those, therefore, who wish it progress will be gratified in hearing that, during the first six months commencing my duties here, there have been admitted no less than 78 patients, of whom 28 were private. This must be deemed to be a very large number of admissions and it appears still larger when compared with kindred institutions. At Hanwell, the largest institution in Great Britain, only 63 were admitted in the past year, whilst 78 are admitted here in six months.

Nesbitt also emphasised the moral aspects of the Asylum:

The bird's eye view of the operations of the establishment would not be complete, did I omit to state that, whilst the bodily health of the patients has been attended to, no means of improving or comforting their mental condition have been neglected. Whilst all acknowledge the difficulty of 'administering to a mind diseased', all will be disposed to hear with gratification that the treatment pursued here towards the afflicted inmates has been characterised by a strict adherence to those enlightened and soothing principles which the merciful spirit of the age insists upon. To control the violence of frenzy, or the passion of excitement, no severer method has been practised than that of withdrawing the patient from the surrounding objects of irritation by placing him in his own room, and even the temporary deprivation of liberty has not occurred without a reference or report to the Superintendent, and without its being registered among the events of the day.

This address, and the report made in October 1846 at the end of his first year, established the pattern of his superintendence. On the latter occasion, Dr Nesbitt emphasised that freedom from bodily restraint was one of the fundamental principles and that not even a strait-waistcoat had been used during the period under review. He however used what he later (January 1850) described as 'therapeutic agents', foremost among them being morphia, which had been found of 'inestimable value'.

Religion played a prominent role throughout. He stated in this report:

The Sunday ordinances of religion have been attended by the average number of 142 patients and nothing can be more decorous than the demeanour and attention of this orderly congregation. The consolation which public worship offers the insane, even if its effects be transient is striking, and affords an incontestable proof of the happy results which follow all well-directed efforts to improve the condition of this afflicted class.'

It was during his superintendency that plans were first considered to erect a chapel for the Asylum.

Nesbitt also considered, like Conolly, that exercise, education, amusements and occupations of various kinds were important factors in restoring sanity or at least in harnessing the energy of the patients. 'Music,' he reported to the Directors, 'has its charms for some, books for others, whilst idleness is discouraged in all.' In supplying entertaining books and means of employment and amusement, he was much encouraged by the Commissioners in Lunacy. Great attention was also paid to diet. When several paupers during the potato famine of 1846–7 'found a difficulty', according to Nesbitt, 'in reconciling themselves to the abstraction of their favourite esculent', and showed physical signs of dietary deficiency, they were quickly restored to health with vinegar, green vegetables or wine in addition to rice.

Before discussing Dr Nesbitt's term of office in more detail, it is important to note the effect of legislation upon the Institution. In August 1845, Parliament under Sir Robert Peel's administration passed two vital Acts. The Lunatics Act (8 and 9 Vict., *c*. 100) made compulsory the building of county asylums for pauper lunatics under the Justices of the Peace. It also established the new Commissioners in Lunacy – formerly the Metropolitan Commissioners in Lunacy – and laid down its composition and duties, including the records which the asylums were to keep; these dealt with admission, diagnosis, escape, cases of restraint or seclusion, transfer, discharge or death, and reports by official and other bodies. The Commissioners included five unpaid laymen, among them Lord Ashley who did so much to help the poor and mentally handicapped, together with three legal and three medical, salaried Commissioners. Their duties consisted of inspecting, licensing and reporting. A legal and a medical Commissioner were to visit each hospital once a year and licensed houses more frequently. They were to inquire about each patient under restraint and could discharge patients on their own authority. The second of the two Acts (8 and 9 Vict., *c*. 126) dealt with the erection and management of the county asylums.

These two Acts arose from a new social conscience, intent on tackling the appalling hardships imposed on the ignorant and poor by the Industrial Revolution; in 1842 it was estimated that one person in eleven was a pauper. They reflected the growing belief that those who could not help themselves should be cared for by the community and that there should be national standards of administration under the control of a central inspectorate.

As a result of this legislation and earlier enactments, the number of county asylums grew rapidly. By 1847, thirty-six of the fifty-two counties had asylums for the care of their pauper lunatics; by 1854, the number had risen to forty-one. This in turn led to a fall in the number of private licensed houses for the insane, as the county or public asylums absorbed an increasing number of patients. The Commissioners in Lunacy had, moreover, agreed in a supplementary report that, with prompt and proper medical and moral treatment, a high percentage of new cases of insanity could be cured; this in turn depended upon the availability of asylums. This view was optimistically supported by the superintendents, of whom Nesbitt was one. The newly emerging psychiatric branch of the medical profession was gaining confidence in its ability to cure. It was, however, frustrated by the continuing reluctance, through pride, of relatives and friends to send patients to the asylums until it was too late, which resulted in the space available being so largely occupied by chronic, long-term cases.

There was also the question of expense. The Commissioners' 1844 report made clear the reluctance of the local authorities to commit themselves to unnecessary expenditure in an age in which the principle of 'self-help' was being elevated as an ideal, and declared: 'Although we have no wish to advocate the erection of unsightly buildings, we think that no unnecessary cost should be incurred for architectural decoration, especially as these Asylums are erected for persons who, when in health, are accustomed to dwell in cottages.' Again staff wages were low and, as a result, so was the calibre of attendants, especially males, who were in general uneducated and on occasion too inclined to use force as a method of persuasion.

The administrative staffs were extremely small; even in the North-ampton Asylum there were only three medical officials, namely the Superintendent, the Matron and the House Surgeon who, with the help of an assistant, had to take care of some 260 patients in 1846; their number had not increased by 1859 when there were 320 patients. The Commission-ers recommended 200 as the maximum number of patients in an asylum but, because of the cost savings which could be achieved by size, the county asylums grew steadily. Here the Commissioners fought a losing battle. The Hanwell and Colney Hatch Asylums in Middlesex were each expanded to accommodate over 1,000 patients. The local authorities were unwilling to pay for small costly institutions, especially when it became increasingly evident that far fewer patients than anticipated were being cured. During the rest of the nineteenth century, the asylums could more and more be likened to warehouses for the incurable.

Against this somewhat sombre background, the Northampton Asylum occupied an unusual position. Many of the landowners in a predominantly agricultural county thought, in 1846, that they would suffer from a fall in corn prices as a result of the repeal of the Corn Laws. They were anxious therefore to avoid the cost of building a county asylum when they already had an Institution to which many of them had generously subscribed. The local Justices, many of whom served as Governors of the Asylum, genuinely wished to see the Asylum flourish, and to make it as comfortable as they thought reasonable, but not at the expense of the ratepayers. Many, accordingly, were in favour of the Institution becoming the county asylum for pauper lunatics as laid down by Parliament.

The Governors of the Institution, both county and borough, were however concerned to maintain a percentage of profitable paying patients which enabled them to introduce improvements and at the same time to retain control; this they would lose if the Institution became just another county asylum. There was strong support for the idea of helping those who were above the pauper class, who had worked to maintain their independence and who, when they became mentally afflicted, deserved better treatment than the pauper; many people believed paupers became so because of their own indolence. This aspect of policy was referred to again and again over the years when the Asylum's future was being debated.

Some counties wished to avoid the expense of building an asylum, preferring to farm out their pauper patients to other counties. Thus, in January 1845, before the passing of the two Acts that August, the Chairman of the Warwickshire magistrates attended a committee meeting in the Northampton Asylum where a proposal he had already made to Dr Prichard about the provision of permanent accommodation for 120–150 pauper patients from Warwickshire was discussed. A Special Court, held in March, to consider this further, thought it inappropriate to effect a union with Warwickshire in advance of the anticipated legislation. Nevertheless, the Warwickshire Magistrates again approached the Management Committee that November for a permanent arrangement.

A Special Court in April 1846 decided not to negotiate further with Warwickshire, which was to build its own asylum in 1854. It agreed to admit the Northampton county magistrates as part-proprietors of the Asylum for the sum of £12,000, providing that there was always accommodation for sixty private patients. The borough was likewise invited to participate, 'the terms to be calculated in proportion to the population of the Borough and the County with reference to the above £12,000'. A Committee was then appointed to discuss how to achieve this amalgamation.

No further progress was made for several years. Then in 1853, Lord Ashley, who had by now succeeded as 7th Earl of Shaftesbury, introduced an amending Act (16 and 17 Vict., *c.* 97). This laid down that a county asylum could be established not only by a single county but by two counties forming a joint authority, or by combining public financing and private subscription. In December that year, the Court of Quarter Sessions recorded that the Directors of the Northampton Asylum were willing either to unite permanently with the local magistrates, to contract for five years, or to continue receiving pauper patients under current arrangements. Moreover, the Asylum had no objection to magistrates being appointed visitors to the Asylum, attending its committee meetings, but they would not be permitted to vote. This was agreed.

In August 1854, the local press advertised a Special Meeting of Directors to elect a committee of five to discuss the admission of paupers with the county and borough magistrates. This arose from a recommendation by a Special Committee, under the chairmanship of Sir George Robinson, that additional accommodation for forty male pauper patients should be erected on terms to be agreed with the county and the borough. By 14 August, however, it had become apparent that the number of pauper patients requiring accommodation was much greater than originally calculated and it was therefore decided to postpone building until spring 1855 to allow time for negotiations. It is worth noting that the number of patients known to the Commissioners in Lunacy rose from over 20,000 in 1844 to close on 36,000 in 1858, the result of the increase in the population and of asylum accommodation but also of the lengthening expectation of life.

The need for more space had been emphasised in October 1854 when some forty paupers had to be sent away to allow alterations to the Asylum buildings. It had been intended to send them to the new Warwickshire Asylum until it was discovered that the weekly charge for each pauper would be 14s. to which several parishes objected. Arrangements were then made for them to go to Haydock's Asylum in Lancashire at a weekly charge per head of 10s.6d. in spite of objection by the Commissioners in Lunacy that they would be too remote from family and friends; this objection was further justified when the Haydock's Asylum raised its weekly charge to 14s., more than that charged by several County Asylums much nearer Northampton. Transport however provided no difficulty. There had been an enormous growth in the railway system during the 1840s and every railway company, according to the Cheap Trains Act of 1844, was compelled to run daily a train, using covered wagons, in each direction, at no less than twelve miles an hour and charging passengers no more than one penny a mile.

1855 saw the continuation of discussions between the Asylum and the magistrates of town and county, including those of the Soke of Peterborough, about sharing the responsibility of running the Institution and the fees to be charged. To provide the additional accommodation needed for all the pauper lunatics would however create severe financial problems. The two new wings required would, according to Milne, cost £10,000. In addition, £614 would be needed for new fixtures and fittings, plus a further £2,000 for a chapel, now considered essential. Altogether some £14,000 would be wanted if an estimated annual bill of £1,320 for wear and tear on the buildings, the equivalent of 3 per cent of the value of the hospital buildings, was taken into account.

It might be possible, the Committee thought, to raise a mortgage on the £14,000 required at 5 per cent; this would cost £700 a year. To pay for this, a weekly charge of 2s. rent per pauper patient, in addition to maintenance costs, might be made to bring in £1,100 per annum, leaving a surplus of £400 for paying off the debt. The sum required could be reduced only by postponing the building of the chapel and perhaps one of the two proposed new wings. The Committee earnestly wished that they could propose a plan 'by which this large sum may be realised, but as the Security which the Directors have to offer is not such as would induce capitalists to lend it either by a Mortgage or otherwise', they considered that it would be useless conferring with the magistrates without further consideration by the Directors.

From the Minutes of the January 1856 Quarterly Court, it appears that the Committee had reached agreement with the magistrates to receive all the county pauper lunatics, charging them each the additional 2s. per week, but the Commissioners in Lunacy objected to the scheme. It was therefore decided to send a deputation, representing both the Asylum and the magistrates, to persuade Sir George Grey, Home Secretary, to accept this proposed amalgamation. A meeting with him, held early in 1856, was followed by one with the Commissioners in Lunacy. The reason for the objection of the Commissioners was now clear; they would not have under the proposed agreement the absolute authority over the Northampton Asylum which they had over the county asylums. While they were unlikely to oppose the proposed arrangement for a five-year period, they would not commit themselves to a permanent union 'unless in the meanwhile', according to a letter from the Commissioners, dated 13 February 1856, 'the Justices of the County shall have taken steps to ensure for their pauper patients all the advantages and protection contemplated by the existing Lunatic Acts'. The Commissioners had, as early as 1853, informed the then Lord Chancellor, Lord St Leonards, that the Asylum offered suitable accommodation for pauper lunatics but they had 'no surety against its deterioration'. In the same communication, they had stated that they did not consider it desirable to exempt Northamptonshire either by a general or a special enactment. 'If the Justices or the ratepayers desire such an exemption they should obtain it by a local Act containing full and proper recitals.'

These meetings and the correspondence referred to above were discussed at length on 26 March 1856. As a result, it was decided to proceed with the erection of one wing only and to inform the Commissioners that the arrangement was to be for five years only and that they would together discuss 'the steps proper to be taken to meet the circumstances of the case at the expiration of the five years'. The meeting doubted whether a permanent arrangement with the magistrates could be reached as the 'stringent and restrictive character' of the legislation would reduce the Asylum to the status of a county asylum and 'render it illegal at least in public opinion for the reception of that Class of Patients by whose payment it had hitherto been so prosperously sustained'. They confirmed that the composition of its patients should continue to be two-sevenths private and five-sevenths pauper.

Progress in reaching agreement with the local magistrates on how to proceed further and what charges should be made for pauper patients slowed to a halt. The magistrates were not attracted, according to the *Mercury* of 2 August 1856 when reporting a Special Court held on 30 July, to the idea of advancing money towards the additional buildings required and then, at the end of five years, to have no property at all. Nevertheless, on the proposal of Sir George Robinson, who that year became the Asylum's Chairman, it was agreed to go ahead with building the additional wing, whose plans had been approved by the Commissioners.

There was no further progress in the negotiations with the magistrates for over two years. At the autumn Quarterly Court of 1858 it was minuted that further consideration of union with the county be postponed. Then in January 1859, at the start of Nesbitt's last full year as Superintendent, a copy of an extract from the Minutes of the Northamptonshire Committee of Magistrates was received. This asked its Chairman, the Hon. F. W. C. Villiers, to find out whether the Directors of the Asylum would agree to unite with the county to bring the Asylum under the provisions of the 1845 Lunatics Acts, 'the terms of the union to be reserved for subsequent consideration.' The Directors replied that they would be happy with such an agreement, 'provided the Committee of Magistrates can frame such terms as the law requires and as will be approved of by the Directors of the Institution.'

In the following month, Mr H. P. Markham, a member of Markhams, Solicitors, sent, as Clerk of the Peace of the County, to the Asylum a copy of a submission made by the county magistrates to the Home Secretary for inclusion in a Bill regarding pauper lunatics:

–   Whereas there are in some Counties in England Lunatic Hospitals erected and maintained by private and voluntary subscriptions which are fully sufficient for the reception of all the Pauper Lunatics of such Counties as well as the Private patients therein maintained, Be it enacted that in all Counties where there is such a Provision for the reception of Pauper Lunatics it may be lawful for the Magistrates of any such County etc. to contract with the Governors and Directors of any such Hospital or Asylum for the reception and care of their Pauper Lunatics provided that such Hospitals (as far as related to the Management of the County Paupers) shall be subject to the provisions of the Acts 8 & 9 Vict., c. 100 and 16 & 17 Vict., c. 98.

This submission recognised that the Asylum wished to retain its independent control with regard to private patients.

In March Mr G. W. Hunt, MP, wrote to say that it was desirable for a member of the Management Committee to give evidence in support of this clause to a House of Commons Committee. The Management Committee therefore asked that Sir George Robinson, Mr Collins or the Rev. H. J. Barton should attend and make clear the Committee's wishes that the county should be enabled to pay a proportion of the pauper patients' charges by way of rent so that the weekly charges imposed on the parishes might be reduced.

No further advance was made in 1859. Sir George Robinson as Chairman drew attention to this in the Annual Report for that year. The magistrates had been informed, he explained, that with the completion of the new building, the Directors were now in a position to undertake and guarantee the care of all pauper patients sent them by the county and borough. The number of private and paying patients had been reduced. They thought it was incumbent upon them to save the county ratepayers the heavy expense of erecting a new asylum. Their charitable intentions were evident from the financial outlay on the new wing, built and furnished to accommodate all the county paupers. Some of the funds for this came from the payments by private patients. He emphasised that, although no more was demanded than the average charge of the six surrounding county asylums, the diet of the Northampton Institution was 'most undoubtedly superior to the average of County Asylums'. To recover some of its out-of-pocket expenses, it was intended to increase the weekly charge of maintaining a pauper to 12s.6d., allowing 9s. for maintenance and 3.6d. for lodging.

Sir George was hopeful that all concerned would co-operate for several good reasons. Firstly, it was a temporary arrangement only until legislation allowed the cost of pauper accommodation to be thrown, as in most other counties, on the county rate. Secondly, no other county charged so little for maintenance as the Northampton Asylum. By voluntarily accepting the majority of the county's paupers, the Asylum had lost probably as much as £700 over the six preceding years. Finally, to quote at length a passage from the Report which reveals the good intentions of the Directors:

Because they [the Directors] strongly and painfully feel that since, by the passing of the said Act [Lunatics Act 1845], the care and cure of the pauper class has become a legal obligation, and ceased to be a charitable duty, they have not been acting up to the intentions of the benevolent individuals through whose liberality the Northampton Asylum was originally built. In accordance, as they believe, with the wishes of those men . . . they have kept steadily in mind the important object of making some adequate provision for bringing the advantages of the Asylum more easily within reach of that which may be called the lower middle-class of our population, such as tradesmen and farmers in narrow circumstances, and others whose means raise them just above the level of the Union Workhouse.

It is our firm belief that by a judicious appropriation of the surplus funds that may come into our hands, an immense amount of good may be effected, for it is known only to the eye of God what distress is occasioned, what heart-rending difficulties are endured, when insanity attacks a parent or a child in that narrow home whose apartments admit no seclusion and no silence, and where every hand is busily engaged in the struggle for daily bread. Your Committee of Management . . . have admitted from time to time about fourteen patients of the class alluded to above, but they earnestly hope that the Magistrates and Ratepayers of the county generally will support them in carrying out their benevolent object to a much greater extent. They cannot do so till they have paid off the heavy debt incurred in building the New Wing for the pauper patients, and that debt will not be discharged till the Ratepayers consent to pay for their patients on something like an adequate scale.

By insisting on their intention of helping 'the lower middle-class of our population' and at the same time maintaining control over the Institution, they forfeited the support of the Commissioners in Lunacy. Some years were to pass before the status of the Asylum was finally clarified.

There was at this time a growing fear among wide sections of the public that individuals were being wrongly certified as insane, often for unscrupulous reasons, and committed to an asylum. This was well illustrated by the activities of the Alleged Lunatics' Friends Society, founded in 1845 'for the protection of the British subject from unjust confinement on the grounds of mental derangement and for the redress of persons so confined'. The Society put considerable pressure on the Commissioners in Lunacy to deal with complaints sent to the Home Secretary by relations and friends of inmates in the Asylum who alleged ill-treatment or unfair confinement. Nesbitt scrupulously investigated each case; some patients were allowed their freedom, perhaps at first on a trial basis, only to be shown on occasion to be indeed insane to the satisfaction of the Commissioners.

In the summer of 1858, the Northampton Asylum came directly under the attack of this Society. Its Honorary Secretary was then Mr John Perceval, a son of the Rt. Hon. Spencer Perceval, who had been assassinated in 1812 while Prime Minister. Perceval had been approached by two former inmates of the Asylum, Trist and Verity, with a number of serious accusations against the Asylum's staff. As a result the Commissioners asked that the Asylum's Directors investigate the charges at the earliest opportunity. They did not consider it necessary for a member of the Commission to be present but agreed with the Directors' proposal to invite Perceval, Trist and Verity to attend in person.

In the event, none of the accusers appeared at the enquiry, the findings of which completely exonerated the Asylum of the charges brought against it. The Commissioners, in forwarding the Directors' report to the Home Secretary at the end of July, recorded their entire agreement with the Governors' conclusions and added that no further attention should be paid to Verity. A letter was sent to Perceval by the Asylum's Secretary, regretting his absence from the investigation and adding that they considered it 'their duty to represent to Mr Perceval the injury he may do to this Institution and the trouble and annoyance he gives to the Managers by encouraging and endorsing charges made by such worthless persons', and that they would not again waste time with statements made by Verity.

Perceval then considered it necessary to vindicate himself and gave a lecture in the Milton Hall, Newlands, in August 1858. The *Mercury* described him as calm, gentlemanly and remarkably self-possessed – bearing interruption with an unruffled courtesy – and exceedingly full of his subject; the lecture lasted four and a half hours. Having once himself been an inmate of an asylum, he was convinced that the accusations by Trist and Verity were true. Mr Collins, who attended this meeting with Nesbitt and the Chaplain, produced convincing proof to the contrary, while Sherlock, a former attendant at the Asylum, shouted out that one of Verity's statements, quoted by Perceval, was a lie. If the meeting was not an unqualified success, it may have raised doubts in the minds of some of the audience. Perceval continued to justify himself in a long letter to the *Herald* in September, while Verity held his own meeting at the Saracen's Head that month, at which Perceval failed to appear, in order to repeat his previous accusations.

Perceval did however pay tribute to Nesbitt on two counts. It was at the latter's suggestion that a doctor had to state, when making out a certificate of commitment, whether he was doing so through his own knowledge or upon hearsay. It was also on Nesbitt's initiative that a doctor had now to indicate whether he had previously known the patient or not.

The strength of the lobby supporting the Alleged Lunatics' Friends Society was further revealed according to the *Mercury* at a meeting held at the end of December 1858 at Milton Hall, 'for the purpose of taking into consideration the present defective state of the laws of lunacy'. The Chairman of the Asylum, Sir George Robinson, assumed that this meeting might be used to attack the Asylum and did not attend, nor did members of the staff. The chair was taken by Dr Charles Pearce, anxious to form a branch of this Society in Northampton, and was supported by Admiral Saumarez, the Society's Chairman. Pearce's arguments, primarily concerned with the property-owning classes, were the familiar ones, that on the request of a relative and with certificates signed by two physicians, an individual, unless a pauper, could be unjustly confined within an asylum. The pauper had greater protection since, in addition to an examination by the district medical officer, the relieving officer was consulted and a local magistrate or the clergyman of the parish called in; the guardian of the parish also usually signed the certificate. What was needed was a decision by a jury before a commitment of a non-pauper to an institution was made.

Dr Pearce's references to local concern about the alleged ill-treatment of inmates in the Northampton Asylum, including those already proved to be unfounded, and his statement that at least one-third of the patients 'in our Lunatic Asylums were curable' brought a vigorous protest in the *Mercury* from Sir George Robinson. He considered that, to release inmates before they were completey cured, would if these unfortunates were to marry lead to the spread of insanity to future generations. Not to be left behind in seeking improvements, Sir George also outlined the idea, long considered by the Management Committee as a result of the problems which had arisen during Dr Prichard's superintendency, that a physician be asked to visit the Asylum and report on conditions, but the Commissioners disapproved of this because it reduced the authority of the Superintendent. As a result, this idea was dropped. The controversy in the local Press rumbled on for some weeks.

The most constructive approach was made by Dr Nesbitt. In the first of two letters to the *Mercury*, he showed that the argument favouring trial by jury, when determining whether an individual should be confined for insanity, would be counter-productive. A person considered, possibly, to be of unsound mind would more likely be kept out of the public eye for reasons of shame and embarrassment than be brought before a jury; this would be turning the clock back to the bad old days when lunatics were kept in garrets and obscurity. He started the second letter by saying 'in justice to the existing law, that it is not in accordance with my experience to have known a single instance of its perversion to improper uses when due care has been taken to observe the provisions of the Statute'. In suggesting changes, he was hoping to obviate possible abuses, not because he felt that these abuses were of frequent occurrence. His main proposals were: that a patient should have the unimpeded right to appeal to the official powers; that the Commissioners should be empowered to empanel a jury to determine questions of insanity if they considered the circumstances warranted this; that the patient should have access to writing materials if he wished to complain; and that every patient be provided with a printed *Guide to Patients* within several days of admission so that he might know the rules of the Institution and how to obtain redress against detention and improper treatment. Overall, the correspondence which arose from the meeting at Milton Hall showed that there were still too many inadequate, bullying attendants, especially males, in the county asylums and that both proper training and better pay to attract a better type of staff were necessary. On several occasions, the Asylum's Minutes record cash rewards given to staff, on the recommendation of Nesbitt, for initiative and good behaviour.

Regarding complaints from and about patients and in matters of inspection, the Commissioners were very active from 1845 onwards. Two Commissioners visited Northampton every twelve to eighteen months, sometimes more frequently, and reported on all aspects of the Asylum, including the quality of the attendants. Their reports were entered in the Visitors' Book. They repeatedly criticised the overcrowding and ventilation in the attics, where the ceilings were very low, and offensive smells in the refractory dormitories. They were far more often than not complimentary on the cleanliness of the patients and the quality of the food. They were also occasionally shocked. In their 1849 inspection they found three females secluded in separate cells in the refractory ward, two of them naked and the third clad in a pair of trousers; apparently they had torn their clothes. This objectionable condition could have been obviated in their view by providing appropriate dresses.

In October 1850, they pointed out the need for a proper drying room – the offensive smells often derived from wet and unwashed bedding – for the enlargement of the airing courts, proper lavatories in the pauper wards, baths to be repaired and rendered more fit for use and the removal of objectionable beds and soiled bedding. The refractory wards were again unsatisfactory – this was all too often the case – and there was a need for a complete code of rules and regulations for the guidance of nurses and attendants. There should also be night nurses. A second visit in December that year, to find out how far the suggestions made in their October report had been carried out, showed much more satisfactory conditions.

There was further criticism in July 1854 about the refractory wards. 'The confined nature of the airing courts and the absence of all the usual articles of furniture and objects, calculated to occupy and interest the patients, tend to promote refractory and disorderly habits, and we recommend that immediate and earnest endeavours be made to improve the condition of the patients in that part of the Establishment by the introduction of better furniture, by affording ... frequent opportunity of taking exercise ... and by greater attention to their dress and general demeanour'.

The February 1855 report recommended the appointment of a Head Attendant on the male side and a night watch organised for both male and female departments. Otherwise the patients were found to be generally tranquil and in fair bodily health. In their September 1855 report, they found that additional furniture and some cheap weekly publications had been provided, a night watch organised but as yet no Head Attendant. Some improvements had also been made in the refractory wards.

A long list of suggestions appeared in the Commissioners' report for June 1856. These included: better ventilation and the plastering of the walls of the single private bedrooms and the refractory wards; the provision of washing arrangements and mirrors in the pauper wards; the enlargement of the principal airing grounds which should be laid out as flower gardens and planted with shrubs and provided with additional sunshades and seats.

Further criticism of the conditions in refractory wards were made in their July 1857 report, especially on the male side. 'Indeed when we consider the very defective arrangements of these wards, the confined nature of the airing courts, the total want of occupation and amusement and the congregation in them of all the worse cases in the Institution, we cannot wonder that their condition should be bad. We again urge upon the serious attention of the Governors and the Superintendent the suggestions made in the several entries in this book.' The 1859 report records that 'tell-tale' clocks had been installed for the night attendants, bedroom windows had been enlarged and the practice of using ordinary house mops to clean up 'dirty' patients discontinued, but there was obviously room for more progress.

In general, the relationship between the Governors of the Asylum and the Commissioners appears to have been good. That progress was not made as quickly as the Commissioners might have wished, must have partly been due in the earlier years to lack of funds, partly to uncertainties about the reception of the county and borough pauper patients and partly through lack of senior staff. This was to some extent recognised by the Commissioners. They wrote to the Asylum in December 1855 that they 'learn with satisfaction that so many of their recommendations have been adopted by the Committee of Management . . . As to the remaining recommendations which the Committee have not thought fit to adopt, the Commissioners forbear from further pressing their views and are satisfied with the fair consideration given to them by the Committee'.

There were a great many other developments in the years under review. In the summer of 1849, the Asylum purchased the adjoining twelve-acre estate, including, a cottage, from Mr James Atkins for £3,625 plus £7.10s. for various shrubs which could not be moved; it was decided to accommodate five private female patients in the cottage. This acquisition ended a quarrel between Mr Atkins and the Asylum. Atkins had complained continuously from October 1847 onwards of the nuisance caused by the smoke from the Asylum's chimneys and of the stench from its pigsties. Much time was spent by the Asylum's Directors in discussing how to overcome these problems, especially after Atkins had successfully taken them to court, but no completely satisfactory solution appears to have been found. Atkins sold the estate to the Asylum to avoid further unpleasant confrontations.

The maintenance and improvement of the main structure and its surrounds were constantly under review. The progress made by the end of 1852, when Nesbitt had served as Superintendent for seven years, was summarised in his report to the General Court of January 1853. Having dwelt at length on the increasing number of patients, he continued by congratulating the Court 'on the extinction of your debt and the brighter auspices under which you now meet as compared with so recently as three

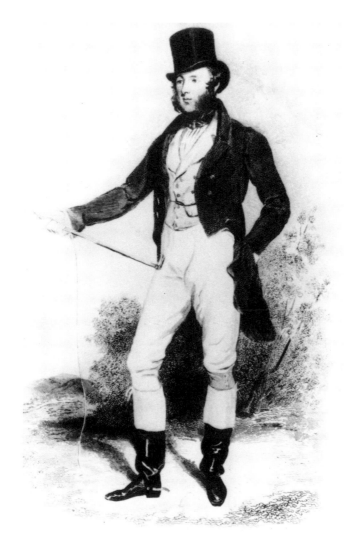

The 3rd Lord Southampton, President, 1866–72 (British Museum).

years since: then you paid £70 a year as interest to your Treasurer for money borrowed; you have now for the first time in the annals of the Asylum received from that Functionary £14 as interest due to you on this year's operation. During the last seven years you have succeeded in extinguishing a debt between £4,000 and £5,000. You have added one-third to the area of your property and will have at no distant time to consider how you shall deal with a surplus. You have accomplished all this whilst you have at the same time encountered heavy building extensions and improvements'. In the past year gas as recommended by the Commissioners in Lunacy, had been introduced 'and diffused its comforts in every part of the House' (but it was not extended to the Superintendent's bedroom until 1855); this was acknowledged as being of great benefit. Much needed extra water had been supplied by deepening the well, while the fitting of an artificial filter had rid the sewage water of impurities. There had also been heavy expenses in providing a new boiler in the laundry and repairing the kitchen ovens.

During Nesbitt's second seven years, the momentum displayed in the first half of his superintendency continued. In 1853 a further twenty-eight acres, belonging to the Rev. John Sergeaunt and lying immediately to the south of the Asylum, were acquired for £4,500. The Asylum's land contained clay suitable for bricks, over a million of which, intended for use in future building, had been made by 1856. Cows were bought and temporary dairy buildings ordered to be erected in 1858. Whenever possible, pauper patients were employed; they were not paid but, as Nesbitt pointed out, the income they produced to some extent balanced the outgoings on breakages.

Nesbitt throughout looked for considerable support from his Chaplains. Thornton resigned in 1847 and it was several months before his replacement was found. According to the *Herald* of 30 October, there was little interest in this post, but in the following month, the Rev. T. A. Manning was appointed on the recommendation of the Bishop of Peterborough at a salary of £125. He retained the post until March 1852 when he resigned through ill-health. The Management Committee then appointed a Sub-Committee of two clergymen (Sir George Robinson and the Rev. Chancellor Wales) and one layman (Mr Allan A. Young) to examine what the Chaplain's duties should be. It was agreed that there should be two services with sermon on each Sunday, and Holy Communion once a month. The wards should be visited daily and religious instruction given for one hour on each of the six week days alternatively in the male and female wards. Nesbitt considered that some patients could benefit by receiving elementary instruction in reading and writing. It was therefore decided as an experiment to employ someone, thought suitable by the Superintendent and Chaplain, to find out what results could be achieved. The greater importance of the Chaplain's post was emphasised by offering an annual salary of £200. The Rev. James McKee was then given the appointment, as usual on the recommendation of the Bishop of Peterborough.

Perhaps the most memorable occasion during McKee's chaplaincy was the report he made to the Annual Court in February 1856. He developed at length what he regarded as the relationship between the mind and the body and the causes of insanity. As reported by the *Herald* of 1 March:

> Every human being, he believed, received from his Creator a mind
> endued with intellectual faculties or powers and capable of a high degree
> of culture. Acquiring knowledge through physical or material organs, its
> attainments depended upon the state of those organs, and their
> malfunctions with imperfect or diseased conditions impaired or
> suspended the operations of the mind . . . But the mind being an
> immaterial, indivisible and incorruptible essence, it could not be subject
> to disease . . . In every case of what was incorrectly called mental
> disease, the cause was invariably a diseased or impaired condition of the
> nervous system . . . He went on to say that it might be regarded as a
> general rule that insanity was occasioned by whatever promoted vice, or
> was opposed to virtue, as by drunkenness, dissipation, infidel and
> revolutionary principles, and false and distorted views of Divine truth,
> which, keeping the mind in a state of feverish excitement and painful
> uncertainty, induced disease of its physical organs.

Of all causes drunkenness was the most awful.

It was an unusually long report and there followed much discussion about whether it should be reproduced in its entirety. As if to defend himself from implied criticism as to its length and contents – the Rev. Wm. Wales said that they did not look for that kind of thing from their Chaplain, but something of a more simple and statistical character – the Chaplain said that it was not half the length of some similar reports he had seen. Every part of it was intimately connected and he considered it would be incomplete if any part were left out. If their Chaplain was to be prevented giving in his report the result of his experience, he was placed in a most unenviable position, and might as well keep his mouth shut altogether. When his report was read at leisure, he felt sure they would not consider that he had wandered so wide from his province as they now seemed to think. Eventually it was agreed by all, including Mr Wales, that the whole report should be printed and circulated.

Nesbitt's initiative in providing occupations and amusements for the patients appeared to have been well supported. During his first month as Superintendent, Mr C. M'Corkell, who organised many concerts on its behalf, offered to sell to the Asylum the organ used for divine service. Because of the then uncertainty about the future, this was not taken up. Instead, a pianoforte then in the Institution was purchased for £31.10s.0d.

In November, an organ was hired for 15s. monthly. Mr M'Corkell's long service to the Asylum was eventually recognised in February 1858 when, having contributed £105 from two concerts, he was made an honorary Director for life.

In February 1847, Mr L. H. Forbes presented a pony chaise 'for the use', according to the Minutes, 'of such of the patients as the Superintendent may think right shall take exercise therein'. Inquiries were put in hand for a pony to draw the cart. In June of that year, fourteen copies of the *Christian Remembrancer* and forty-two numbers of Colbourn's *New Monthly Magazine* were acquired for the library for five guineas. At the Quarterly Court in January 1848, Nesbitt announced that 'a handsome bagatelle table had been added to the gentlemen's gallery and a very considerable accession of standard books to the library. Three daily newspapers are circulated in the house, in addition to various weekly publications and magazines of more or less ephemeral character'.

On the 19 January 1850, the *Herald* published the following paragraph under the heading of 'Northampton Lunatic Asylum':

On Tuesday evening last, about 160 of the patients, the officers, attendants and servants met together and, after tea, amused themselves with dancing; after which dissolving views, etc., were exhibited by Messrs Greville and Stenson to the gratification of all present. On the last picture, the portrait of Her Majesty, being shewn, the company rose and sang the National Anthem with éclat, accompanied by an efficient band. All seemed delighted by the evening's entertainment.

According to the *Mercury*, the ball ended at midnight by dancing the 'Sir Roger de Coverley'.

These dances, which became a regular feature of the Asylum's activities, were an exception to the usual strict segregation of the sexes. In 1859 a brass band played regularly once a week in summer. By then, a wider range of books, newspapers and magazines, which had received the approval of a Sub-Committee, were available. The education experiment, started with female patients, was proving satisfactory. Efforts were being made to improve the appearance of the wards with maps, pictures and furniture. As recommended by the Commissioners, patients with the necessary skills were being encouraged to make and mend the Asylum's clothing and footwear and a list of items made in the Asylum was included in the Annual Reports. In general, male patients were occupied with outdoor work until the making of clothes and footwear was introduced; female patients were ordinarily engaged in needlework, knitting, the

TABLE VII.

A RETURN OF ARTICLES

MADE AND REPAIRED IN THE ASYLUM,

DURING THE YEAR 1859.

MALE SIDE.

Made in Shoemakers' Shop—
Men's Blucher Boots (pairs) . 97
Women's Cashmere and Cloth
Top Boots (pairs)........... 91
Women's Leather Boots
(pairs) 44

Repaired in Shoemakers' Shop—
Boots and Shoes (pairs) 577

Made in Tailors' Shop—
Tweed Coats.................... 8
Fustian Jackets 55
Cord Trousers (pairs) 79
Fustian Waistcoats 32

Caps 166
Stocks 59

Repaired in Tailors' Shop—
Coats........................... 179
Jackets 261
Trousers 587
Vests 353

Made in No. 2 Male Ward—
(The whole of the hair being also
cleaned and picked.)
Horsehair mattresses 185
Sofa Mattresses and Cushions 18
Bolsters......................... 19

FEMALE SIDE.

Male Clothing—
Aprons 2
Flannel Vests 16
Neckerchiefs................... 37
Shirts—Day 109
,,   Night 12
Shrouds......................... 20
Stocks 15

Female Clothing—
Aprons 180
Bonnets......................... 6
Bonnet Trimmings 84
Chemises 133
Day Caps 185
Flannel Petticoats 135
Flannel Vests 19
Gowns 119
Hats 2
Night Caps 24
Night Gowns.................... 166
Pinafores 68
Pocket Handkerchiefs......... 87
Neckerchiefs—Cotton 48
Upper Petticoats 68

Bedding—
Bed Cases...................... 14

Blankets 172
Bolster Cases 343
Bolster Ticks 87
Mattress Ticks................. 32
Pillow Cases................... 13
Pillow Ticks................... 25
Sheets 185

Furniture—
Bed-side Carpets 16
Coffee Bags 14
Counterpanes 48
Cushion Cases 10
Cushion Ticks 10
Dusters 202
Long Curtains 11
Muslin Blinds 43
Pincushion Covers 12
Shaving Cloths................. 22
Tea Bags 2
Tea Cloths...................... 196
Table Cloths................... 3
Toilet Covers 112
Towels—Bath 67
,,   Round 18
.,   Toilet................. 21
Window Valences.............. 29

List of work done by female patients, 1859.

83

TABLE VI.

DIET TABLE.

PAUPER PATIENTS.

BREAKFAST.

Males— 6 oz. of Bread, ½ oz. of Butter, and 1 pint of Coffee.
Females—6 oz. of Bread, ½ oz. of Butter, and 1 pint of Tea.

DINNER.

Sundays,
Tuesdays
and
Thursdays.
}
Males—11 oz. of Uncooked Meat, 12 oz. Uncooked
  Vegetables, 3 oz. of Bread, and ¾ of a pint of Beer.
Females—9 oz. of Uncooked Meat, 12 oz. Uncooked
  Vegetables, 3 oz. of Bread, and ½ a pint of Beer.

Mondays
and
Fridays.
}
Males—1¼lb. of Irish Stew, 3 oz. of Bread, and ¾ of
  a pint of Beer.
Females—1lb. of Irish Stew, 3 oz. of Bread, and ½ a
  pint of Beer.

Wednesdays
and
Saturdays.
}
Males—16 oz. of Meat Pie or Suet Pudding, and ¾
  of a pint of Beer.
Females—12 oz. of Meat Pie or Suet Pudding, and
  ½ a pint of Beer.

SUPPER the same as Breakfast.

SCALE FOR ARTICLES UNDERMENTIONED.

PER GALLON.

Tea—1 oz. of Tea, 3 oz. of Sugar, and ½ a pint of Milk.
Coffee—3 oz. of Coffee, 5 oz. of Sugar, and ¾ of a pint of Milk.

PER POUND.

Meat Pie—2oz. of Uncooked Meat, 12 oz. Uncooked Potatoes, 5 oz. Flour, with Dripping.
Irish Stew—2 oz. Meat, 10 oz. Uncooked Potatoes, seasoned with Pepper, Salt and Onions.
The liquor of the previous day's boiled meat is added to the Irish Stew.
Suet Pudding—4 oz. of Bread, 2½oz. of Flour, 2oz. of Suet, ¼ a pint of Milk, and 1 oz. of Sugar.

The diet of pauper patients, 1861.

laundry and housework.

The pace of improvement in the provision of amenities for the patients did not however always satisfy the Commissioners. In their report, dated 8 June 1858, they recommended that:

> a better description of comfortable furniture be provided for the sick, such as small bedside tables, leaning chairs, sofas, etc.; and that a lighter kind of movable furniture, more washstands and blinds and curtains, be introduced generally. We further recommend that objects of interest and amusement be supplied to every ward, regard being had to the classes of patients occupying them. We would suggest, among other things, cheerful Illustrated Publications (as the *Leisure Hour*), prints, maps, statuettes, chimney ornaments, flowering plants, singing birds and domestic animals. We also suggest the introduction, for the amusement and instruction of the Inmates, of Stereoscopes, a Magic Lantern, Cheap Microscopes and Kaleidoscopes. The patients also would, we think, much enjoy many games, as Les Graces, Carpet bowls, Ninepins etc.
>
> A much larger number of Patients than at present should, we think, be taken out to walk beyond the limits of the Institution, and no Patients should be restricted for exercise to their walled Airing grounds.
>
> It is essential, in our opinion, that persevering efforts be made to induce all Patients capable of employment to occupy themselves. We suggest, among other occupations, mat making, straw plaiting, hat and bonnet making, basket making, netting and spinning.
>
> A more systematic arrangement for the supply and distribution of instructive and entertaining books and periodicals throughout the wards appears to be much needed and we suggest that, for the purpose of quiet reading and occasional social intercourse, the Committee room might beneficially be made available.
>
> As respects the Male Pauper Patients, we think it desirable that they should be provided with more varied dress and a better suit for Sundays.

There was also some criticism for the first time during Nesbitt's superintendency of the diet.

The administrative efficiency of the Asylum was also improved during the 1850s, largely due to the commercial acumen of Mr Collins. In 1852, he was highly critical of the stock-taking and accounting procedures. There were, for example, no accounts kept of the Asylum's farm produce. According to the *Herald* of 28 February, he told the Court that:

> The institution was never enough considered in the light of a large

mercantile concern which it really was. They had 270 ledger accounts with patients, and what was wanted was a check to ensure that they were charged with all that they should be and an account of stock taken yearly. They might then obtain a correct statement of their position at the end of each year.

Collins considered the management of the stores and the keeping of proper accounts too much for one person. He added that the accounts were kept in a way which made an analytical and comparative review of the Institute's progress impossible. He challenged an accountant to make anything of them for the past five years. He also argued that the Management Committee should have a regular Chairman. While these comments aroused the ire of the honorary auditors, the Directors agreed that his recommendations on book-keeping be seriously considered.

In 1855, Collins called attention, at the Annual Court, according to the *Mercury* of 1 September, to the extremely irregular attendance by members of the Management Committee. When Sir George Robinson pointed out how far some members had to travel, Collins emphasised how serious the situation was becoming in view of the amount of work facing them; he did not see how they were to function efficiently without something like a continuous committee. Sir George admitted the force of Collins's argument and pointed out that, although this was an Annual Court, they had no statement of accounts and no progress report on the Institution; it emerged that two years' reports were published together. A regular Chairman and Vice-Chairman were elected from 1856 onwards.

Starting with 1858, there was an Annual Report, which in addition to statements by the Chairman of the Management Committee, the Superintendent and the Chaplain, contained much statistical and other information. That of 1860 included lists of deceased benefactors, anonymous donors, living benefactors and Directors; an annual balance sheet; salaries; statement of income from pauper patients; contract prices for provisions, necessities, etc., and a summary of provisions used and their cost; abstract of the farm account, a diet table and an account of work done by patients. There were also tables showing the assistance given to private patients of small means and a return of structural additions and alterations carried out during the year.

Certainly the Finance Committee went to considerable effort to find the most efficient accounting system for the Asylum. In 1856, the Rev. H. J. Barton had for this purpose visited the asylums in Buckingham, Oxford, Gloucester, Worcester and Leicester. Convinced that the Leicester methods were the best, he had gone there again with Mr Collins and the

Rev. Mr Wales and, as a result, that system had been operating for a year in Northampton when in March 1858 a Special Court of Directors met to consider combining the offices of Secretary and House Steward. The duties of the Secretary were said to be largely nominal, the greater part of them being the House Steward's responsibility. There was much to be said for one person keeping the accounts. The opportunity for doing this arose from the resignation through ill health of Mr Harday, who had been Secretary to the Asylum since its inception; he was granted a pension of £60 per annum. At the same time, Hetherington, the House Steward, had been dismissed for misconduct, so the way was clear for this move which the Court unanimously approved. In the following month, John Godfrey of Leicester was selected by a clear majority to fill the new position of Secretary-House Steward. Godfrey had been clerk in the office of Mr Frere, a Leicester solicitor, who was Clerk of the Leicester Asylum. Godfrey had been responsible for its accounts, the whole of which had devolved upon him; in fact the Leicester system had been suggested by Godfrey. He was also Secretary of the Leicester Young Men's Association. His annual salary was, after much discussion, fixed at £200.

Throughout his superintendency, Nesbitt appears to have insisted on the respect he considered due to his position and himself. In October 1846, he received a sharp rap over the knuckles by a junior employee of the Commissioners in Lunacy for failure to make certain returns. His lengthy reply, making clear that the omissions were the fault of his predecessor and not himself, was so worded that he received a handsome apology from the Commissioner's Secretary. He was firm in his politely expressed opinions and occasionally clashed without disadvantage with individual Directors. His good reputation pulled him through the mischievous attack made on him in 1857.

In October of that year, the Commissioners received several letters accusing the Superintendent of drunkenness. These letters were accordingly forwarded to the Asylum in November, where they naturally aroused considerable perturbation. The Management Committee immediately investigated the charges and on 25 November instructed the Secretary to reply, pointing out that 'they are all written on the same description of paper and apparently in the same though a disguised handwriting'. The letter continued:

It is clear that a Gentleman in the official function which Dr Nesbitt holds may sometimes in the imperative discharge of duty expose himself to the ill-will of Servants, as well as of patients, and it may be of their friends and that the greatest inconvenience might arise were it generally understood that the ear of the Committee is readily open to complaints.

At the same time it is due both to Dr Nesbitt and the wellbeing of the Asylum that grave charges such as those conveyed through the Commissioners should receive the serious and best attention of the Committee. They have accordingly examined the Chaplain, House Surgeon, House Steward, Deputy House Steward and Secretary, these being parties with whom Dr Nesbitt is in constant daily communication and they deeply regret to state that the conclusion to which they are brought (though upon the evidence of the House Surgeon alone) is that, while Dr Nesbitt may not have exceeded the bounds of temperance so as to disqualify him for the discharge of his duty, there have been times of distant date when by the use of wine he has exceeded the bounds of discretion.

The House Surgeon was a Mr George Smith whose request for a salary increase in October 1854 had been turned down; he resigned in May 1858 and later became an active Director of the Asylum.

Still however when the Committee remembers the service which Dr Nesbitt has rendered during the twelve years that he has been Medical Superintendent of this Asylum and when they also take into consideration that for the last between three and four months he has abstained altogether from the use of alcoholic or fermented liquors and expresses his intention permanently to do so, they are unanimously of the opinion that the necessities of the case will be met by reading this letter to him and admonishing him from the Chair of the certain and serious consequences to himself of charges similar to the present being substantiated.

The Committee postponed returning the original letters until such time 'as the purpose for which they wish to retain them shall have been accomplished'. This purpose was achieved when, at the General Court in January 1858, it was decided to dismiss Hetherington, the House Steward, for forging the letters; this was confirmed at a Special Court in the following February.

On that occasion, the Chairman, Sir George Robinson, told the meeting how the case against Hetherington had been built up. One of the letters had said: 'Ask Mr Hetherington, the House Steward; he, at least, dare speak the truth'. Hetherington, however, had refused to tell anything about Nesbitt, except on oath; as nobody had the power to place him on oath, he escaped the responsibility of saying anything. From that moment, the

Chairman had concluded that the House Steward was not worthy of confidence. On questioning other officers, it transpired that Harday, the Secretary, had heard Hetherington say that he would have his revenge on Nesbitt. On being questioned, the House Steward replied: 'I did not use the word "revenge". I said, "satisfaction".'

At this stage in the enquiry, the Chairman thought it proper to ask the Commissioners to see the original letters. The Commissioners gladly agreed as there was a suspicion of forgery; 'on comparing the several communications, it was evident that they proceeded from the same source'. The originals were then compared with Hetherington's books: they were also sent to a handwriting expert who, having examined them against orders written by Hetherington, had not the slightest doubt that they were all written by the same person. The Rev. William Wales understood that Nesbitt was prepared to have him back but, in spite of Hetherington's protests of innocence, the Court unanimously decided that he should be dismissed.

The Commissioners, in acknowledging the Management Committee's letter, were not sympathetic. They considered it highly dangerous 'that the habits which appear to have been proved against Dr Nesbitt should be held to be in any form, however modified, compatible with the discharge of a duty so delicate and so responsible as that which is entrusted to him, they can only offer to the Committee a hesitating and qualified concurrence. They cannot but feel that Dr Nesbitt's conduct has been viewed with extreme leniency, having regard to the nature of the practices charged and established against him'. They hoped that Nesbitt's future conduct would justify 'the consideration and tenderness with which he has been treated'.

There can be little doubt that, as in the case of Prichard, the ever-growing responsibilities of the Asylum put Nesbitt under enormous pressure. Added to this there was his wife's growing and understandable concern with bringing up their large family, which was housed in the asylum building, itself a contributory factor to his decision at the end of September 1858 to resign. In spite of having 'exceeded the bounds of discretion', his record and achievements at the Asylum had evidently retained the respect, even the affection, of the Asylum Directors. In view, no doubt, of the confidence they showed him, he was persuaded to rescind his resignation, 'feeling satisfied', as he wrote on 26 October, 'that, whilst I devote myself to the faithful discharge of my duties, you will always respond to the just and legitimate influence which the Superintendent of this important hospital should possess. It only remains for me to say that whilst Mrs Nesbitt would have preferred to exercise the more strictly domestic duties of Life, she is willing to continue in the position she fills . . .'. It might be assumed that in writing thus he felt himself to be in a position of strength. Certainly there had been no accusations of the neglect of patients, as in the case of Dr Prichard, nor any hounding by the local press. His contribution to the controversy aroused by the supporters of the Alleged Lunatics' Friends Society probably increased his standing.

The Directors, however, seemed unable to comprehend the load under which Nesbitt worked. They did not understand the warning implicit in his reference to his wife in his letter of 26 October. At the Quarterly Court in April 1859, Nesbitt called attention to the overcrowding of the male quarters of the Asylum. Nevertheless, he did not recommend the addition of a wing, such as had recently been completed for female patients, but instead the use of his family accommodation in the Asylum for patients and the provision of his own house. His current accommodation was inadequate: he often had to surrender his dining room to allow patients to be visited by friends while his family took refuge in their bedrooms. In any case it had become the practice at modern asylums to provide houses for Superintendents. The cost of such a building was estimated to be about £1,200.

Nesbitt may have been encouraged in making this request by the speed with which the Secretary had been provided with a small house in the grounds; the proposal was made in July 1858 and the structure virtually completed by the following January. No response, however, to Nesbitt's letter is recorded in the Minutes.

Then on 27 July Mrs Nesbitt handed in her letter of resignation:

Allow me most respectfully to ask your permission for the Doctor to reside with myself and family without the walls of this Institution.

The continual anxieties and responsibilities of my office are now telling fast upon my constitution and I feel it due to my own family to tender my resignation before it be too late to retrieve the effects of the long strain that has been imposed on my energies.

I would not on any account inconvenience the Directors unnecessarily but if agreeable to them I should wish to move in October next before the winter sets in when I shall have completed my fourteenth year of official life in your Asylum.

The Court, chaired by Lord Euston, later 6th Duke of Grafton, accepted her resignation with regret but decided that neither the Superintendent nor the Matron should reside outside the Establishment nor were they prepared to make any alterations in the Statutes on the subject. Nesbitt accordingly handed in his own resignation at the next Management Committee meeting. At the same time he advised the Committee that it needed to print the regulations, some of them newly revised, as these would need to be available for candidates for his office. There was currently only one copy of the Statutes, last printed in 1851.

The regret which the Superintendent's resignation occasioned was made abundantly clear at the Quarterly Court on 25 January 1860, the last which he attended as Superintendent. William Smyth, according to the *Herald* of 28 January, said that he did not wish as Chairman to take the initiative but he felt strongly that the services of Dr and Mrs Nesbitt had been very great and deserved the thanks of the Directors. There may have been faults at different times, but anyone could see that the Asylum's interests had been greatly promoted by their devotion. A formal resolution thanking them for their zeal and ability was passed unanimously. Nesbitt had decided to establish his own asylum but made it clear that he was taking no attendants with him and exerting no pressure on private patients to follow him. Satisfaction was expressed at that statement.

In conclusion, it might here be asked how effective was the Asylum in achieving cures during the period under review. Nesbitt in his report covering 1856 and 1857 was cautious on this point. He made it clear that fair comparison between Northampton and such major institutions as Bethlem and St Luke's was not possible as these, unlike his own Asylum, excluded 'epileptics, paralytics and those whose malady has been of longer duration than six months'. However, over a ten-year period, he calculated that on average 33 per cent of the cases were cured, which he regarded as as high as could be expected and therefore a satisfactory result.

Chapter Six

DR EDWIN WING (1860–1865): THE
BUILDING OF THE CHAPEL

*T*he Directors met to discuss the appointment of a new Superintendent in October 1859, an occasion on which Dr Nesbitt was told that any recommendation he might wish to make would be welcome. The main point at issue was whether the new Matron should be the wife of the Superintendent. Mr Smith, the former House Surgeon, said there were decided objections to this. The Superintendent and Matron, when husband and wife, made a formidable combination and no one dared speak; moreover, this arrangement put too much power in their hands. It was accordingly agreed that the Superintendent should be married but that the Matron should not be his wife.

It was also generally considered that the new Superintendent would probably want to be far more independent domestically than his predecessor had been. He would wish to be provided with his own servants and kitchen. Mr James Mash said that a gentleman must see his friends and such arrangements would no doubt be more agreeable to him. Sir George Robinson, however, advocated just offering a salary of £400 plus apartments, board and attendance; further details could be discussed with the successful candidate if they were raised. In the event, the new Superintendent was given an extra £150 per annum, instead of board, and the use of a separate larder; he was allocated a housemaid and provided with vegetables from the garden. The question of accommodation outside the main asylum did not arise.

At the Special Court, held in December, there were five candidates both for the superintendency and for the post of matron. It was an unusually large meeting attended by fifty-five Directors. Because many of them were not well-acquainted with the way the Asylum functioned, Mr Collins, with the approval of his colleagues, expatiated on the qualities required of a Superintendent. He also referred to the question of the accommodation available, which was not commodious enough for an official with a large family. This immediately ruled out one candidate with a family of ten. After further discussion, fifty-three votes were given in favour of Dr Edwin Wing, Medical Superintendent for ten years of the Fisherton Lunatic Asylum, Salisbury. Prior to this, he had been Superintendent of the Wyke House Asylum, near London, and Resident Manager of the Longwood Asylum, Bristol.

Of the candidates for the post of matron, Mrs Grant had testimonials from, among others, the Mayor of Northampton, the Rev. Mr Wales and from Henry Terry, the surgeon to the local jail. Mrs Grant had been deserted by her husband, who had embarked with a Miss Spencer for America and it was thought they had lost their lives when their ship had gone down. Mrs Grant was therefore virtually single – a plain, honest, intelligent, kind-hearted woman, according to one supporter, with a good knowledge of common life. Many Directors present knew her and the voting gave her a clear majority. The Superintendent was given two living rooms, one each side of the ground floor main entrance and five bedrooms on the second floor; the Matron was allocated a living room on the ground floor and a bedroom on the second. Perhaps because she had only two rooms, the Management Committee refused to allow her two sons to spend part of the Christmas holidays in the Asylum. Six other rooms not in use on the second floor were reserved for male private patients.

During the years of Dr Wing's superintendency, the number of patients steadily increased. In January 1860, the year he took office, there were 321 on the books; the number at the year end was 342. By the end of 1861 there were 357 patients; by the end of 1862, 371; by the end of 1863, 406; and by the end of 1864, as many as 414. The total number of pauper lunatics in Northamptonshire as on 1 January 1861, according to a report published by the House of Commons, was 510; 258 of these were in the Northampton Asylum with 11 in other institutions, while 107 were in workhouses, 122 resided with relatives and the remaining 12 boarded out.

Continuing attention was accordingly given to increasing the accommodation. Early in 1860, new offices and storerooms were provided for the Secretary-Steward, Mr Godfrey, on top of which were constructed rooms for male pauper patients, giving what was then thought to be an ample supply of new beds for sometime to come. There were other improvements.

The No. 3 Refractory Ward, so often criticised by the Commissioners in Lunacy, was entirely remodelled, making a spacious and airy day-room. The kitchen's facilities were improved; the exercise yards were enlarged and fitted workshops provided.

Wing was undoubtedly a man of intelligence and energy, determined on making a favourable impression. He took over from the Nesbitts on 1 February 1860, and on the following day inspected the Asylum. He found the female wards neat and clean but had criticisms to make of those on the male side. He disapproved of the way the bedding was folded up at the foot of the bed in a manner calculated to conceal its condition. This system he immediately altered. He also objected to the long-standing custom of horsehair being picked for blankets in Ward No. 2 as this caused litter and dust. A workshop was soon allocated to mattress-making and hair-picking. The shoemakers were also removed from the wards for similar reasons. He remarked on the shortage of urinals and the state of some of the water-closets, matters which were later remedied. He also ordered that gas lights should not be left burning unnecessarily, and that all should be turned off by 10p.m. except in the officers' room.

Another step taken in his first year was to separate the accommodation of the private from the pauper patients as far as he considered desirable. The two groups met at Divine Service, saw each other during their outdoor occupations and occasionally at their recreations. It was sometimes argued that private patients felt degraded by being placed under the same roof as paupers. This, as shown in his first Annual Report, he believed to be purely a theoretical objection. In any case, some of the paupers had started life in far more favourable circumstances, only becoming impoverished through their illness. It was his opinion that there was 'an animation and cheerfulness if not an efficiency, in the mixed Asylums not met with in the exclusively pauper or private Institutions'.

By 1863, the Asylum, according to Wing, was becoming overcrowded but it was not until 1864 that an addition to the female side provided thirty-one extra beds, a schoolroom and other useful space. A separate building was also commissioned for fifty patients. The Mayor and Town Council of Northampton objected to the siting of this new building adjoining the Billing Road.

> Such a step [they wrote] will in our opinion be very prejudicial to the comfort of a large class of respectable people living in that neighbourhood. The Hospital as it now exists is nearer to the Road than it should have been as the cries and noises from the Patients on the present premises are occasionally most distressing and indeed

occasionally alarming to passengers using the Billing Road, which we
need scarcely say is fast becoming the most desirable locality for
residents in the town of Northampton.

It was pointed out to them that this would not be the case. Other
improvements during these years included a further enlargement of the
kitchen, additional lavatories and urinals, new floors and ceilings, extra
boiler accommodation, an enlarged brewhouse, and terraced walks and
flowerbeds in some of the airing courts and much redecoration. A new,
much taller chimney was also authorised as the original one was found to
be in a perilous state.

Wing believed that all efforts for the recovery or improvement in health
of the patients should follow three general principles. The first step to a
sound mind was a sound body. This should be promoted by encouraging
the proper performance of the various bodily functions through correct
diet, good clothing and lodging, pure air, exercise and judicious medical
treatment. Secondly, for comfort and ease both of body and mind, all
sources of discomfort and irritation should as far as possible be removed.
'In pursuing this object we may sometimes appear to lean to the luxurious
rather than the useful; but in the case of the insane, that which with others
might appear a superfluity and extravagance is, in truth, but a powerful
remedial means'. Thirdly, everything possible should be done to divert the
mind away from morbid brooding by directing its attention 'into new and
more healthful channels, by rousing the torpid, stimulating the listless and
apathetic, soothing and comforting the timid, nervous and apprehensive,
and by calming and tranquillising the restless and excited; in short, by the
employment of the various means ranged under the general heading of
moral treatment'. The absence of restraints is not mentioned: by now this
was no doubt taken for granted. Nevertheless, forced feeding was occasionally considered necessary, as in the case of a female patient who in
February 1860 had refused food for several days. A pint of beef tea with two
eggs in it was given her via a tube passed through the nose into the
stomach.

Patients who appeared to be well on the road to recovery were allowed
out when practical and with the approval of the Management Committee
for trial periods, rather than discharged as completely cured. To follow the
latter course would artificially raise the number of cures and at the same
time the number of admissions, when patients released prematurely were
returned to the Asylum because they were not yet capable of coping
independently. Wing more than once protested, as his predecessors had
done, at the practice of sending patients to him only when they were dying

ARTICLES.		First Quarter.		Second Quarter.		Third Quarter.		Fourth Quarter.	
		s.	d.	s.	d.	s.	d	s.	d.
Bread	Per 8lbs.	1	0½	1	0½	0	10¾	0	10½
Flour	Per 20 stones.	45	0	44	0	38	0	40	0
Ox Beef—Sides	Per stone	3	6	3	8	4	1	3	8
Wether Mutton	Per stone	3	11	4	6	4	1	3	8
Arrowroot	Per lb.	1	4	1	0	1	0	1	0
Butter	Per lb.	1	1½	1	1½	1	1	1	1¾
Candles { Moulds	Per dozen lbs.	8	0	8	0	8	0	7	4
Candles { Composites	Per dozen lbs.	11	6	11	0	...		...	
Candles { Dips	Per dozen lbs.	6	3	7	0	6	6	6	4
Cheese	Per lb.	0	7½	0	7	0	7	0	6¾
Coffee	Per lb.	1	4	1	2	1	2	1	1¼
Eggs	Per score	2	0	...		1	6¼	...	
Mustard	Per lb.	0	10	0	10	1	0	1	0
Pepper	Per lb	1	2	1	2	1	2	1	2
Rice—Patna	Per cwt.	26	0	20	0	18	0	18	8
Snuff	Per lb.	5	0	4	9	4	9	4	9
Soap	Per cwt.	42	0	40	0	38	0	38	0
Soda	Per cwt.	8	0	6	0	6	0	6	0
Starch	Per lb.	0	5½	0	4½	0	4½	0	4½
Stone Blue	Per lb.	1	6	1	3	1	3	1	3
Sugar { Loaf	Per lb.	0	5¾	0	5½	0	5½	0	5½
Sugar { Moist	Per lb.	0	5	0	4¾	0	4¾	0	4¾
Tea	Per lb.	3	0	3	0	2	10	2	9
Tobacco	Per lb.	3	5	3	6	3	6	3	6
Malt	Per bushel	8	3	8	3	8	3	8	0
Coals	Per ton	14	3	14	3	14	6	14	6

Contract prices for the principal articles of consumption for the four quarters of the year 1861.

or completely beyond hope of recovery.

Perhaps Wing's philosophy is best summed up in his 1861 Annual Report where he stated:

I would desire most earnestly to remove the impression, which all too extensively prevails, that a Lunatic Asylum is merely a place for the safe custody and detention of the dangerous and troublesome, and to substitute the knowledge that it is a hospital specially arranged for the medical treatment, cure, and relief of a class of diseases the most

disastrous with which man can be afflicted, and that all the means and
appliances used have this end solely for their object, and nothing will be
found inconsistent with the highest philanthropy.

He went on to quote from the most recent report from the State Asylum
of Pennsylvania:

It is now so well established that the most liberal provision for restoring
the citizens of a State to a sound mental health and usefulness, in a
reasonable period of time, is vastly more economical than any
arrangements, however humble their character, which look only to the
permanent security and support of the same class as incurable, that no
further argument on this branch of the subject can be necessary. Many
incurable cases cost the community more thousands of dollars than
restored patients do hundreds, or parts of hundreds, while the latter
become productive members of society. Nor is it less well established by
universal experience that, in a large majority of cases, insanity can be
treated with the highest degree of success only in its early stages, and in
institutions especially arranged for its treatment, with abundant
provision for classification, occupation and amusement, under the
direction of competent medical officers, and with a great variety of
means and appliances that can hardly be got together but by the
patronage of the state, or extraordinary efforts of private liberality.

The Court was sufficiently impressed by Wing's statements and quota-
tions to agree to have them printed and sent to the county gentry, clergy
and Guardians of the Poor on the recommendation of the Rev. Lord
Alwyne Compton, a member of the Management Committee, who was the
fourth son of the 2nd Marquess of Northampton; he later became Bishop of
Ely.

Wing appeared to be sensitive to all aspects of a patient's reaction to
circumstances. There was, for example, the question of attire. A greater
variety of wearing apparel was introduced, including the provision of
Sunday suits. Clothing the insane was not, he declared, a simple matter:
much depended upon knowledge of their habits and feelings. Unsuitable
raiment could cause considerable irritation, not easily soothed. 'Many are
in the habit of destroying their clothing; but it would be a great mistake to
dress all these in strong and coarse materials, or to suppose that old, worn,
or shabby garments are good enough for them. On the contrary it often
happens that, when supplied with good neat and comely clothing, they
respect and prize it; the vicious propensity is broken and finally forgotten.

Loss of self-respect is a prominent feature among many of the insane, and to be well dressed is a powerful means of reviving it'. In his monthly report for July 1862, Wing asked permission to carry out a recommendation made by the Commissioners, that male paupers should have two shirts a week instead of one.

Wing also placed great emphasis on recreation. He allowed as much liberty as was consistent with security. When feasible, patients were allowed out of the Asylum's grounds on parole and without attendants. Others were taken out in large or small parties for walks or occasional drives in the surrounding countryside. Picnics were organised in summer and outdoor games encouraged. A bowling-green was laid out in the grounds and footballs and skittles provided.

There were even grander occasions. In July 1862 there was, according to the *Mercury*, a cricket match between members of the asylum staff and a team drawn from various local clubs. A large concourse of visitors took tea with the teams, and there were speeches and toasts. While this was going on, the patients assembled on the adjoining bowling green, where they 'regaled themselves *ad libitum* with tea, plumcake, etc., their appetites being sharpened by the strains of the Asylum brass band'. After tea, there was the following programme:

Dance: Hands Across
A hurdle race for men
A Comic Scene by two black men
Dance: Polka
A flat race for old women
A song and chorus by the Asylum Glee Club
Dance: Quadrille
Bobbing for tobacco and buns dipped in treacle
Game: drop handkerchief
A comic song by two old female itinerants
A wheelbarrow race blindfold
Dance: Scottische
Jumping in sacks
A flat race for women under forty
Dance: Triumph

Prizes for the races, including a full tobacco box or tie for men, and gowns or handkerchiefs for women, were supplied by Dr and Mrs Wing and the House Surgeon.

Indoors there were facilities for bagatelle, billiards, cards, chess, draughts and other games. On two evenings a week, two-hour recreational meetings were held under the guidance of one of the Officers; there would be dancing, singing, music, magic lantern shows, lectures and readings – sometimes by the Chaplain – from Shakespeare, Dickens and other authors. There were also conjuring shows, one of them performed by 'a professional illusionist, Herr Dobler', an entertainer sufficiently well known to have his name mentioned in the Annual Report. These occasions were enlivened by the brass band formed from among the staff of the Institution.

On New Year's Eve 1860, the new room of No. 3 Male Ward was the scene of a party attended by over a hundred patients, who were allowed to invite relations and friends. There were two Christmas trees, hung with thoughtfully chosen presents for individual inmates. This party was also attended by one or two Directors, several clergy and medical men and 'other respectable inhabitants' of the neighbourhood, 'who cheered us by the sanction their presence gave to our proceedings'. Wing also reported that many objects of interest, especially 'pictures, birds, gold and silver fish, guinea pigs, white, black and spotted mice, fancy poultry, etc.' had been introduced into the Asylum to interest the patients. At the same time, every effort was paid to discipline, cleanliness and regularity, all of which influenced the mental climate: 'None but those accustomed to witness them can fully appreciate the evil effects upon the insane of a want of punctuality, disorder in arrangements, untidiness, broken furniture and numberless other matters, an attention to which is indispensable to comfort and to make life agreeable.'

The appointment in April 1861 of a new House Surgeon, a Dr Summerhayes, aged twenty-six, previously Medical Officer at the Surrey Dispensary, allowed Dr Wing to introduce the custom of male and female private patients 'of the first class', selected by him, dining each evening with the House Surgeon and Matron, their meal being served with every attention.

> This mixing of the sexes, which, in our recreation meetings, is carried out on a much larger scale, is attended with the best effects and has the most civilising influence in promoting habits of self control. Those whose language and deportment in the presence of their own sex alone are most offensive, learn to behave themselves with perfect propriety in the society of the opposite sex.

Summerhayes, incidentally, proved to be idle and ineffectual. Having failed to report three attendants for bullying and neglecting one John Jayes, who was badly injured as a result, he was reprimanded by a Special Committee in January 1862, whereupon he resigned and left at once. His successor, Duckworth Williams, aged twenty-two, six months acting Assistant Medical Officer at Gloucester Asylum, where his father was Superintendent, was of a very different character. At his selection, it was agreed in principle that the post of House Surgeon be open to all practitioners in medicine and surgery, including those with Scottish and Irish qualifications and not, as previously, confined to members of the Royal College of Surgeons of England and licentiates of the Apothecaries Company.

Wing in 1861 brought forward a further development.

Female influence is about to be brought to bear in another way in the establishment, and in this I am glad to have the full sanction of the Commissioners in Lunacy, women having been engaged to nurse the very aged, the helpless and the sick men. Nursing is the natural province of woman; her superior delicacy and tact are universally acknowledged, and in all our civil hospitals and infirmaries, as well as in many of the military ones also, females are employed to tend the men. A few Lunatic Asylums have followed the example, with which it is a pleasure to number our own.

There were excursions in 1860 and 1861 to the Parks of Castle Ashby and Althorp, to Blisworth Gardens by rail, to Wombwell's Menagerie and to Hamilton's Diorama of a continental tour shown in Northampton, to flower shows at Easton Neston and Kingsthorpe Hall, and to religious meetings and services. There were other amusements, occasionally unexpected. A fox strayed into the large men's airing group, was chased, caught and petted; the fox subsequently broke loose and escaped but after a few days 'voluntarily returned to his quarters and quietly submitted to his loss of liberty, thus showing that the care and attention bestowed upon him while with us had made a grateful impression upon him'.

It was in June 1862 that the first expedition to Llandudno, North Wales, took place; it was made with the full support of the Management Committee and with the approval of the Commissioners. In his report for that year Wing wrote:

The benefits to be derived from change of air and scene, from the interest created by the novel and the beautiful, the relief from the monotony of the daily routine of life, and the invigorating agency of the sea breeze, are universally acknowledged and eagerly sought for by the sane whose means place these advantages at their command. They frequently form the first means resorted to on the appearance of mental derangement in the higher class of patients, and there can be no question of their beneficial tendency upon the mental and bodily state of asylum residents, provided the cases are selected with judgement.

It was a well-organised expedition.

In his April report, Wing explained that he had been offered a large and commodious house in Llandudno and that the Railway Company had agreed to a considerable reduction in fares and to provide special carriages to go all the way without changing. He had been in touch with the friends of the patients he wished to take and they were prepared to pay the extra expenses. He merely asked the Management Committee to allow a sum equivalent to the cost of maintaining the patients as if at home in the Asylum. Thirty-five patients, all private except for one female pauper, made the journey. The party spent a month at Llandudno and the holiday was considered an outstanding success.

The reaction of the inhabitants of Llandudno was at first less than friendly. According to an indignant report in the *Mercury* of 2 August, 'The benighted views of a century back were still prevalent amongst them, by which affliction was considered as a crime and its unfortunate subjects loathed, execrated and shunned. Had an uncaged menagerie been taken to the place, greater consternation could not have been produced.' A public protest meeting was held, strong language used and forcible expulsion threatened. John Godfrey, the Asylum's Secretary, who organised and accompanied the excursion, wrote to the Rev. John Morgan, one of the Improvement Commissioners of Llandudno, that while Dr Wing wished:

to pay every proper deference to lawfully constituted authorities, he
cannot, on the other hand, lose sight of the serious responsibility entailed
upon him of protecting the legitimate rights and interests of those
committed to his care; legally, he cannot for one moment doubt his
position . . . Taking, therefore, the circumstances of the case into
consideration, the ill effects that might follow upon the hasty removal,
after so long a journey, to several of the party who are old and infirm,
and the hopes of absolute restoration to health a sojourn at the sea-side
would give to many others, Dr Wing desires most respectfully, but yet
most firmly, to inform the Improvement Commissioners that their views
cannot be acceded to. At the same time he would reiterate the assurance
that every precaution has been, and will continue to be, taken to make
the stay at Llandudno as little noticeable as possible.

The Commissioners in Lunacy were informed, gave Wing their full support, and their letter was forwarded to Dr Morgan. In 1862, a slightly smaller party spent the month of September peacefully in Southsea. During their stay, they were visited by the superintendents of several asylums who were obviously interested in the possibilities of these holidays. Several years, however, were to elapse before further such vacations were taken.

The occupation of the patients was as important as their recreation. In his report for 1860, Wing commented on the considerable increase in the number of patients employed in various tasks, amounting to a daily average of over fifty. The Matron was congratulated on the high quality of the articles made in the female department and the Steward likewise complimented on the results of the tailors' and shoemakers' efforts in the new workshops. The work out of doors also increased and would have been reflected in the farm's profits had there not been a severe frost the previous winter.

In 1861, the average daily number employed in various ways had increased to between 230 and 240; these figures did not include private patients who occupied themselves with such pursuits as reading, drawing, painting and music. All the boots, shoes and articles of clothing required by the patients were now made in the Asylum's workshops, producing a useful profit. Likewise, the farm provided the patients with good, fresh and early vegetables at a very moderate cost, 'luxuries which many of the private patients can fully appreciate and to which they are justly entitled.' Even if these enterprises were unprofitable, which they were not, the advantages of providing the inmates with occupations fully justified them. Wing had personally run the farm without a bailiff which enabled him to regulate the work of the patients according to their dispositions and mental states. 'In addition to the more ordinary labour of cultivation, hay time and harvest give rise to occupations which may almost be classed with recreations, in which many women and patients of the higher classes join; they afford, too, opportunities for festive gatherings productive of much happiness and keen enjoyment.'

In his 1864 report, his last, Wing showed his willingness to experiment with new methods of treatment. Great attention had been paid to epilepsy, which he regarded as the most grievous of the complications associated with insanity. Dr Williams, the House Surgeon, had given bromide of potassium, a new medical preparation, careful and extensive tests with excellent results, which had been reported in the medical Press as 'exhibiting industry and a talent for research most creditable to him'.

Wing, like his predecessors, always gave credit where it was due. For this, among other reasons, his superintendency must have been popular. It was not affected by the occasional suicides, accidents, escapes and bullying by attendants; every case appears to have been carefully investigated and swift retribution taken against inadequate employees. There was certainly no shortage of staff. In 1862, junior nurses started at a wage of £9 per annum, including board and lodging, while more senior female staff earned up to £20. On the male side, attendants earned from £20 upwards with uniform provided. The hall porter was paid £27 per annum, but had to find his own uniform. The attendant who looked after the farm received £33 per annum. Wages were regularly reviewed and increments given.

The House Visitors' Report Book recorded the comments of the Management Committee who visited the Asylum in rotation. Nearly all of their remarks were favourable although the water-closets and urinals were sometimes adversely mentioned. The cleanliness and general contentedness of the patients were often noted. The Visitors' genuine concern for the patients is very clear. James Mash in April 1861 'examined the meat, bread, cheese and butter which appear to be of good quality. Also tasted the Port Wine and Porter which is very good'. Several visitors that year thought that the beer might be improved. In September 1861, C. E. Crawley was not satisfied with the want of cleanliness in the kitchen, more particularly in the larder, store rooms and basement. The cook was overworked and needed help. He found the iron stove alarmingly overheated and the floor of the washroom sunk in places; immediate attention was needed in both cases. Such criticism was comparatively rare. The entries were read out regularly at the monthly meetings of the Management Committee and usually acted upon.

The visits of the Commissioners in Lunacy were also recorded in the House Visitors' Report Book. In 1860 and 1861, while generally well-satisfied with the work of the new Superintendent, they advanced a number of recommendations; these included inspection of bedsteads and the withdrawal of those which seemed dangerous, the disuse of corded sacking as the cords offered facilities for suicide, better ventilation in the dormitories and more care in serving and distributing the food. Subsequently, they gave increasing credit to Wing. In February 1863, they wrote: 'We highly approve of the efforts on the part of Dr Wing to cheer and amuse the patients and relieve the monotony of their existence and the good results of his labours are to be found in the general tranquility and contentment which prevails among them . . . We had no complaints of harshness or ill-treatment on the part of the Attendants, who on both sides (male and female) seem to be respectable and well-conducted.' Their report for March 1864 was equally flattering although, 'while the whole of the inmates gave evidence of kind and careful treatment', efforts might be made to bring the male wards up to the very high standard of the female wards. Wing was again warmly complimented both in 1864 and 1865.

The Asylum was now entering a period in which its financial problems were lightened. By March 1860, no agreement had been reached with the county and borough Justices about the housing of their pauper lunatics. The Management Committee under Sir George Robinson therefore decided to raise the weekly charge to the Workhouse Unions for paupers from 11s to 12s.6d. and to ask for the magistrates' co-operation in making the Boards of Guardians appreciate the situation. This increase was to be temporary until the introduction of legislation which could impose the expense of lodging and repairs on the counties instead of on the parishes, as was done in respect of the county lunatic asylums.

The county magistrates quickly responded. In a letter to Sir George Robinson, Mr Villiers suggested that an attempt be made to have a clause inserted in a Bill concerning the management of asylums, then thought to be in preparation, to allow the magistrates of Northamptonshire not only to contract from time to time with the Northampton Asylum, notwithstanding previous legislation to the contrary, for their pauper lunatics to be cared for by the Asylum, but also for the county to be empowered to raise the necessary funds for their lodging. To this, the April Quarterly Court of 1860 unanimously agreed.

The Guardians of the Unions accepted the increased charges but asked that the lodging costs be paid for by the county. William Smyth, Vice-Chairman of the Management Committee, spelt out in a paper which was circulated to the Unions the details of the agreement reached between the Asylum and the magistrates, together with the instructions, based on this agreement, which had been sent to the Members of Parliament representing the county and the borough.

It was not until the autumn of 1862 that the hoped-for legislation was passed. The Lunatics Law Amendment Act (25 and 26 Vict. 111) of that year contained a provision legalising a contract between a lunatic asylum and the County Justices for the former to accept the county pauper lunatics and for a sum, not exceeding a quarter of the total cost of maintaining and caring for a pauper, to be charged on the county rate. A Committee of Magistrates, led by Mr Villiers, accordingly met the Management Committee with Lord Euston, later the 6th Duke of Grafton, in the chair and decided to work out a detailed agreement. At a further joint meeting in the following February, the Asylum agreed for a three-year period to reduce its weekly overall charge for pauper patients from 12s.6d. to 12s. or less, leaving it to the magistrates to decide how this sum was divided between the county and the parishes. The Commissioners in Lunacy gave their somewhat grudging approval, subject to minor alterations in the wording and to the Justices becoming responsible for the full payment for those pauper lunatics whose parish could not be established.

The Asylum Directors were delighted. They had achieved the best of both worlds, namely the right to provide accommodation and care for the county pauper lunatics, and at the same time to take in private patients, whose revenue allowed them to look after those unfortunates, described as members of the lower middle classes, whom the Management Committee had always desired to help.

> That desire [as the Management Committee stated in their Report for 1862], they had every reason to believe, will very speedily be gratified, and they may now look forward with confidence to having an increasing surplus each succeeding year, from the payments of the high-class patients, which may be devoted to the relief of those in humbler and poor circumstances, who are now received at the lowest charge as private patients.
>
> Their wishes in this direction have been hitherto necessarily restrained by the heavy expenses entailed upon them for the reception of all the county pauper lunatics. Large sums of money have been annually expended on building and furnishing for that purpose . . . These expenses will now cease, and your Committee have much pleasure in announcing that they have entered into a contract with the County Justices to take charge of all their lunatics for the next three years at a weekly maximum charge of 12s per head for their board and lodging; their cure, if possible, their care at all events.

In their 1863 report, the Management Committee could 'use no other language but that of congratulation' when commenting upon the current and future prospects for the Asylum. Having generously thanked the Asylum's officials for their achievements, they drew particular attention to the Institution's financial prosperity.

> The year began with a balance due to the Treasurer of £1837.13s.7d. It ended with a somewhat diminished balance of £1771.7s.7d, a difference in favour of the last year of £66.16s.0d, but to this small difference we must now add: For mortgage debt paid off, £2000; for the contribution to chapel, £942.16s.0d; for new buildings, £797.12s.10d; for extra furniture, £310.15s.1d. These together give us a surplus, beyond the ordinary expenditure, of £4117.19s.11d. If no sudden emergency should call in the present year for a greatly increased expenditure, we confidently expect

that to our successors on this Board of Management will devolve the grateful task of reducing the charge for the maintenance of Pauper Lunatics.

The current rate of charges on the ratepayer was lower than the lowest of the neighbouring Asylums of Leicester and Rutland. In addition, £642.9s.0d. had been paid out charitably to support the needy.

This new legislation of 1862 also gave Management Commitees the power to demand maintenance payments for patients out on trial. 'Patients on leaving an Asylum,' according to the Superintendent's report for the same year, 'have much difficulty in procuring employment; their friends are too poor to support them and the customary grants from Poor Law Funds are inadequate to their requirements, the consequences of which are frequent relapses from poverty and hardship.'

The Management Committee had not, of course, waited until the legislation had been enacted to give financial help to deserving members of the lower middle classes. Their report for 1860, signed by Sir George Robinson and William Smyth, Chairman and Vice-Chairman respectively, stated:

> It is feared that an impression has gone abroad that this Institution does not administer the amount of charity that many of the Subscribers would desire to be supplied to that class of private patients whose friends are hardly able to pay the sum of £1.1s.0d a week for their maintenance, which is the lowest rate of payment for private patients. The Committee, therefore, desire to call public attention to a Table, appended to the Report, which will show that, by the reduction of this charge in the cases of thirty-eight of the poorer class of private patients, a sum of between £600 and £700 has been this year remitted or given in charity.

The generosity of the Asylum in this respct has been consistent throughout its history.

In view of the sums regularly spent on helping the poorer private patients, it was formally agreed at a Special Court of Directors, held after the July Quarterly Court of 1861, that the 1852 resolution, 'that all Donations and Legacies be funded and the interest applied to such charitable uses as may be approved by the Directors', be rescinded. It was decided to ask the Trustees for their consent to the money being transferred to the Institution's general account.

There were other matters of interest worth recording. Mr Collins, seconded by the Rev. H. J. Barton, proposed in February 1860 that, at

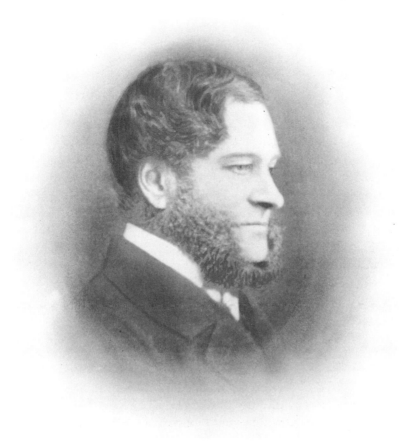

William Smyth, Esq., Vice-Chairman 1856–65, Chairman 1965–70.

meetings of the Management Committee, they should have a preliminary private sitting without the presence of the Asylum's officials; this was agreed. Godfrey, the Secretary-Steward, on being asked for £100 security, offered his life policy for £400 and his furniture; these were accepted. A Committee was formed in 1861 to discuss with the Commissioners of Taxes a revision of the Asylum's assessment. A reduction was promised but the £1,000 demanded in September 1862 was double what had been agreed at the meeting. Collins investigated the matter and reported that, while on a three-year average the amount due was less than £1,000, it was over this sum for 1861 and 1862. It was therefore agreed to pay what had been assessed on the understanding that there would be no further charges for several years to come.

General Everard William Bouverie, the son of Edward Bouverie, who had played a prominent part in the early years of the Asylum's history, was by now taking an increasingly active part on the Management Committee as was W. H. I. Mackworth Dolben, who also became a member of the Finance Committee. Sir George Robinson and William Smyth remained Chairman and Vice-Chairman respectively throughout this period. In 1863, it was agreed that a Sub-Committee be appointed to visit the patients and inspect the buildings once a month. In April 1864, Mr Collins referred to the quantities of wine and malt liquor consumed on a scale far greater than at Leicester and Birmingham Asylums, but the Superintendent was able to show that the percentage of patients in Northampton who recovered was greater than in the other two institutions!

It was decided by the Management Committee that from August 1864 the Medical Visitation Book, the Superintendent's journal, the House Surgeon's diary and the Secretary-Steward's day book should be regularly inspected and signed. It also became a serious breach of the rules if food unconsumed at dinner was not returned to the larder.

Perhaps the outstanding event during Dr Wing's superintendency was the building of the chapel. That one should be erected was forcefully recommended by the Sub-Committee which had been appointed in April 1852, when Dr Nesbitt was the Superintendent, to consider what the additional duties of the Asylum's Chaplain should be. It had become increasingly difficult to accommodate the number of patients wishing to attend Sunday service in the No. 1 Male Ward. The Sub-Committee emphasised, from their own experience and from the observations of the Superintendent, that they were satisfied 'that a building of an Ecclesiastical character for the solemnization of Public Worship would not be without its cheering and solacing as well as sanitary effect upon the minds of the unfortunate persons who might be assembled therein'.

At the General Court, held on 26 January 1853, it was formally resolved that a chapel was desirable. The Rev. J. P. Lightfoot, later to join the Management Committee, pointed out that not only was the Institution then out of debt but before long should have a large sum to its credit. They could not do better than by devoting their first favourable balance to the building of a house for the honour and service of God. Mr Young thought that the use of a gallery for worship did little to soothe the mind or solemnise the occasion. Ecclesiastical architecture was a most important factor in achieving the right response and he hoped that a first class ecclesiastical architect would be employed. Dr Nesbitt emphasised how inconvenient it was to assemble patients in a gallery 'where smoking and other propensities connected with the insane polluted the atmosphere.

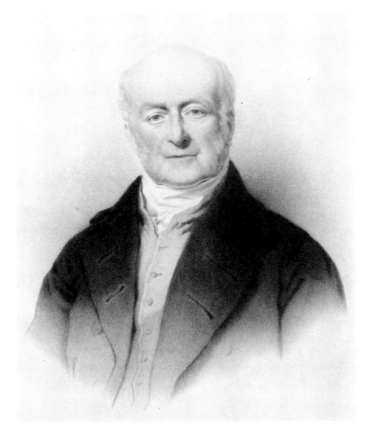

General Everard Bouverie, son of Edward Bouverie of Delapré Abbey.

At an Occasional Meeting later held under the chairmanship of Mr Edward Bouverie, it was decided to recommend that a chapel be erected between the Billing Road and the male airing ground and that it should be connected by a covered way with the main building. On 11 May, it was decided to seek legal advice whether the consecration of the chapel, although on private ground, would entitle the public to be granted admission; if so, confusion might be created. It was also decided to engage Mr George Gilbert Scott to produce the necessary plans.

Scott's first plans were examined in detail at a Special Court in July 1853 and were adopted. Scott was also asked for specifications to enable the Committee to go out to tender; the date for completion was to be left to the Committee, guided by the architect.

George Gilbert Scott (1810–77) was the leading exponent of High

Victorian Gothic. Knighted in 1872 on the completion of the Albert Memorial, he built up an enormous, mainly ecclesiastical, practice. Among his best-known works are St Giles, Camberwell; St Mary Abbots, Kensington; St Mary's Cathedral, Edinburgh; the Martyrs' Memorial, Oxford and St Pancras Station Hotel. He was in his early forties when approached by the Directors and at the height of his powers.

The chapel was not however completed until 1863. The reason for the delay had been lack of funds, in spite of Lightfoot's hopes, and uncertainty whether satisfactory arrangements could be reached to house the county's pauper patients. At the General Court of October 1855, it was reluctantly recommended that the building be postponed, although this would 'seriously interfere with the spiritual comfort and instruction of the class patients in the Asylum'. Accordingly, in December it was decided to ask Scott to send in his charges for professional attendance and his plans, which then would have to await a more favourable climate.

In January 1858, Dr Nesbitt again reminded the Management Committee of the need for a chapel. It was therefore decided to create a Special Fund for this purpose, allocating to it part of the income derived from private patients and placing in it sums contributed as the qualification for new directorships. In March, the Annual Court accepted the recommendation that a Committee, consisting of Sir George Robinson and Messrs Nethercoat, Wales, Barton and Nesbitt, be formed to raise the necessary funds. It was agreed to approach the nobility and gentry of the county and the relatives of patients in the Asylum, each letter of appeal to be accompanied by a lithographed plan of the proposed building and the information that every donor of £20 or more would qualify as a life Director.

The report of the Chapel Committee was given priority in the Annual Report for 1858. It regretted that 'they have not met with that cordial support which they had anticipated ... Compared with the wealth and extent of the County of Northampton, the amount of subscriptions hitherto promised or given (about £1,000) is lamentably small'. In the hope that the public would make up the deficiency once the work had begun, they were taking steps to complete the work if possible before next winter. 'They have requested Mr Scott to come down and inspect the site, that he may be prepared with specifications and working drawings without further delay.'

The invitation was sent to Mr Scott in March 1859. He was unable to comply with an immediate appearance as he was completing his designs for the government offices in Whitehall, originally planned in the Gothic style but altered, on Lord Palmerston's insistence, to a Renaissance treatment. As for the money required, Sir George Robinson was strongly of the opinion that it should not come from the Asylum's general funds but from special contributions by churchmen. He also pointed out that several subscriptions had been made on condition that the chapel was consecrated; there were difficulties here which it was hoped could be overcome but, if not, those contributions, which were dependent on consecration, would have to be returned.

Little progress financially appears to have been made in 1859. 'The same complaints, the same regrets, are still expressed on all sides, and expressed hitherto in vain.' The new Superintendent, Dr Wing, was said to have been as anxious as Nesbitt for the provision of a chapel, because of its immense importance 'in the moral treatment of the insane'. Wing, according to the report, continued: 'The assembling in a proper ecclesiastical edifice has quite a different effect from gathering in an ordinary room or ward. The preparation for going – the walk there – the meeting in an appropriate place – the more solemn and impressive character of the service – the return, etc., all exert a beneficial influence, while there are positive disadvantages in the use of a ward, irrespective of a want of due reverence and solemnity. It makes confusion, untidiness and disorder in apartments where quiet order and neatness ought to prevail'.

Nevertheless, the Chaplain was encouraged by the attendance of patients at Sunday services and daily prayers; 'Quiet decorum of behaviour and devotional attention have invariably characterised them', according to his 1859 report. 'In institutions like this', he continued, 'much more is attempted, and, I think I may say, much more is effected, than many persons unacquainted with the internal discipline and economy have any idea of. It is not only that under skilful medical treatment we here give strength to the infirm, health to the sick, and relief to diseases of the mind, but, by bringing before our afflicted brethren the soul-striving influences of the blessed Gospel on every fitting opportunity, we also lead "the weary and the heavy laden" from their temporal to their spiritual physician, and through this means bring their souls to God.'

In 1860 the Chapel Sub-Committee to which William Smyth, H. O. Nethercote and the Rev. Thomas James of Thebbingworth, Rugby, had been co-opted and from which Dr Nesbitt had retired, issued a further appeal. In it the Committee reminded their readers that they were 'pleading for those who cannot plead for themselves ... It may seem to some that the estimated cost of the chapel is excessive, and that a too ornamental building is contemplated, but it must be borne in mind that the very object of the present attempt is to place before the Patients a CHURCH-LIKE building, which by its outward dignity and associations may influence their minds to good ... At the same time the Committee are prepared to resist the erection of an extravagant or elaborate fabric as inconsistent with the nature of the Charity and Buildings to which it will be attached. They have requested Mr Scott to furnish a simple and substantial design.'

There followed a list of subscribers and the amounts donated by each individual. The list was headed by H. O. Nethercote who raised £145 through a flower show at Blisworth, followed by the Duke of Buccleuch who gave £100, by the Duke of Cleveland, the Marquess of Exeter and the Marquess of Northampton, each of whom gave £50, by the Duke of Bedford who gave £25 and by the Earl Spencer and Lord Southampton who each gave £21. The Committee members canvassed vigorously and in the surviving correspondence are several letters asking for copies of this list before subscribing.

The reference to those, who might find the estimated cost of the proposed chapel excessive, may have been a reaction to the Commissioners' report after their inspection in May that year: 'The estimated cost, as we are given to understand, is very large and much more than required for the structure of adequate dimensions and sufficiently ornamental character. We are induced to make this observation by the consideration that all the available funds of the Institution could be advantageously applied to other additions and improvements'.

This appeal was a success. Over £2,000 was raised to which was added a percentage from the payments by private patients which had been voted in 1855 for that purpose. 'This sum', according to the Annual Report for 1860, 'has been considered sufficient to justify the commencement of the work. A very beautiful design has been obtained from G. G. Scott, Esq.' The decision to proceed with the building, which was to have 204 fixed seats with room for a further 58 movable seats, was taken by the Management Committee in September 1860. Tenders were invited by the architect later in the year, the names of local contractors having been supplied by the Asylum's Secretary; these were formally opened at a Special Chapel Court in January 1861. The winning tender, which was for £2,750, was submitted by C. Ireson, Snr., a local builder, whose work Scott had always found satisfactory. This sum was for the chapel only: a further £180 was asked for the building of a crypt but the Court decided against it. A formal contract with the builder was signed on 20 February 1861. The chapel was to be completed by 24 June 1862. In the meanwhile, some patients were allowed by Dr Wing to attend various churches and chapels in and around the town of Northampton – 'a privilege highly valued by them' – while the attendants and servants of the Asylum, according to a new rule, gathered every evening under the Superintendent for family prayers and readings from the Scriptures.

Wing in his report for 1861 wrote that the chapel was now rapidly being built and that, when finished, 'so beautiful an edifice, daily present to the eye, cannot fail to be productive of beneficial impressions upon the minds of those who contemplate it, if only as a work of art, independently of the feelings it is calculated to engender so favourable to the purposes for which it is designed'. The Chaplain, the Rev. Halford Burdett, was equally pleased: 'When so much is being done, and being done well too, to attract the outer senses of our unhappy friends around us, it is delightful to contemplate that the liberality of those blessed with health and wealth without these walls is contributing to rear up a House of God where, when all external objects shall cease to afford interest or enjoyment, the troubled spirit of the poor afflicted one may join his fellow-worshippers in common prayer, or hear that Word of God read and preached which alone can impart abiding peace to the troubled soul.'

The chapel was not however completed in 1862 as originally planned. In April 1861, Gilbert Scott wrote personally about the problems of sand on the site. Referring to a letter from Ireson, he said: 'They seem to think they shall have to go to a very considerable depth as the sand seems too loose to be trusted . . . Mr Irvine, the Clerk of Works, tells me that the sand could be sold at a good price. Perhaps it would be best to dig throughout the entire surface and sell the sand if it will pay for digging out by the patients – we could then have a wood floor excepting for the altar space below which is a crypt. The slipping of the sand mentioned by Mr Ireson would be a good deal obviated by this course.' In spite of this encouragement, a crypt was not built, nor was there a public ceremonial laying of the corner stone, which Scott expected.

It was however decided to face the interior with finely dressed stone. This pleased Scott as shown by his letter of 30 July 1861, in which he wrote: 'I think it well worth the money'. He went on to answer a criticism. 'I do not think you will find the irregularity in the side windows in any degree disagreeable, but the reverse. There is reason for all the deviations from uniformity. The finest old church of this description in existence, that built by the Hospitallers or Templers at Temple Balsall in Warwickshire, is still more irregular in its windows and looks *admirable*. I presume if there is no public ceremony then there will be a private one at the laying of the stone. It seems but proper in commencing a Christian work that it should not have *less* religious sentiment expressed than in commencing one for secular purposes.'

The problem of consecration had yet to be resolved. A draft resolution had been prepared, requesting the Duke of Buccleuch, the Earl of Cardigan

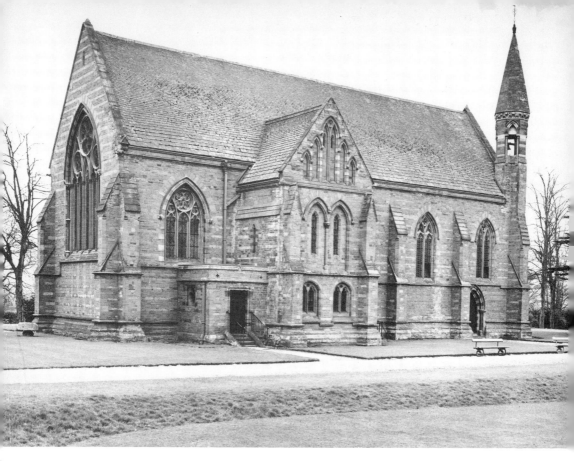

The chapel.

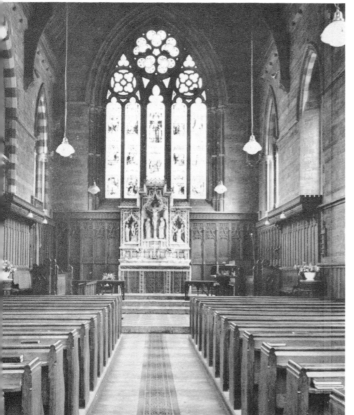

The Hospital chapel was designed by Sir Gilbert Scott in his favoured Gothic style and was built by C. Ireson, a local builder.

LEFT: *The interior of the chapel.*

and Lord Southampton, the Asylum's trustees, to convey the site of the chapel to the Archdeacon to enable it to be consecrated. It was felt however that if consecration enabled the general public to attend the patients' services, it might be better to be content with the Bishop's license alone. This was done in June 1863, deferring the question of consecration to a later date, two eminent counsel having disagreed on this question of ecclesiastical law. In the meanwhile, the Superintendent had contacted ten other asylums to find that only one of their chapels had in fact been consecrated.

A further problem was that of heating. A letter of 25 March 1862 from a member of Scott's staff regretted that 'the *flue* had been neglected: it must be cut out of the wall. I have written to Irvine about it. Mr Scott advises that Mr Haden's system of hot-air or hot water be adopted, the latter is the best but most expensive. Godfrey apparently had other ideas, as shown by a letter from Scott of 5 April: 'Mr Godfrey has shewn and explained to me his proposed system for warming the chapel, which seems to me to be very good and economical both in first outlay and future use. The only things to be made sure of are the retention of the heat of the steam during its passage from one building to the other and the introduction of a sufficient quantity both of steam and of piping.'

There were still one or two minor flaws to be corrected. In April 1863, the architect's atttention was drawn to defects in the woodwork; there were also faults with the glazing, which were speedily rectified. In February 1864, payment to the builder was held up because the windows did not all fit properly, so that cold air was let in, cancelling out the warmth from the steam heating which was provided by the boilers in the main building. This again was quickly put right. In 1873 there was renewed correspondence between Godfrey and the architect, now Sir Gilbert Scott, about the heating. Godfrey's system, at first successful, was no longer providing the required warmth and the addition of a chimney to the chapel had become essential. Plans were promptly provided. The covered way from the Asylum to the chapel was never constructed so that the elegant gothic chapel, built of dark golden stone, today stands largely unaltered externally from the time of its completion.

If, as they would appear to have every right to be, the Asylum authorities were pleased with the result, not everybody was equally satisfied, judging by a letter which appeared in the *Mercury* of 29 July 1866, over the name of 'Viator':

Like all Mr Scott's work [it read], this chapel has many beautiful features, but we cannot admire everything about it. Almost all the windows, for instance, are spoilt by that plate cusping which, because in some cases the effect is good, is made just now to obtrude itself everywhere, botching the tracery as if some lazy mason had left his work half done . . .

The building is long and high and if the brains rather than the interests of the patients had been consulted, instead of placing it among the trees on the north side, where the appearance and situation would have been admirable, the managers of this business appear to have conceived that they were erecting some sort of curtain to a quixotic fortification; for it shuts in the lawn and deprives it of its views and airiness – casting a gloom where cheerfulness is so essentially necessary . . . What formerly looked like a magnificent mansion when viewed from a distance, now, by the erection of a monster chimney, has the appearance of a manufactory, and the chapel, from its form and contrast in colour, would be taken for a large hayrick. The town of Northampton, once the glory of the middle counties, has been quite sacrificed as to its picturesque appearance.

The Commissioners in Lunacy, however, thought the chapel building to be of 'very elegant design and appeared to be finished in the best manner'.

The chapel was eventually opened on 12 July 1863. The Superintendent reported that there had been 'a marked improvement in the reverential bearing of the congregation to what prevailed when the services were conducted in the wards . . . '. The Chaplain, in the Annual Report for 1863, congratulated the Directors upon the completion of the chapel, 'a noble building that does honour, not only to Him for whose service it is erected, but to all who have had the privilege to take part in its execution'. He reported that the Committee had provided Bibles, Prayer Books and hymn-books, while the Society for Promoting Christian Knowledge had given a Bible and Prayer Book for the lectern and reading desk and two copies of *Communion and other Services* for the Communion table. The Committee of the Architectural Society for the Archdeanery of North-ampton, of which the Rev. J. P. Lightfoot was the Honorary Secretary, went to considerable trouble to recommend the decorations and fittings which would best harmonise with the chapel's interior, all of which were accepted by the Management Committee in January 1864. Only an organ was now wanted.

Suddenly in September 1864 there began a series of tragedies. In the middle of the month, the Rev. Halford Burdett died unexpectedly and a special meeting was convened on the 21st, under the chairmanship of the Rev. H. J. Barton, to decide what steps should be taken. Burdett's annual salary had by then risen to £250 but he had a large family and no emoluments. It was decided to appoint a successor at the Quarterly Court in October and, in the meanwhile, to accept the offer of the Rev. Mr Lawson, the late Chaplain's son-in-law, to take the services at the Asylum. A sum of £100, to be administered by the Chairman and the Vice-Chairman, was eventually granted for the benefit of the widow who was left with six children and totally unprovided for by her husband; she had only £50 per annum of her own with a further £50 from her father. Some Directors felt that such a grant might be regarded as setting a precedent, while Mr Collins, according to the *Mercury*, was not sure whether a gratuity in this case was not a premium on improvidence; Burdett should have taken out life insurance. After some months more generous counsel prevailed.

There was the usual large gathering at the October Quarterly Court when the Rev. Samuel Charles Haines, aged thirty-five and married, was elected Chaplain on the fifth count. He was then curate of Long Sutton, Lincolnshire and had previously served in the Canadian Mission, not with the Indians but with immigrant Irish and Scottish backwoods settlers, described as a rough population, scattered over 600 miles. His salary was to be £250 per annum.

Haines approached his task with energy. He took up residence on 22 November and in the following week at the monthly Management Committee meeting presented a long letter, pointing out a number of shortcomings. Singing practice in the chapel was popular and well-attended, but there was no music; he accordingly requested a small grant for books and music. Again, there were no reading, spelling or copy books nor writing materials for the classes which he hoped to hold for males and females on alternate days.

The library was also poorly stocked and virtually the only reading material were often incomplete sets of magazines. He asked permission to acquire a selection of entertaining, instructive and religious works published by the Society for the Promotion of Christian Knowledge. 'Some persons', he continued, 'have asked me for *Uncle Tom's Cabin*, *The Wide-Wide World* and books of that character – as these could be purchased in a cheap form and are decidedly better than the modern sensation novel'. He then tactfully added, 'I cannot pretend to point out what additions should be made to the Library, as I am sensible that I am addressing those who know far more about the matter than I do myself and from whom I myself desire to learn, but I am sensible of a great want in this respect'. He was successful in his appeal. Ten pounds was granted for the purchase of church music and for books and materials for the school and a further £10 for the library, the books to be chosen jointly by the Superintendent and the Chaplain.

It is unlikely that Dr Wing was able to help in selecting the books as he that month fell ill, the second tragedy of that year. He wrote the Superintendent's monthly report for December 1864, but those for the first five months of 1865 were the work of Williams, the House Surgeon, Wing having been given three months leave of absence in February. The June, July and August reports were signed by Wing who returned for a few weeks that summer, but at the monthly meeting on 26 July it was announced that he was resigning through ill health but would continue his duties until the end of September. He died in the middle of December at the age of forty-seven. In the Annual Report for that year, it was recorded that 'he had ministered to the afflictions of its inmates with great kindness and with a medical treatment which the large amount of recoveries fully proves to have been most successful'.

In the November 1864 monthly report, an outbreak of typhoid fever among the domestic staff was recorded; three nurses were affected and were promptly isolated for treatment in the ladies' cottage. Another nurse, Catherine Soden, who had also been ill of the fever but was now convalescent, was allowed 10s. to take a fortnight's change of air and given two bottles of wine.

At the beginning of January 1865, there was further trouble for smallpox broke out among the male inmates; twelve were affected as well as one attendant but, according to the House Surgeon, 'in the greater number the disease has been greatly modified by vaccination'. In Wing's absence, the House Surgeon was empowered to find temporarily a professional assistant and engaged Mr James Snook at £10 a month with board and lodging. Stringent measures were taken to prevent the disease from spreading; the male patients did not attend chapel and the Chaplain held divine service in their wards; entertainments also ceased while a temporary building was set up in four days on the farm where the infected were isolated. This building, for whose design the Secretary was credited, was mainly of wood, consisting of an outer and inner wall, with straw stuffed in between to retain warmth; there was one room of 50 ft by 16 ft and two of 16 ft square. This structure was to remain there for some years.

Later in January, the Committee decided to engage a doctor to attend exclusively the smallpox victims and to hire nurses from the London Smallpox Hospital. The Asylum's Secretary accordingly enrolled a Mr Broom, described as 'a duly qualified Practitioner both in medicine and surgery' at £12.12s.0d. a month plus board and lodging. Unhappily no nurses were obtainable from the Smallpox Hospital because of the great many cases there. Broom's services were only required for a month as it was reported at the February Committee meeting that there had been no further smallpox cases; gratuities of from £3 to £5 were given to the attendants who had coped with this epidemic.

Williams told the Committee at its meeting on 29 March that he had planned to send the smallpox victims, who were now all convalescent, back to the main buildings on 8 April. As, however, one more case had appeared as recently as 9 March, it was decided to keep them isolated until 15 April. All the victims recovered. As late as the 29 April, it was decided, on account of the prevalence of smallpox in Northampton, to prohibit visitors except in an emergency.

On 26 April, Williams asked for a short leave of absence on the advice of Dr Francis of the Infirmary because of ill-health. The pressures on, and the responsibilities of the House Surgeon, aged only twenty-four, must in the absence of the Superintendent have been enormous; not only was there the normal running of the Asylum with over 400 patients, but there was in addition the smallpox epidemic. His only assistant, Snook, was temporary. Leave was given to Williams and the Commissioners in Lunacy asked to suggest a suitable medical officer to take over acting control. In the meanwhile, the physicians of Northampton Infirmary, Drs Francis and Webster, were requested to visit the Asylum.

The Commissioners in Lunacy promptly suggested a *locum tenens* in the absence of Wing and Williams, but there was a snag. As explained in a long letter from Drs Francis and Webster, which was read to the Committee on 29 April, Snook declined to work under another temporary official. The doctors themselves felt strongly that Snook was so good at his job – intelligent, industrious, painstaking, kind and considerate: he knew the names and the mental peculiarities of nearly all the inmates – that he should be retained. They themselves would be happy to continue visiting the Asylum daily and to help in every way 'to relieve the Directors of the temporary difficulty in which they are placed'. The Committee accepted the situation.

Williams had hoped to return to duty early in May but his health did not improve. At the end of that month, the Superintendent, briefly back, was asked to arrange for him to take a holiday as early as possible and a gratuity of £100 recommended as a reward for his extra responsibilities during the previous six months. In spite of this, Williams resigned his position that July with immediate effect. The testimonial he received from the Committee showed how much he had gained their respect:

the Committee have much pleasure in certifying that during the three and a half years he has been connected with the Institution he has performed his duties of the Office in a manner to reflect the highest credit upon himself and the Institution. For more than six months during the illness and absence of Dr Wing, Dr Williams acted as Medical Superintendent and in that capacity displayed much discretion and ability and received the thanks of the Committee for his services with a gratuity of £100. The Committee have much cause to regret that the official connection of Dr Williams with the Institution has ceased, but he has their best wishes for his future success in life.

Chapter Seven

JOHN CLARE (1793–1864)

*O*n 21 May 1864, the death occurred of the most distinguished inmate known to have been cared for by the Northampton General Lunatic Asylum. John Clare, the peasant-poet, whose *Poems Descriptive of Rural Life and Scenery*, published in 1820, had brought him fame at the age of twenty-seven, was confined in the Asylum for the last twenty-two years of his life; this however did not check his lyrical outflow which welled-up like a perpetual spring until almost the end. Some of the most important of his great output of poems, both pastoral and semi-mystical, were composed during this period.

Clare was born on 13 July 1793, in Helpston, a small, straggling Northamptonshire village, some seven miles north-west of Peterborough and about a mile to the west of the road leading from there to Market Deeping, just over the border in Lincolnshire. To the north and east of the village was fenland, which originally stretched to the Lincolnshire coast and the Wash; to the south and west were woods and heathland, the area which most inspired him.

Clare's parents were simple, uneducated peasants. His father, Parker Clare, was the illegitimate son of John Donald Parker, a Scott who was for a time the village schoolmaster, but who disappeared before he was born; Parker was of powerful build, well-known locally as a wrestler and a singer of ballads at village feasts. His son's boyhood and youth coincided with a period of intensive enclosure of commonlands. While this led to much-needed improvements in providing food for the country's growing population, the cottagers and farm labourers lost their traditional grazing and

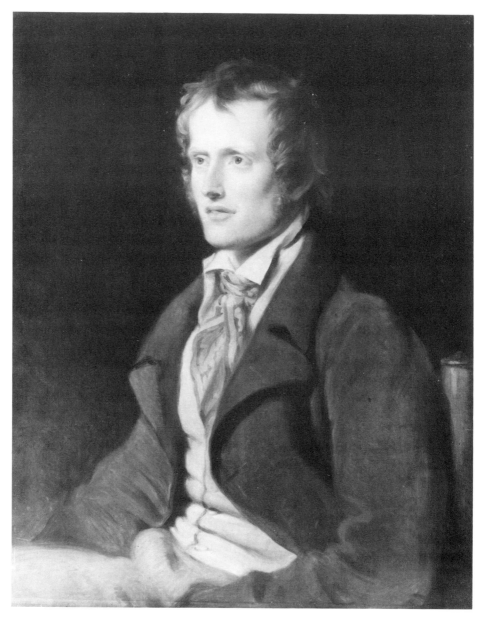

John Clare as a young man on his first visit to London, from a painting in 1820 by William Hilton (National Portrait Gallery, London).

other rights on the commons with little compensation. Parker, while in the prime of life, earned a meagre but regular living as a thresher, but with advancing age became increasingly crippled with rheumatism and eventually dependent upon what little he could get from the Poor Law Guardians. As a result, John Clare became increasingly responsible for keeping his parents as well as, in due course, his own family. Their diet often consisted of bread and potatoes with meat as a rare treat.

John Clare was the elder of twins; his sister, though seemingly stronger at birth, died within a few weeks. A second sister died young but a third lived with her parents until the 1820s. Although Parker Clare and his wife were illiterate, they had ambitions for their son to acquire some learning. He was sent first to a dame school in Helpston and then intermittently, from the age of about seven until twelve, to a school in nearby Glinton. Here, when he was not helping his father on the land, he learnt simple arithmetic and to read and write. His father's failing health made it impossible to continue at day school because the boy was needed to earn to support his father. He did however attend night school at Glinton for two or three more years. By this time he had already started to write verse, perhaps inspired by his father's ballad singing and later to a considerable extent by Thomson's *The Seasons*; when he was about fifteen he managed to find the few pence necessary to acquire a copy from a bookshop in Stamford, five miles away.

John Clare was fair-haired, small, frail, with piercing blue eyes. He suffered from repeated illnesses, some of which were referred to as 'fen ague', which may have been malaria. He was also a timid, fearful boy, much preoccupied with witches, ghosts and hobgoblins, so that walking home at night often aroused great trepidation; at the beginning of the nineteenth century, the medieval world of witchcraft and spirits still lingered faintly in such remote places as Helpston. He was also a solitary boy, happiest when roaming, perhaps with an intimate friend or on his own, through the fields and woods to the south-west of Helpston. His observations of the countryside were the basis of his poetry. He once said he found his poems in the fields and only wrote them down.

At the age of sixteen, Clare saw a man fall off a haycart and break his neck. So moved was he by this incident that he 'swooned away' and for years suffered fits in spring and autumn. Later in *Sketches in the Life of John Clare by Himself* he wrote:

> The ghastly paleness of death struck such a terror on me that I could not forget it for years, and my dreams was constantly wanderings in churchyards, digging graves, seeing spirits in charnel houses, etc., etc.

In my fits I swooned away without a struggle, and felt nothing more than if I'd been in a dreamless sleep after I came to myself; but I was always warn'd of their coming by a chillness and dithering, that seemed to creep from one's toe ends till it got up to one's head, when I turned senseless and fell. Sparks as of fire often flashed from my eyes, or seemed to do so, when I dropt; which I laid to the fall. These fits were stopped by a Mr Arnold, MD, of Stamford, of some notoriety as a medical gentleman, and one whom I respect with grateful remembrances; for he certainly did me great benefit, tho' every spring and autumn since the accident happened my fears are agitated to an extreme degree, and the dread of death involves me in a stupor of chilling indisposition as usual, tho' I have had but one or two swoonings since they first left me.

While still a boy at school, Clare had fallen in love with a young girl, Mary Joyce, the daughter of a prosperous farmer.

My regard for her [according to his *Sketches*] lasted a long time after school days were over, but it was platonic affection, nothing else but love in idea, for she knew nothing of my fondness for her, no more than I did of her inclinations to forbid or encourage me had I disclosed afterwards. But other Marys, etc. excited my admiration, and the first creator of my warm passions was lost in a perplexed multitude of names, that would fill a volume to calendar them down, ere a bearded chin could make the lawful apology for my entering the lists of Cupid. Thus began and ended my amorous career.

By the age of sixteen, he was idyllically in love with Mary but she apparently realised that Clare, son of a poor labourer, had no prospects and broke with him. She haunted his thoughts to the time of his death. She died unmarried in 1838.

On leaving school there were at first hopes that he might gain employment as a clerk, but in this he was unsuccessful. Instead he worked as herdsman and ploughman, under-gardener for a time at Burghley and, in spite of his short stature, served briefly in the Northampton Militia. By the time he was twenty-three, he had become completely responsible for his parents' upkeep. He depended upon casual work from neighbouring farmers and from a nearby brick-kiln. Nevertheless, he continued to write verses and his ambition to achieve publication grew.

In 1819, through a Stamford bookseller, his work came to the attention of John Taylor, the London publisher who had befriended and published Keats. Taylor was much impressed both by Clare and his work and in

January 1820 published *Poems Descriptive of Rural Life and Scenery*. Thanks in part to a well-planned publicity campaign and in part to the public's interest in 'working-class' poets at that time, the book was a great success, went into four editions and attracted considerable critical interest and acclaim. Clare visited London for the first time and was lionised by literary society. The shy, diffident, socially awkward poet found this a great trial, but managed to control his social phobias by dosing himself with alcohol. In spite of his shyness and quaint rural accent, it would seem that he was regarded with respect by some of the leading authors and artists of the day.

Not only did literary London take him up but also some of the great landowners in Northamptonshire. Lord Milton, who succeeded his father as the 5th Earl Fitzwilliam in 1833, invited Clare to call on him and received him kindly. Henry Manvers Pierrepont, third son of the 1st Earl Manvers and elder brother of P. S. Pierrepont of Evenley Hall, North-ampton, invited him to Burghley, the home of his father-in-law, the Marquess of Exeter.

Admiral Lord Radstock, a son of the 3rd Earl Waldegrave, took the greatest interest in the poet. He wrote to Lord Milton asking him to grant Clare a cottage and land free for life, a plea which brought a response some years later. He also helped raise funds to provide Clare with a settled income. He himself collected £100 and Lord Fitzwilliam sent in an equal sum. The 2nd Earl Spencer promised an annuity of £10, Lord Exeter one of £15 and there were also contributions by John Taylor and other friends. As a result of this generosity, Clare had an annual income of £43.15s.0d. It was by no means adequate in view of his commitments, but it was a symbol of hope.

This provision was most timely as he was married on 16 March, two months after the publication of *Poems Descriptive of Rural Life and Scenery*. Three years earlier, while working at the lime-kiln, he had been attracted to Martha, or 'Patty', Turner. Although he still yearned at times for Mary, attraction developed into love, which was returned. The courtship was a difficult one as his prospects were poor, but Patty's parents, who had seen better days, became more amenable after the appearance of his poems. There was also a question of honour as their first child was born within three months of the wedding.

In some ways Clare wished that he had married earlier, for:

Temptations were things that I rarely resisted; when the partiality of the
moment gave no time for reflection, I was sure to seize it, whatever
might be the consequence. Still, I have been no one's enemy but my
own. My easy nature, either in drinking or anything else, was always

ready to submit to persuasions of profligate companions, who often led me into snares, and laughed at me in the bargain when they had done so; such times as at fairs, coaxed about to bad houses, those pained pills of poison by whom many unguarded youths are hurried to destruction like the ox to the slaughter house, without knowing the danger that awaits them in the end. Here not only my health but my life has often been on the eve of its sacrifice, by an illness too well known, and too disgusting to mention. But mercy spared me to be schooled by experience, who learned me better.

In 1821, a second collection of his poems was published under the title, *The Village Minstrel and other Poems*. This was not so successful as it came out at a time when the market was swamped by works from such major writers as Scott, Byron, Shelley and Southey. With his growing family responsibilities, his need for money was becoming pressing. Nevertheless, in 1822 he paid a second visit to London, staying about a month, in which he much enjoyed meeting his literary friends, but found difficulties developing with his publishers. On returning to Helpston, he began writing large numbers of poems in the hope of selling them as penny ballads, but this scheme failed. So, in spite of the small income from the trust fund, he began to feel desperate. It is likely that at this time he suffered from chronic malnutrition.

Towards the end of 1823 Clare developed increasingly severe mental symptoms. Details of these can only be gleaned from references in the letters of Mrs Emmerson, whom he had met in London through Lord Radstock, and who became a devoted friend; his 'mind was dead', he spoke of how he 'had lost his memory – was nearly blind, and he was certain he was dying'. She recorded that he was suffering from 'high, nervous debility, which is of all diseases the most painful to the poor patient'.

In April 1824, he decided to go to London again in order to consult Dr Darling, a Scottish physician who had been Keats's doctor, and whom he had met socially. As he acknowledged in his autobiography, '*Sketches in the Life of John Clare by Himself*', 'the complaint lay in my head and chest. I was very ill when I first went but I gradually received benefit'. The benefit was physical, not mental. He also suffered at this time with night terrors which he attributed to an incident in his youth when he had been frightened by a foal in a lonely lane.

He unhappily found that his anxieties and fears were as tormenting in London as in Northamptonshire and he would not venture far unaccompanied. As he later explained:

I used to sit at night till very late because I was loath to start not for the sake of leaving the company but for fears of meeting with supernature [agents] even in the busy paths of London and tho' I was a stubborn disbeliever of such things in the daytime, yet at night their terrors came upon me tenfold and my head was as full of the terribles as a gossip's – thin death-like shadows and goblins with saucer eyes were continually shaping on the darkness from my haunted imagination and when I saw anyone with a spare figure in the dark passing or going on by my side my blood curdled cold at the foolish apprehension of his being a supernatural agent whose errant might be to carry me away at the first dark alley we came to.

He remained in London for three months and on his return home in August 1824 he wrote to Thomas Inskip:

> I have been in a terrible state of ill health six months, gradually declining and I verily believe that it will upset me at last I was taken in a sort of apoplectic fit and have never had the right use of my facultys since a numbing pain lies constantly about my head and an aching void at the pit of my stomach keeps sinking me away deeper and deeper.

He continued to receive pills and prescriptions from Dr Darling.
   That same month he wrote to John Taylor:

> I think the doctors none of them know the cause of my complaint I feel now a numbness all over me just as I should suppose a person to feel when bitten by a serpent & I firmly believe I shall never get over it be as it will I am resigned for the worst my mind is placid & contented and that is something for when I first took God forgive me I had hard work to bear up with my malady & often had the thought of destroying myself & from this change in my feelings I satisfactorily prove that Religious foundation is truth.

Sometime late in 1825 Clare had a liaison with a woman whose name remains unknown. He confessed this affair to Mrs Emmerson in letters, the content of which can only be derived from her replies. On 11 January 1826, she wrote urging him to give up the relationship and remain with his wife and children. Clare himself was full of guilt and remorse, and very concerned that he might have contracted venereal disease. He was later assured that this was not the case.
   During the next few years he struggled against his illness and continued

to write essays and verses, some of which were published and brought in a tiny income, but never enough to relieve him from financial worry. He also embarked upon his *Sketches* and kept a journal in which he recorded his depressions. In 1827, Taylor published his third book, *The Shepherd's Calender; with Village Stories, and other Poems*, but it did not sell.

There was a fourth visit to London early in 1828 to collect payments for accepted work and to find new commissions but the vogue for poetry about nature and the rustic way of life was rapidly waning. Clare found himself slipping ever deeper into debt, not helped by a fall in interest rates in 1831. As a result, his health continued to fluctuate over the next few years; periods of lethargy and despondency alternated with brief intervals of activity and enthusiasm, usually with an exacerbation in spring and autumn.

In 1831, Lord Milton came to understand Clare's plight and allowed him to rent for £15 per annum a newly built cottage on his estates at Northborough, lying between Helpston and Market Deeping, together with five acres, which, with two cows, he could work profitably. This was a great improvement on the overcrowded shack in which he lived with his parents, wife and children at Helpston. Although the new home was only some three miles away, he viewed the move with deep despondency. He eventually went in January 1832, but only after considerable persuasion, having several times put off leaving his childhood home.

Some idea of the impression he made on visitors at this time appeared three years later in the *Druid's Magazine*:

> The first glance at Clare would convince you that he was no common man; he has a forehead of a highly intellectual character; the reflective faculties being exceedingly well developed; but the most striking feature is his eye, light blue, and flashing with the fire of genius; the peculiar character of his eyes are always remarked by persons when first they see him; his height is rather below the common. His conversation is animated, striking, and full of imagination, yet his dialect is purely provincial; his ideas being expressed in the most simple manner, you can compare his conversation to nothing but the line of Goldsmith –
> 'Like a fair female, unadorned and plain!'

In March 1831 Clare wrote to Taylor, asking him to get some prescriptions from Dr Darling:

> it is now necessity for I am ill & very ill & as I cannot get a frank soon enough (for Lord Milton is not in parliament) to write to Dr Darling I

trouble you to tell him & I hope you will write to tell me you have done so – I was taken 3 weeks back or more – with a pain at the stomach which would not go off & as it affected my head very much I felt alarmed & took a part of Dr Ds last prescription which checked it & subdued the humour in some measure but whenever I attempted to walk friction brought it on as bad as ever & the pain at my stomach started again as bad as ever & I then finished the packet of powders & on last Saturday night by the recommendation of Mr Mossop (having nothing left of my last prescription) I took a blue pill & on monday morning I walked with a dreadful burning humour in my lisks & a contraction so as almost prevented me from making water on Monday I commenced a second course of Dr Darlings medicine & the humour tho abated is not subdued – for I awoke this morning with a burning heat in my fundament where the humour again made its appearance with prickly pains in my head arms & shoulders and they are as bad just now – I fear I shall be in the same state I was in last summer – for unlike last night I got tolerable rest but the pain at my stomach was more frequent in its attacks & I awoke in a dreadful irritation thinking that the Italian liberators were kicking my head about for a foot ball – my future prospects seem to be no sleep – a general debility – a stupid & stunning apathy or lingering madness & death – my dreads are very apprehensive & uneasy I dislike this prickly feel about the face & temples worse than anything & a sobbing [dialect for throbbing] or beating when I lay my head down on the pillow was first felt last night for a long time – my appetite was gone & from monday to this morning 4 eggs & a bit of bread have been the whole of my food – it never attacked my appetite before as I know of & I am so alarmed & so anxious to get better that if I cannot in no other way I will draw upon or sell out my fund money (if it can be done without extravagent loss) & take lodgings in a humble way as near Dr Darlings as I can & the steam bath in great Marlboro Street which did me uncommon benefit in 1827 & would do me as much benefit again I write this not as a resolution but for your advice as a friend for I want to get better & Dr Darling in his last letter ordered a steam bath but there is no such thing here.

Throughout his struggle to meet his financial obligations, he remained determined to continue writing. In October 1831, he wrote to Taylor:

All I want to go on is a stimulus an encouraging aspiration that refreshes the heart like a shower in summer – instead of that I have nothing but drawbacks & disappointments I live in a land overflowing with obscurity & vulgarity far away from table & books & friends . . . I see things praised that appear to me utterly worthless & need criticism in the periodicals when I do see them that the very puffers of Blacking & Bearsgrease would be really ashamed of – & I lay my intentions aside having no heart to proceed but I am resolved to show them I can judge for myself & whatever remarks I may make on the ryhmes [*sic*] of others they shall be done honestly & with as little vanity as possible.

If the mental strain lifted from time to time, it was never far away. In November 1832, he wrote to Mrs Emmerson: 'I was delighted to see your handwriting for I have been in such an excess of melancholly that I was obliged today to send over to Deeping for some medicine which I have commenced taking for last night my very brains seemed to boil up almost into madness & my arms & legs burnt as it were with a listless feebleness that almost rendered them useless . . . it is a sad thing to feel such a debility that will neither bear rest or fatigue long together . . . ' In January 1835, a letter to Taylor gave some idea of the constant pressures of his responsibilities: 'I am so very afflicted that I am scarcely able to get across the house . . . I am happy to say that the children are all well but we have had the loss to bury the youngest my father has also been very ill all the winter & under medical advice but he is now better'. (Parker Clare lived on at Northborough until 1846).

In 1835, *The Rural Muse*, the last volume of Clare's poems, was published: it was dedicated to his benefactor, Earl Fitzwilliam, formerly Lord Milton. It was well-received but the first edition did not sell out, so there was no money from it. There was however a gift of £50 from the Literary Fund which left him with a little in hand after paying off his debts. The 2nd Earl Spencer had died in 1834, but his successor kindly renewed the annuity of £20. The clouds lifted a little but briefly.

By the autumn of 1835 he was ill again. In a letter to Dr Darling, he wrote:

I am very unwell & though I cannot describe my feelings well I will tell you as well as I can – sounds affect me very much and things evil as well (as) good thoughts are continually rising in my mind I cannot sleep for I am asleep as it were with my eyes open & I feel chills come over me & a sort of nightmare awake I got no rest last night I feel a great desire to come up but perhaps I shall not be able & I hope you write down directly for I feel you can do me good & if I was in town I should soon be well so I fancy for I do assure you I am very unwell & I cannot keep my mind right as it were for I wish to read & cannot – there is a sort of numbing through my private parts which I cannot describe & when I was so indisposed last winter I felt as if I had inflamation (?) in the blood & at other times such a sinking as if I were going through the bed – & though not so bad now I am really very uneasy in fact I have never been right.

From this it was apparent that the move to Northborough was not a success. That December his mother died.

During 1836, Clare's mental state seems to have both deteriorated and changed. In November, Taylor called, bringing with him a doctor from Stamford:

> We found him sitting in a chimney corner looking much as usual. He talked properly to me in reply to all my questions, knew all the people of whom I spoke, and smiled at my reminding him of the events of past days. But his mind is sadly enfeebled. He is constantly speaking to himself and when I listened I heard such words as those pronounced a great many times over and with great rapidity - 'God bless thcm all', 'keep them from evil', 'Doctors'. But who it was of whom he spoke I could not tell . . . The medical man's opinion was that Clare should go to some asylum. His wife is a very clever, active woman, and keeps them all very respectable and comfortable, but she cannot manage to control her husband at times; he is very violent, I daresay, occasionally.

Nothing was done, however, until June 1837. Taylor had published a book, *Essays on the Classification of the Insane*, by Dr Matthew Allen, advocate of the non-restraint method of treating the mentally ill, who had established a private 'madhouse' at High Beech, near Epping. Taylor therefore arranged for Clare to be taken there for treatment. According to Allen, quoted by June Wilson in *Green Shadows* (1951), Clare arrived:

> exceedingly miserable, every instant bemoaning his poverty, and his mind did not appear so much lost and deranged as suspended in its movements by the oppressive and permanent state of anxiety, and fear, and vexation, produced by the excitement of excessive flattery at one time and neglect at another, his extreme poverty and over exertion of body and mind, and no wonder that his feeble bodily frame, with his wonderful native powers of mind, was overcome. I had then not the slightest hesitation in saying that if a small pension could be obtained for him, he would have recovered instantly and most probably remained well for life.

Later Allen wrote:

He is at present in excellent health, and looks very well, and is in mind, though full of many strange delusions, in a more comfortable and happy state than he was when he first came. It is most singular, that ever since he came, and even now at almost all times, the moment he gets a pencil in hand he begins to write the most beautiful poetic effusions. Yet he has never been able to maintain conversation, nor even in writing prose, the appearance of sanity for two minutes or two lines together, and yet there is no indication whatever of insanity in any of his poetry.

In Clare's general conversation, however, more florid delusions began to appear. He expressed the idea that he was a prize fighter. He wrote to Elizabeth Phillips in 1841 from High Beech, that:

having been cooped up in the Hell of a Madhouse till I seem to be disowned & even forgot by my enemies, for there is none to accept my challenges which I have from time to time given to the public I am almost mad in waiting for a better place & better company & all to no purpose. It is well known that I am a prize fighter by profession & a man that never feared anybody in my life either in the ring or out of it – I do not much like to write love letters but this which I am now writing to you is a true one – you know that we have met before and the first opportunity that offers we will meet again – I am now writing a New Canto of Don Juan.

The delusion that he was a prize fighter was also mentioned in an account of Clare by Cyrus Redding, Editor of the *English Journal*, which appeared in that magazine's edition of 15 May 1841:

The principal token of his mental eccentricity was the introduction of prize fighting, in which he seemed to imagine he was to engage, but the allusion to it was made in the way of interpolation in the middle of the subject on which he was discoursing, brought in abruptly, and abandoned with equal suddenness, and an utter want of connection with an association of ideas which it could be thought might lead to the subject at the time, as if the machinery of thought were dislocated, so that one part of it got off its pivot and protruded into the regular workings, or as if a note had got into a piece of music which had no business there. This was the only symptom of aberration of mind we observed about Clare.

'Don Juan' was the first verse of Clare's to show any evidence of mental disturbance:

I have two wives and I should like to see them
both by my side before another hour
If both are honest I should like to be there
For both are fair and bonny as a flower;
And one, O Lord – now do bring in the team, mem!
Were bard's pens steamers such of ten horse-power,
I could not bring her beauties fair to weather,
So I've towed both in harbour blest together

The delusion that he had two wives, Patty and Mary, his childhood's first love, became more and more prominent. Moreover, the forms of his letters as well as their content began to change. He took to starting every word with a capital letter and some were written in a curious shorthand in which vowels were omitted. His sense of personal identity also began to break down, and he started to claim that he was Lord Byron.

On 20 July 1841, he absconded from High Beech and made his way back to Northborough on foot, taking four days to cover the eighty miles. His only food and drink during that walk was a pennyworth of beer on the second day, grass on the third day 'which seemed to taste something like bread', and two pennyworth of bread and cheese and a pint of ale on the fourth. He wrote a full account of the journey on reaching Northborough.

Clare remained at home for some five months. He was probably now out of touch with his friends after four years at High Beech, but his notebooks show that his inspiration still flourished. Much of the time was spent wandering in the surrounding countryside. He fought hard against the insanity which was closing in on him, but it must have been a difficult time for his wife, Patty, especially as visions of Mary were often uppermost in his mind. So in December 1841, Dr Skrimshire of Peterborough certified him as insane, testifying that the disease was 'hereditary', and he was removed to the Northampton Asylum. Lord Fitzwilliam, who had generously contributed earlier in the year to another appeal to provide the poet with a living, paid for his keep for the rest of Clare's life.

The Superintendent, Dr Prichard, classified Clare as harmless and allowed him almost complete freedom to wander in the neighbourhood, including the town. Clare took full advantage of this, returning to the Asylum only for his meals and bed. A result of his confinement was that his bodily health greatly improved. One visitor, Spencer T. Hall, who saw him in 1843, recalled in his *Biographical Sketches of Remarkable People* (1873) that, instead of the spare, sensitive person he appears in the portrait of him from Hilton's painting [John Clare, 1820, by William Hilton, RA, in the National Portrait Gallery] . . . found him rather burly, florid, with light hair and somewhat shaggy eyebrows, and dressed as a plain but respectable farmer, in drab or stone-coloured coat and smalls, with gaiters, and altogether as clean and neat as if he had just been fresh brushed for market or fair.

Another description appeared in the *Northampton Mercury* on 30 April 1842:

He writes frequently and beyond a doubt composes many more poems than he puts on paper, if indeed his life is not passed in one almost unbroken poetic dream. He may be seen any fine day, walking, with a rapid step and an abstracted manner, about the grounds of the Asylum, one hand in his pocket and the other in the bosom of his waistcoat, easily distinguishable by the most careless observer as no ordinary man. His stature is short, his limbs muscular and well knit, his forehead ample and the head generally of a very intellectual character. Outwardly there is nothing to indicate insanity. It needs a closer acquaintance to discover that there are chords jarring and out of tune in that excellent piece of Nature's handiwork.

In November 1843 Prichard wrote: 'Poor Clare is in good health, but his state of mind has not improved. It rather appears to become more and more impaired: he used at one time to write many and very good pieces tho' he scarcely ever finished them. He now writes but little and in a coarse style very unlike his former compositions. I much fear that the disease will gradually terminate in dementia'. Clare was much impressed by Prichard who, he believed, had supernatural powers and had therefore to be strictly obeyed. Later, in 1845 or 1846, someone in Northampton made him drunk so he was subsequently confined to the Asylum's grounds.

G. J. De Wilde, editor of the *Northampton Mercury*, visited him and wrote later to Clare's first biographer, Frederick Martin (25 February 1865), to describe Clare's confusion about his own personality:

He would talk rationally enough at times, about poetry especially, but on one occasion in the midst of a conversation in which he betrayed no signs of insanity, he suddenly quoted passages from 'Don Juan' as his own. I suggested, gently, that they were usually attributed to Byron, upon which he said that was true; but he and Byron were one; so with Shakespeare; and turning round upon me suddenly he said 'perhaps you

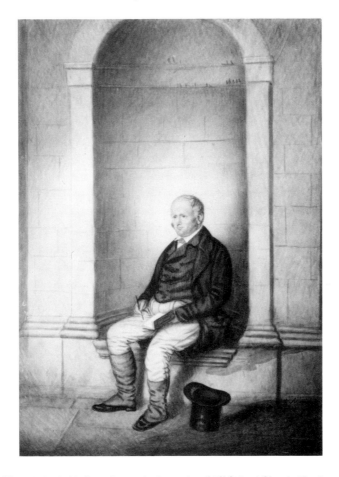

John Clare sitting in his favourite spot in the portico of All Saints' Church, Northampton,
painted by George Maine in 1848.

don't know that I am Jan Burns and Tom Spring?' [prize fighters]. In
fact, he was any celebrity whom you might mention. 'I'm the same
man', he said 'but sometimes they call me Shakespeare and sometimes
Byron and sometimes Clare'. Later he fancied himself to have witnessed
the execution of Charles 1st and to have served as a naval rating with
Neslon at the Battle of the Nile, both of which he would describe
graphically and in much detail.

Clare was lucky, and so indeed has been posterity, with the appointment
in April 1845 of W. F. Knight as Steward to the Northampton Asylum.

Himself a writer of verse, he took a keen interest in Clare and transcribed over 800 of his poems. Knight noted in his transcripts of these poems in the Northampton Public Library:

> Copied from the Manuscripts as presented to me by Clare – and favoured with others by some Ladies and Gentlemen, that Clare had presented them to – the whole of them faithfully transcribed to the best of my knowledge from the pencil originals many of which were so obliterated that without referring to the Author I could not decipher. Some pieces will be found unfinished, for Clare will seldom turn his attention to pieces he has been interrupted in while writing – and in no instance has ever rewritten a single line.

Knight, in addition to giving Clare sympathy and encouragement, attempted to collect together a selection of poems with a view to publication, but nothing came of this, perhaps because in 1850 he took up an appointment in Birmingham. Nevertheless, they continued to correspond. On 8 July 1850, Clare wrote: 'I am still wanting like Sternes Prisoners Starling to "get out" but cant find the way . . . Write me when you can for I am very lonely by times – I am without Books or Amusements of any kind I have got nothing to kill time.' Knight's reply, dated 11 July, promised Clare some tobacco. He continued: 'I am sorry that you do not string together some more poetry – for that that I have in pencil of yours I am getting copied – and I like it better and better. Let me persuade you, dear Clare, to strive to amuse yourself by your favourite occupations – your time will not seem so heavy on your hands – and in all respects you will be much happier.'

In April 1851, Clare again referred to his confinement

> I would try like the Birds a few songs i' the spring but they have shut me up & gave me no tools & like the caged Starnel of Sterne 'I cant get out' to fetch any so I have made no progress at present but I have written a good lot & as I should think nearly sufficient . . . I love the 'rippling brook' – & 'the singing of Birds' – But I cant get out to see them or hear them – while other people are looking at gay flower Gardens – I love to see the quaking bull rushes & the broad lakes in the green meadows – & the sheep tracks over a fallow field & a land of thistles in flower – I wish I could make a little book of Songs worth sending but after some trials I cant do it at present – 'the Chat of Books Poetry and Poets' are what I want now.

His longing to return home keeps cropping up in the few letters he wrote from the Northampton Asylum. He warned Charles, his youngest and favourite son in a letter dated June 1847, that Frederick and John, Clare's first and second sons, 'had better not come unless they wish to do so for its a *bad Place* & I have fears that they may get trapped as prisoners as I hear some have been'. In a letter of the following February, he emphasised, 'There is nothing like home'. In July 1848, he told Patty, 'I have not written to you for a long while but here I am in the land of Sodom where all the brains are turned the wrong way I was glad to see John yesterday & should like to have gone back with him for I am very weary of being here – you might come & fetch me away for I think I have been here long enough . . . I think it is about two years since I was first sent up to this Hell & not allowed to get out of the gates – There never was a more disgraceful deception than this place'.

There are hardly any letters after 1852. The last, written in March 1860 to a Mr James Hipkins, an unknown enquirer, read: 'Dear Sir, I am in a Madhouse & quite forgot your Name or who you are You must excuse me for I have nothing to communicate or tell of & why I am shut up I dont know I have nothing to say so I conclude – yours respectfully, John Clare'.

There are two descriptions of Clare in his last years. A lawyer, Robert Walton, author of *Random Recollections of the Midland Circuit*, who visited the Asylum in about 1860 'was attracted by the appearance of a man who sat on a stone bench, his hands clasped before him, his eyes looking listlessly towards the ground. Inquiring who he might be, I was told it was no other than John Clare, formerly well known as the "Northamptonshire poet".'

Another visitor in 1860, Agnes Strickland (co-author of *The Lives of the Queens of England*), described a conversation she had with Clare: 'I am glad you can amuse yourself by writing'. 'I can't do it', he replied gloomily, 'they pick my brains out'. I enquired his meaning. 'Why', he said, 'they have cut off my head, then picked out all the letters of the alphabet – all the vowels and consonants and brought them out through my ears; and then they want me to write poetry; I can't do it.' 'Tell me which you liked best, literature or your former avocation?' 'I liked hard work best,' he replied, with sudden vehemence, 'I was happy then. Literature has destroyed my head and brought me here.'

Clare's last days, as described in Superintendent Wing's casebook, reveal his slow physical and mental decline as cerebral artery disease increased:

August 29th 1861

Mr Clare in getting up immediately after dinner today fell, probably from a slight apopleptic seizure, of which he has had several, hit his head against the sharp edge of the table, causing an irregular jagged wound of about 3 inches in length and in depth through the integument to the periosteum which was uninjured – the wound was dressed with dry lint and plaster and he was put to bed.

February 1st 1863

Became very giddy and appeared to lose the use of his legs just before dinner time today, so he was put to bed. His delusions about his personal identity are as strong as ever, sometimes fancying himself Lord Byron, at others a Sea Captain, etc., His language is at times very bad.

April 8th.

His habits are becoming very dirty and scarcely a day passes without his having to be changed on this account – otherwise he is much the same.

July 2nd.

Is a trifle stronger than he was in the winter and he is occasionally taken out amongst the flowers to view the beauties of that nature of which he was wont to be so fond, but without apparently awakening any pleasurable emotions.

October 1st.

Was somewhat improved in general health lately, but mentally there is but little change, phantoms still haunt him and he will often swear most coarsely at the creatures of his own disordered fancy, his left side being usually where they locate themselves.

He wrote his last poem some time that winter, about six months before his death:

Tis Spring, warm glows the South,
Chaffinch carries the moss in his mouth
To filbert hedges all day long,

And charms the poet with his beautiful song:
The wind blows blea o'er the sedgey fen
But warm the sun shines by the little wood
Where the old Cow at her leisure chews her cud

The casebook continued:

Jan. 11th 1864

Remains in much the same condition as on the last entry; improved on
what he was 9 months ago, but yet very helpless and quite childish.

April. 5th

His general health has not been so good lately and the right side had
more than once shown distinct sings of paralysis. His language is still
often very bad indeed and he sometimes becomes so excited when
swearing, that always having a quid in his mouth the piece finds its way
into his larynx which brings on a dreadful fit of coughing and his face
and head become perfectly scarlet and give strong fears of a sudden
apoplexy.

May 16th

A boil is forming near the anus, so he is to remain in bed for a time.

May 20th

He has appeared to feel the present excessively hot weather extremely
and the perspiration would roll off him in streams as he lay in bed. This
morning on being visited he was found to be completely comatose and
never rallied but died quietly late in the afternoon.

His death certificate, signed by Dr Irving, stated: 'John Clare aged 72
years died on May 20th, 1864 at 4.55pm in the presence of myself and
others, the cause of death being apoplexy'. He was taken in his coffin on his
only train journey to be buried in Helpston churchyard as he had wished.
    Dr Wing reported the poet's death in the Asylum Annual Report for
1864:

John Clare, who though ailing for sometime, yet not in a degree to excite serious apprehensions of immediate danger, was suddenly cut off by apoplexy on the 20th May. It had been my purpose, had space and my physical strength permitted, to have written somewhat at length on the character of his insanity, and to have pointed out the frequent connection between mental aberration and genius, and especially as illustrated by some of our most noted poets. Latterly his intellect had become sadly clouded, yet there were periods when the shadow would be temporarily lifted. There are some verses, written long after his admission into the Asylum (probably between 1846 and 1848), that I cannot forbear to introduce, as showing the deep melancholy under which he must have laboured at the time they were written. They are entitled

I AM

I am – yet what I am none cares or knows
    My friends forsake me like a memory lost;
I am the self-consumer of my woes,
    They rise and vanish in oblivions host
Like shadows in love – frenzied stifled throes
    And yet I am, and live like vapours tost

The third and final stanza reads:–

I long for scenes where man has never trod,
    A place where woman never smiled or wept;
There to abide with my Creator, God,
    And sleep as I in childhood sweetly slept;
Untroubling and untroubled where I lie,
    The grass below – above the vaulted sky.

Wing of course, did not live to describe Clare's insanity. Dr Nesbittt, Wing's predecessor as Superintendent, however, wrote from The Friars, Acton, on 15 April 1865 to Frederick Martin:

I was always led to believe that his mental affliction had its origin in dissipation. It was characterized by visionary ideas and hallucinations. For instance he may be said to have lost his own personal identity as with all the gravity of truth he would maintain that he had written the works of Byron, and Sir Walter Scott, that he was Nelson and Wellington, that he had fought and won the battle of Waterloo, that he had had his head shot off at this battle, whilst he was totally unable to explain the process by which it had been again affixed to his body. He was generally docile and tranquil, but would brook no interference – anything approaching to this last would excite his ire in a torrent of ejaculation of no ordinary violence in which imprecations were conspicuous; but this was an exceptional state of things. Seated on a bench and with his constant friend a quid of Tobacco, he would remain silent for hours. He was a passionate lover of the beauties of Nature – wild flowers being especially objects of interest to him. He was once asked how he had contrived to write his pretty poetry – his reply was that it came to him whilst walking in the fields – that he kicked it out of the clods.

If there was one subject more than another that he had an aversion to it was biography – he designated it as a pack of lies – but the beauties of poetry he could always appreciate and was never more at home and at his ease than when the productions of one of the time-honoured bards was placed in his hands.

He was essentially a kind-hearted, good-feeling man with unusually large cerebral development – possessing great breadth and altitude of forehead – such as we are in the habit of associating with men of the highest order of Intellect.

A more recent description of Clare's illness by Dr Thomas Tennent, Superintendent from 1938–62, was published in the *Journal of Mental Science* for January 1953. According to J. W. and Ann Tibble, authors of *John Clare* (1972 edition), Tennent 'described Clare's "epileptiform" attacks or loss of consciousness under stress in his adolescence; the creative fury which drove him to write for days on end, scarcely stopping to eat or sleep; the "blue devils" of depression in the ensuing years following frustration over the publication and non-sale of his poems; his later delusions of identity. "In my opinion", wrote Dr Tennent, "this was a cyclothymic disorder, and not a schizophrenic one as suggested by one of his recent biographers, [Geoffrey Grigson in his introduction to *Poems of John Clare's Madness*, 1949]. Apart from the actual symptomatology, the excellence of much of his poetry written in hospital and the slow development of deterioration support this diagnosis." Dr Russell (later Lord) Brain agreed with this diagnosis in *Some Reflections on Genius* in 1960. Clare endured this form of insanity, Dr Brain wrote, in common with Smart, Cowper, Newton, Goethe and Samuel Johnson. It is a disorder 'to which men of broad general views coupled with a sensitive imagination are naturally exposed'.

The idea that Clare's illness was manic depression is hard to sustain. The descriptions given by people who visited Clare strongly suggest that

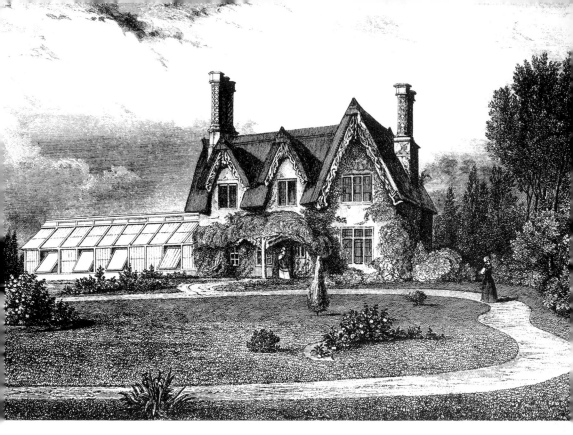

The Cottage Ornée, with conservatory attached, in the grounds of the Hospital, c.1860. It was then used for the reception of female patients.

his delusional ideas were present all the time even when his mood seemed normal and appropriate. The ideas he expressed were grandiose, persecutory and nihilistic, concomitantly not sequentially, as might be expected in a cyclical condition.

Cyrus Redding's description of how the delusions cropped up suddenly in the middle of an unrelated subject also argues against a condition in which the abnormal thoughts stem from a persistent mood state and reflect the view of the world dictated by the sufferer's affective condition. The clinical description fits more easily with a diagnosis of schizophrenia. Yet this is also not a totally satisfactory explanation.

In psychiatry it is often difficult to achieve a precise diagnosis even when the patient is available for repeated examination, when friends and relatives can be questioned at length and special investigations can be performed. With the passage of time and the sparcity of records, the position becomes almost impossible. Equally in psychiatry, a single diagnosis is not always appropriate as many factors may combine to produce a clinical picture unique to the individual. Such a formulation in Clare's case must take into account the following aspects.

He was a frail anxious child who was treated differently from most of his peers in terms of education. In adolescence he developed 'blackouts' of some kind which occurred regularly for some years but then only rarely in adult life. He had marked mood swings which occurred regularly at least until his admission to the Asylum. At times he drank excessively. He was given to womanising and on a number of occasions was convinced that he had contracted venereal disease. He was markedly hypochondriacal. At about the age of forty-three, the nature of his disorder changed and he became deluded and hallucinated to an extent that his family could no longer cope with him. He became increasingly apathetic and inert over the later part of his life. He died as a result of cerebrovascular disease.

The early part of his life can be explained in terms of personality development and his response to the stresses of his life are understandable. The illness of his middle life cannot be accounted for in the same way. It strongly suggests a 'biological' rather than a 'psychological' illness. The

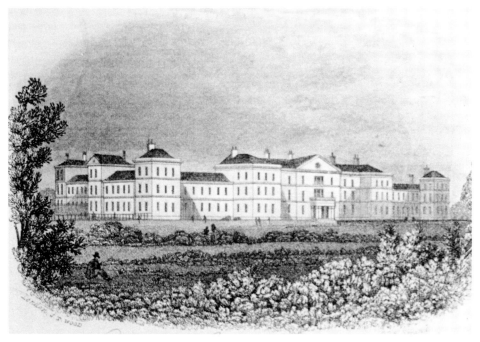

An engraving of the Hospital by J. T. Wood, which was used as a heading for writing paper, c.1860.

possibility of schizophrenia cannot be ruled out but other possibilities must be considered. One such possibility is cerebral syphilis.

At the time Clare was admitted to the Asylum, general paralysis of the insane was a common cause for admission. Its link with syphilis was not then known, though a connection with 'loose living and dissipation' had been postulated. The full clinical picture would have been recognised by any competent asylum doctor of the time. What was not then, however, appreciated was the protean ways in which cerebral syphilis can manifest itself. Probably only half of those who develop the condition show classical signs of general paralysis. The diagnosis of the condition only became more certain with the development of tests which demonstrate the presence of antibodies to the spirochaete in the spinal fluid.

Another fascinating aspect in Clare's case is the fact that he suffered repeatedly from malaria (the fen ague). In 1927 malaria was deliberately induced in patients with cerebral syphilis and this technique remained one of the few effective methods of treatment until the discovery of penicillin. It is reasonable to assume that, if Clare did suffer from cerebral syphilis, the course of the disease might well have been substantially modified if not arrested by his repeated high fevers.

There is unfortunately no way of proving or disproving this theory.

Chapter Eight

DR JOSEPH BAYLEY (1865–1876):

THE FATE OF THE PAUPER PATIENTS

*A*t the July 1865 meeting, it was decided that the post of Superintendent be advertised in *The Times*, *The Lancet*, *The Medical Times* and the *British Medical Journal*. The salary was to be £650 per annum, together with furnished apartments, service, coals, gas, vegetables and washing. There were forty-seven applicants, itself an indication of the growing prestige of the Asylum. Five of the candidates were short-listed and at a Special Court in September, under the chairmanship of William Smyth, Dr Joseph Bayley was elected.

The new Superintendent was then thirty, married and with two children, the younger of whom was only two months old. He was a graduate of King's College Hospital, London, a Member of the Royal College of Surgeons of England and a Licentiate of the Society of Apothecaries of London. After service in the Crimean War as a naval surgeon, he was appointed an Assistant Medical Officer, first at the Leicester City Asylum and afterwards at the Salop County Asylum, which housed over 400 pauper patients under Dr Oliver, whom he succeeded as Superintendent for two and a half years and whose daughter he married. He was to remain Superintendent at Northampton until January 1913 when he died in harness. The Annual Report for 1912 was to state after his death that he had throughout 'devoted all his energies to the promotion of the welfare of the Institution, and its present high state of efficiency is mainly due, under Providence, to his exceptional power of organisation and judicious management. To the members of the Committee he was always a kindly, courteous and genial friend, to work with whom was a privilege and a

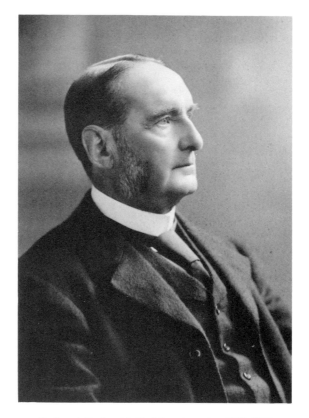

Dr Joseph Bayley, Medical Superintendent 1865–1913.

pleasure, and whose memory will ever be treasured by them with affection and respect'.

Bayley's forty-seven years as Superintendent may conveniently be divided into two periods. The first stretched from 1865 until 1876, when the fate of the pauper patients was finally settled with their removal to other pauper asylums and eventually to a newly built county asylum for Northamptonshire at Berry Wood. The second, from 1877 until his death in 1913, was one of consolidation during which he raised the Hospital's already high reputation to place it among the most distinguished mental institutions in these islands. This chapter deals with the first.

From the time of his appointment, even before he took up his duties in December 1865, Bayley imposed his personality upon all with whom he came in contact. At the time of his election, he made it clear that he would not be happy with accommodation in the Asylum's main building, but would require his own house in the grounds. It would be disagreeable for the Superintendent to have his wife and children living inside the Institution. Remembering perhaps the circumstances of the joint resignation of Dr and Mrs Nesbitt in 1859, the Court appears to have agreed to this. In November, it was decided that the cottage ornée in the grounds, which had been allocated to ladies of the private class, should be made habitable for the Superintendent and his family. It is clear from that year's Annual Report that the Directors were anxious to provide him with adequate privacy and comfort. He was given an allowance of £30 in lieu of using the furniture in the cottage as he had his own. He was also granted £75 per annum instead of service as he intended to employ his own staff. A further £25 was allowed him to arrange for his own washing. It was, however, nearly three years before he was able to take possession of the completed building.

The reason for the delay was expense. Every effort in 1866 was being made to keep additional costs to a minimum because of the extra building which would be required to accommodate all the county's pauper lunatics, should agreement be reached with the county and borough magistrates and with the Commissioners in Lunacy. Mr Law, who had replaced Mr Milne as the Institution's architectural consultant, had estimated that the additions to make the cottage a home would cost £1,400 but the lowest tender was £1,765, so the whole question had to be re-examined. Bayley wisely agreed that, because of the expense, the decision be postponed until the following year.

This question was again discussed at length at the Annual Court in February 1867. Mr Collins pointed out that it was not only the question of the higher tender but the extra requirements which had not been covered by the tender; these included a washhouse, a laundry, a coach-house, a stable and a man's apartment connected to the stable, presumably for a coachman, all of which might amount to £2,500. There was also the question of the architect's fees. It had at one stage been suggested that a plan, drawn up by Mr Godfrey, be adopted, and the work carried out by pauper labour, but Law had strongly advised that labour be employed by a contractor. In any case, the Commissioners in Lunacy had condemned one building of Godfrey's, presumably the isolation ward, as being unsuitable for its purpose. By this time, there was a growing feeling that the Superintendent should be appropriately housed, as indeed had been promised, and the tender of £1,765 for converting the cottage into a suitable house accepted; nevertheless, the final decision was again postponed for another year.

At the March 1867 monthly meeting, a reply from the Commissioners in

Lunacy to the question put to them, whether or not the Superintendent should be resident in the Asylum, was read. The Commissioners thought that he should, provided that 'proper accommodation and due privacy can be secured'. Bayley in a written statement, included in the Minutes, declared himself fully in agreement with the Commissioners' recommendations and then convincingly persuaded the Directors that the cottage was by far the most workable solution. From then onwards, the problem was not the cost but the speed with which the house could be built. Later additions, redecorations and repairs were to be accepted as an expense on the Institution.

By early 1868, pressure was being put on Law and through him on Iresons, the builders, to complete the house. This was only achieved to Law's satisfaction by the end of that July. Even then there were faults. Through a workman's carelessness, a gas-pipe in one of the bedrooms had been accidently severed and an attempt at mending it made with paper and cement. The room had become filled with gas when it was turned on and an explosion narrowly averted.

Bayley's first monthly report as Superintendent was highly critical. While the female galleries were excellent and the female refractory wards a credit to the Matron, he considered the male galleries and day rooms dirty, untidy and very crowded. He objected to the men being allowed to smoke everywhere, including in the kitchens, and at all times. The water-closets were in a poor state and in the worst private patients' ward there was no closet at all – merely a patent earth night stool. While the female clothing could be warmer, the male clothing was good, but 'the men generally have a slovenly appearance, most of them wear their hats indoors and the dirty boots are not changed; they are constantly lounging about, smoking and spitting over the walls and floors'.

He did not consider the kitchens well-conducted and more supervision was desirable; here women, not men, should be employed as cleaners. He also thought it objectionable that males should work in the laundry under female direction; the women should wash the linen and 'fine things', while the men did the heavy work.

More water-closets were necessary. The workshops were too small, the farm buildings needed to be improved and all patients capable of working should be found employment, but under qualified staff tradesmen, who knew the Asylum's rules, not under casually employed labourers who were ignorant of what was expected of them and who ill-treated the patients.

Bayley was obviously displeased that many of the staff, employed by the Secretary-Steward, did not appreciate that the Superintendent was in overall control. Moreover, 'The Steward is doing the work of the

Superintendent, Matron, Head Gardener, Architect and Builder, while the duties which properly belong to his office are done partly by two clerks, partly by the Superintendent, partly by the Brewer and Chief Attendant.' Frequently he found work being carried out of which he had no knowledge, only to find that it had been ordered by the Steward. He made these remarks in 'no spirit of ill-feeling towards the Steward, nor with any wish to underrate his services; he is no doubt a very valuable officer, but I feel it is my duty to point out these things to your committee because I am certain that it is impossible that I or any other person can under existing circumstances conduct this Institution in a satisfactory manner'.

There was no question of Dr Bayley not getting his way, nor is there any evidence of conflict between him and the zealous, hardworking Godfrey, who had been coping with much of the Asylum's administration for so long in the absence of any established superior. It was merely a question of re-establishing a proper chain of command, which was apparently quickly achieved. In the Annual Report for 1867, the Directors refer to the 'able and judicious management of Dr Bayley'.

Bayley at once set about putting things in order. A priority was to ensure that those capable of working did so. In the Superintendent's report for 1866, he stated:

Although at first some difficulty was experienced in getting many of the patients (who for a long time had done nothing) to employ themselves, it is now quite the exception for any patient to be unemployed, unless on account of sickness or infirmity. The result is that the bodily health of all and the mental condition of many of the most violent and hopeless among the male patients have much improved, the wards are rendered less crowded and offensive, and are kept much cleaner. For those patients who, although not on the sick list, are too old or infirm, or too demented to work on the farm or garden, picking and cleaning hair for bed-making in the upholsterer's shop has been found a most useful and suitable occupation, from 20 to 30 being regularly employed in this way; two or three patients are also being instructed by the upholsterers in making door mats with the old coir matting which has become worn out in the galleries.

Meanwhile bathrooms, water-closets, galleries and other improvements rendered necessary through the building expansion were added. In 1866 the cost of these works came to just on £1,430. In 1867 the bill amounted to £1,800 as a result of making the apartments of the male private patients more comfortable, of erecting a conservatory, a hothouse, a potting shed and other amenities for the kitchen garden and of putting the roofs of the Institution in good repair. In the latter Annual Report, Bayley stated that the male patients were now far more comfortable and that the new billiard and smoking-room was much used and appreciated. He looked forward to being able to report satisfactorily on improvements, most of which had already been sanctioned, then being carried out in the other wards.

From the start of his superintendency, Bayley made an excellent impression on the Lunacy Commissioners. Overall, however, they were happy neither with the Asylum's dual role of looking after the county patients and at the same time catering for private patients, nor with the independence of its Directors. They noted that the number of county or pauper patients had been steadily increasing. In 1857, the average number in the Asylum had been 172; by 1866, they had almost doubled to 336. By contrast, the average number of private patients had fallen slightly over the same period from ninety-one to eighty-five. The Commissioners recorded in the latter year that, while no county patients had been refused admission, the Asylum was becoming very full. In August 1867, they stated that the Institution was full and that the pauper patients were encroaching on the private. 'In these circumstances the question of providing adequate statutory permanent accommodation for the pauper lunatics of the County and Borough becomes one pressing for consideration on the part of the Justices and Governors.'

In July 1868, Bayley reported that the number of patients had reached 450 and, much against his inclination, he had had to allow some lunatics to go to the workhouse. He had only just over 400 cubic feet for each patient instead of the 550 cubic feet as laid down by the Commissioners. On the male side he had a total of 243 persons to accommodate, including twenty attendants, for whom he had only 237 beds. The female side was worse with 255 people crowded into space which should only hold 240. This overcrowding had been commented on by the House Visitors. Under current circumstances it was impossible to classify patients properly as to whether they were clean, dirty, noisy, quiet, epileptic, idiotic, violent, old, feeble, etc., as all had to be mingled together. The maximum number of patients in each ward should be no more than fifty – and only forty in refractory wards – but under conditions then appertaining there were as many as sixty to seventy. It was unfair to expect each ward's Chief Attendant to cope with every type of insanity under these circumstances.

The Superintendent then outlined a plan for more wards with the minimum of building, except for raising the roof to allow for a third floor by stages. As a result, the Court unanimously resolved that authority be given to spend £2,900, the sum involved on these improvements. Thus in the

1868 report, Bayley was able to give details of further additions sanctioned, including a three-storey building projecting from the centre tower on the male side to contain a general bathroom for county patients in the basement, a boot-room and a bath for recently admitted patients on the ground floor, a dormitory for nine beds on the third floor and improvements to the private patients' quarters. The kitchen facilities had also been improved, making the area 'free from the clouds of steam and disagreeable smells which used to be so much complained of'.

The whole future of the Asylum in connection with the county patients came to a head in 1869 when the renewal of the contract with the magistrates came up for consideration. In 1863, the Asylum had agreed to receive all the county lunatics for an inclusive payment of 12s. each per week; this contract was renewed for a further three years in 1866 at the rate of 11s.8d. per week. In the meanwhile, additions had been made to the Asylum on a scale much greater than anticipated in order to fulfil this obligation. In doing so, the Directors had been compelled to reduce very considerably the charitable aid given to the more impecunious private patients and had thereby incurred some criticism.

At the March 1869 monthly meeting with Mr William Smyth in the chair, it was pointed out that the rate of 11s.8d. had been unremunerative and was less than what was being paid by the surrounding counties. Accordingly, Mr Villiers, who was both Chairman of the county magistrates and a Director of the Asylum, proposed that the contract be renewed for a further three years at 12s.4d. per week. A Committee was nominated to discuss these terms with the magistrates, when it would be pointed out that the Institute was £3,000 in debt through its building programme to accommodate the county lunatics.

In May, the Committee of Justices considered 12s.4d too high and Mr Villiers, seconded by the local Member of Parliament, the Rt. Hon. G. Ward Hunt, proposed that the Asylum accept 12s. per week for each county patient. The Asylum's Vice-Chairman, the Rev. Lord Alwyne Compton, moved an amendment that the Asylum receive a total of 272 county paupers at 12s. per week each or, alternatively, be paid 12s.4d. per week for each patient in order to provide for the necessary additional building. This amendment was carried and the magistrates informed accordingly.

At the June monthly meeting, attention was given to a letter of 19 May from the Lunacy Commissioners, which was in reply to one from the magistrates, asking if there was any objection to the proposed renewal. In it, the Commissioners reiterated their opinion that, as the pauper patients in the Asylum had increased from 170 to 360, the Justices should with the

least possible delay 'carry out the positive requirements of the Legislature ... the Commissioners would point to the cases of the Stafford,
Gloucester and Nottingham Asylums as illustrative of the advantages of an
entire separation of the private from the pauper branch and the establishment of separate institutions for the patients of the former class'.

There followed a letter, dated 29 May, from H. P. Markham, acting as
Clerk of the Peace, calling the Asylum's attention to the Commissioners'
letter and asking for a meeting when it would be proposed 'that the Trust
Deed, Reports and Accounts of the Asylum and other documents affecting
the same from its foundation to the present time shall be submitted to some
independent person with a view to ascertaining whether the County,
Borough or Liberty (of Peterborough) may equitably or morally claim any
and what interest in the property of the Institution'. The rebuff from the
Management Committee was unanimous. The Duke of Grafton, seconded
by Lord Alwyne Comptom, repeated the offer to receive 272 pauper
patients at 12s. weekly but withdrew the proposal to receive all the county
patients at 12s.4d. until the Justices could give some assurance that the
necessary outlay for additional buildings would not be rendered useless by
subsequent arrangements to house the county patients elsewhere. The Rev.
H. J. Barton, seconded by the Rev. William Wales, then gained full
support for declining to provide the documents for the purpose requested.

The proposed meeting with the magistrates took place on 5 June, when
the county magistrates asked the Asylum Directors to reconsider their
refusal to go to arbitration. A letter dated 4 June, was produced from the
Commissioners, addressed to H. P. Markham, which read:

> Sir,
> I am directed by the Commissioners to acquaint the Justices for
> Northampton present at the meeting to be held tomorrow at the County
> Hall, that Messrs Ward Hunt and Smyth had an interview with this
> Board on the 26th ult. and that the Commissioners' sanction was then
> given to a temporary renewal of the present Contract for the reception of
> Northamptonshire Pauper Lunatics into Northampton Hospital (i.e. the
> Asylum) pending the conclusion of arrangements for the sale of the
> Hospital to the County upon equitable terms.

In the margin of the Minute Book, William Smyth wrote: 'There was a
suggestion from the Commissioners that an arrangement should be made
between the County and Hospital but I do not remember an understanding
that the County were to buy out the Directors of the Hospital.'

After this meeting, the Committee of Management resolved unanimously that the county patients be taken for one year only at 12s. per week. By this time, there was strong feeling in the county on both sides, as shown by the following extract from a letter, dated 17 June 1869, addressed by Sir George Robinson, who had very recently stepped down as Chairman, to his old friend, the Rev. H. J. Barton, who caused it to be published in the local Press. Robinson hoped:

> never to enter the Asylum gates again, unless it is as a pauper lunatic, which, after all, is no unlikely end for any of us. It seems the fashion at the present to strike at all property, whether in Ireland or the County of Northampton, which has been devoted to pious and charitable uses; but when disestablishment and disendowment have achieved their objects, in these and similar cases, and have transferred the estates of the Irish Church to the Roman Catholics and those of our Asylum to the county and borough ratepayers, the turn of the landed gentry will come next . . .
>
> I was very fortunate in having resigned the chair of the managing committee in time to escape the present scuffle, and I most heartily wish that all the directors, with whom I have acted so pleasantly for so many years (with some of them, as with our excellent friend Mr Collins, for as many as 35), would resign their connection with the Institution, instead of standing helplessly by to witness their property sequestered, their good works desecrated, and themselves bullied and insulted by Lord Shaftesbury and his colleagues on one side, and the Chairman of the Quarter Sessions [Ward Hunt] with his coadjutors on the other.

On 26 June, there was a lengthy meeting between the Asylum Directors and the county magistrates, at which Lord Southampton, Lord-Lieutenant of the County presided, to discuss the proposition that the Asylum's documents be submitted to independent arbitration. Mr Villiers expounded at length that the Asylum had been started by the county, which had derived great benefits from it and was entitled to great benefits from it because it had originally been founded by the county. He was having to put this case because the magistrates had been pushed into a corner by the Commissioners and by no act of their own, and therefore needed to know where they stood. It would appear that some magistrates, many of whom were also Directors of the Asylum, were embarrassed at being put in this position but, with the growing threat of having to make the ratepayers finance a new asylum for the county paupers, the stakes were high.

In reply, the Rev. H. J. Barton insisted that the Asylum was a charity and denied the right of the magistrates to participate in the management of its funds. He however apologised for having published Sir George's letter.

Ward Hunt for the magistrates considered that, if the whole question could be examined by a person of high character 'and if that person said the magistrates had no moral or equitable interest in the Asylum, their mouths would be shut for the future'.

Mr Smyth regretted, as Chairman of the Asylum, having to oppose the Chairman of the Quarter Sessions. The Asylum Directors had a divided duty, to receive on one hand the pauper lunatics and on the other the poorer class of yeomanry and tradesmen, who were admitted at reduced payments in proportion to their means. The magistrates had escaped all these years the necessity of building a separate county asylum and if they could enable the Directors of the Asylum to erect buildings which would satisfy the Commissioners without requiring the county to build, he thought the interests of the county would be well looked after. The meeting apparently ended amicably with agreement, later confirmed by the Management Committee, to direct Mr Hensman, Snr., who had succeeded Mr H. P. Markham as legal adviser to the Asylum, to examine all the relevant documents and to report 'upon the whole question legal and equitable of the existing relations between the County and the Hospital' by the end of the following month.

During the course of this meeting, Ward Hunt had charged Sir George Robinson of having used harsh words towards him. In a long friendly letter published in the *Mercury* on 10 July, Robinson took Hunt to task for the way he had tried to make out that the Asylum Directors had committed a breach of trust in the way that they had conducted the Asylum, a charge 'insinuated against us . . . by three gentlemen, two of whom have never, or scarcely ever, been in the Boardroom when any really hard work was to be done, while Barton, who has been so singled out for censure, has laboured at the oar in season and out of season, at his own very heavy cost in money and trouble'. Sir George's opinion was that:

> the best plan the Magistrates can adopt for getting themselves out of "the corner" is to remove their pauper patients altogether to a distance out of town. The objection to this is, of course, the expense, but setting this objection aside, how great the advantages. All our present disputes and difficulties would be terminated; the town would be relieved from what I am told is now a great annoyance to the residents in the district; property in the immediate neighbourhood of the Asylum would be increased in value; the Asylum grounds and gardens would be kept for the use of class patients, whose more civilized and quiet habits would give no offence, and I am not sure that, under certain restrictions, and at

certain hours, when the patients are within doors, our beautiful grounds might not be a source of recreation and pleasure to the inhabitants of Northampton.

He ended by apologising for any words in his letter to Barton which Hunt may have thought hard or discourteous. Sir George died in 1873.

A feeling that the interests of the private patients had become increasingly neglected through devoting their profits to the county lunatics emerged clearly at a meeting of the Quarterly Court on 28 July, Mr J. H. B. Whitworth drew the Court's attention to a resolution of 1860 to increase the amounts spent charitably on private patients from £600 per annum, then considered insufficient, to at least £1,000. Instead, the sum had shrunk to £150. 'Considering the charity was founded for the relief of the middle classes, they had the greatest claim on the Institution. Now, however, they were driving people into the pauper class who would not have become paupers, if the profits of the Institution had been devoted to their relief . . . If additional buildings were required for pauper patients, they should be paid for out of the county rates.'

The Chairman, William Smyth, thanked Whitworth for raising the matter. A difference had arisen between the Asylum and the magistrates as to whether an extra four pence a week should be laid out for each pauper patient for the purpose of paying the cost of the additional buildings which were needed to house them; this the county had refused to do. He personally would not be a party to the laying of another brick, except for internal alterations, unless some arrangement could be made by which the county should bear its full share of the expense.

That the feelings expressed at this Court were so forthright were no doubt influenced by the report Hensman had made earlier that morning to the Management Committee. It was a long report, going in detail through all the relevant events in the Asylum's history. His conclusion was that the ratepayers had no claim 'which a Court of Equity would recognise against an Institution, founded by voluntary subscriptions, and where some of the objects of the charity are now provided for by law'. The Charity Commissioners moreover had no jurisdiction over the Institution under the Charitable Trusts' Act.

On the strength of this finding, the Directors decided that they could not consent to submit their interests to arbitration or their documents to some independent person whose views would be regarded as morally binding, but they would be happy to allow a representative of the magistrates to examine the deeds at the latters' expense to enable him to advise the magistrates; they would also be ready to consider any offer the magistrates might wish to make.

A Special Meeting on 18 August then examined a proposition made by the magistrates that five Justices and five Directors should meet, with the Lord-Lieutenant presiding, 'with a hope of bringing the question of the pauper lunatics to a friendly decision'. This was agreed to by the Directors but the terms they were prepared to offer were unequivocal. They maintained their absolute property in the Asylum and the entire control of its management; they would be willing to help the county by accepting a limited number (say 150, 200 or 250) pauper patients at 12s.4d., 13s. or 14s. per week, depending upon their ability or inability to work; they were reluctantly convinced that the Asylum had not sufficient space to cope with the current number of paupers, much less the yearly increase in numbers; they also considered it their duty to add to the number of private patients.

At the October Quarterly Court, a letter from the magistrates was read, stating that they had submitted certain papers, together with Counsel's opinion, to the Charity Commissioners, asking if they could be counted on to support a Bill in Parliament for transferring the Asylum to the county as suggested by the Commissioners in Lunacy. Mr Villiers, who was present on behalf of the magistrates, was obviously hoping to manoeuvre the Directors into a position in which a compromise favourable to the magistrates might be reached. The Directors however at once resolved: 'That the Commissioners have no jurisdiction over the Hospital, which had been founded entirely by voluntary contributions, and that it was trusted the Charity Commissioners would not lend the sanction of their Board to any Act of Parliament to be proposed by the Magistrates, without the knowledge or consent of the Directors.' The Charity Commissioners replied that their consent for introducing such a Bill would not be required and that the whole matter was outside their sphere of duty.

At this stage, the Directors were sent, at their request, a copy of the legal opinion, prepared for the magistrates by Messrs Hunter Rodwell and G. D. Begg.

The conclusion to which we have arrived [they stated], after the perusal of the reports and documents laid before us, is that the ratepayers of the County of Northampton have not such an interest, *legal or equitable*, in the Lunatic Asylum at Northampton as entitles them to appropriate any portion of the building to County purposes, as to institute it a County Asylum within the meaning of the Act of 1853 and over which the Lunacy Commissioners might exercise control . . . The evident intention of the founders was to supply a want not then provided for by express legislation, and it was contemplated to carry out a voluntary act of charity, and not to satisfy a legal obligation. And although in the course of events the Institute has become a substitute for a County Asylum, the original purpose has never been lost sight of. It does not appear that in any of the communications and negotiations which took place from 1809 to 1862 between the County and Directors the former ever claimed the right of property in the institution.

Counsel went on to say that:

we cannot but think that the ratepayers have or ought to have a quasi beneficial interest in the fabric which has grown out of contributions not from the county rate, but mainly from the voluntary donations of individual landowners and residents in the County, which morally entitles them to participate in the advantage of the institution. And to repudiate such a right now is a departure from the principle which actuated the Directors at the periods to which we have referred.

Ways of dealing with the problem, which was compensation rather than a question of legal right, might be to consult some eminent public man about introducing a private Bill, aimed at transferring the Asylum to the county. If the Asylum Directors opposed this:

the County, might with the sanction of the Charity Commissioners, prepare a Bill for the transfer of the institution to the County upon terms and for vesting the proceeds in the hands of the Directors for the carrying out of the charitable purposes of the Institution, other than the maintenance of pauper lunatics. We need hardly add that in the event of the Bill failing, or being withdrawn, the cost of promoting could not be paid out of the county rates. In order that the requisite Parliamentary notices may be given, if it is intended to apply for a Bill next session, no delay must take place.

As the Charity Commissioners had already stated that the whole question was outside their province, the magistrates did not venture to promote a Bill. Sir George Robinson had meanwhile consulted J. P. De Jex, an eminent equity lawyer, who advised 'That neither the county nor the borough could equitably or morally claim any interest in the property of the asylum'. The magistrates had no alternative but to build their own mental hospital.

On 29 December, the Superintendent reported that there were now 467 beds in the Institution, but to accommodate this number it had been found necessary to use the schoolroom, various passages and even a bathroom. Because of this overcrowding, and bearing in mind the private patients' need for space, it was decided that, in future, no more than 150 pauper patients of each sex should be admited. The payment by the unions for maintenance should be the average rate paid to the seven neighbouring asylums. The contract for lodging paupers from June 1870 should be for three years only.

The 1870 Annual Report declared that the magistrates had given up claims on the Asylum and it had been agreed to receive 300 patients up to June 1873 at the rate of 12s.5½d. per week. Villiers on behalf of the magistrates tried to get this rate reduced but was unsuccessful.

> The Committee much regret that it was not in their power to receive all the county patients and that 32 women and 12 men have been removed by the county to the Asylums of Leicester and Worcester. This measure was rendered necessary by the overcrowded state of the house, which was a subject of complaint by the Commissioners in Lunacy, to which the Committee felt it to be their duty to give effect.

The year's financial results had been good but the debt, although reduced, was still £2,687 and it was important, with the proposed removal of the county patients, to pay this off and to build up a sum to meet further contingencies. The report ended:

> It is too early at present to make any definite plans or propositions for our future conduct, but there is a general feeling (and one strongly urged by the Commissioners in Lunacy) of the great want of an Asylum where Middle-class patients can be received at more moderate rates of payment than are now usually required; and to this view the Directors will probably feel it their duty, as Trustees of a large Charity, to direct their special attention.

The Management Committee was now able to plan the Asylum's future, untroubled by the need to provide ever more space for the pauper lunatics. In July 1870, the Directors told the magistrates that they were prepared to accept 320 paupers, divided equally between the sexes, for three years on condition that all the beds were paid for, whether or not in use; this was afterwards modified, allowing a reduction in the number of beds required if given three months' notice. Northampton town was allocated space for twenty-three of each sex and Peterborough twelve of each. The borough agreed to accept the Directors' terms in a letter from the Clerk of the Peace of 22 September, the second paragraph of which read:

> I have at the same time to say that I was instructed by the Mayor and Magistrates to ask whether the Directors will allow a few more Boro' Paupers to be sent to the said Asylum in case accommodation for more than forty-six be required, and at the same time to intimate that this would be deemed a favour to the Borough Magistrates and save them trouble and inconvenience, and also prevent the hardship to the Lunatics and their friends which would be caused by the former having to be sent to a distance from Northampton.

The Directors agreed to help when possible, 'but they cannot pledge themselves to any definite increase in the numbers already fixed'.

With their eyes on the future, the Directors in January 1871 approved an advertisement to be inserted in the Press of the neighbouring counties about increasing their facilities for private patients. In their Annual Report for that year, they stated that their debt was about to be extinguished 'and that they may reasonably look forward to making the Hospital one of the grandest charities in the Kingdom for the reception of Private Patients, and especially of the middle class of sufferers, at moderate rates of payment'.

In July 1872, the magistrates approached the Asylum for what was to be the last contract for pauper patients. The Finance Committee recommended that the period be either for one year, or for a term not exceeding three and a half years; that the numbers start at 230, 'that this number be reduced by thirty at the end of each half year in equal proportions as to sexes; and the question of payment be deferred until the Justices have decided upon the terms for which they would prefer the Agreement to be made'.

The 6th Duke of Grafton, Chairman since 1970 in succession to William Smyth, who had died suddenly in March, commented soberly in a letter on the suggested terms as follows:

> I take it for granted that the new General Lunatic Asylum cannot receive Pauper Patients before three years from now, and I don't hesitate to say that it is the duty of the (present) General Lunatic Asylum to continue to accommodate them up to that time, or longer if necessary. I don't think it will be advisable to arrange the rate of payment for so long a period owing to the uncertainty which prevails in rate of wages and provisions. It will be only acting fairly to ourselves and justly towards the County to agree to terms of payment for one year. With the opinion I

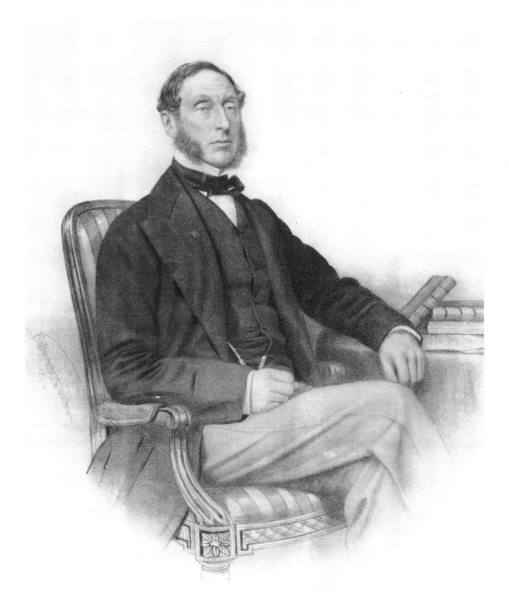

The 6th Duke of Grafton, Chairman 1870–1882.

hold of our duty towards the County I am inclined to think it will be difficult to reduce the number of Pauper Patients by thirty every six months, for I am at a loss to say where these afflicted people are to find a domicile.

160

After some discussion, agreement was finally reached in March 1873 for a new contract, which was to run for three years from 1 July. The Directors agreed to accept 180 paupers for the first year, 150 for the second and 120 for the third. The payment was to be 13s. each per week for the full number, whether or not all places were taken up. Reduced numbers would be accepted on six months' notice. The Asylum was to provide clothing and medical treatment in addition to lodging and maintenance.

From then onwards, the final withdrawal of the paupers was only a question of time. Little difficulty was anticipated in replacing the paupers with private patients, the growth in whose numbers was noted in the report for 1872. The Asylum's ability to achieve cures would, it was claimed, increase as the paupers left. The total number of patients in the Asylum still ranged from 410 to 440. In 1874, the Institution was described for the first time as the Northampton General Lunatic Asylum for the Middle and Upper Classes, but it was only in July 1875 that the overall numbers began slowly to decline as the paupers started to leave. By July 1876, they had dropped significantly to approximately 272 from a total in the previous month of 390. In that year's Annual Report, the Directors announced that the last pauper patients had left in July – actually the final three departed that September – while the number of private patients was rapidly approaching the desired total of 300.

The Directors now decided to convert the workshops into luxury apartments for wealthier patients. One patient was already paying £400 a year for good accommodation and a Commissioner in Lunacy, who had remarked that he had found a patient paying £700 elsewhere for much inferior rooms, promised to recommend the Asylum to others prepared to pay liberally.

Apart from the problem of the pauper lunatics, the Lunacy Commissioners' reports were generally favourable to the Asylum, and were usually included in the Annual Reports from 1869 onwards. They analysed in detail the number of patients admitted, discharged and died, and noted among other matters the cleanliness of the wards and of the patients' clothing, the quality of the food, and the number of attendants, the recreations provided and details of restraint and seclusion. Almost invariably they ended with complimenting Bayley. When an occasional cricitism was made, it was usually noted in the succeeding report that corrective action had been taken. They felt compelled to note, however, in some detail an outbreak of typhoid fever in September 1875, which was not included in the Annual Report for that year.

There had been several cases of typhoid in November 1864, and in March 1866 Bayley reported widespread diarrhoea; this he thought may have been caused by the foul condition of the main water tank, which had afterwards been thoroughly cleaned. He warned that there could be further outbreaks, a prophecy which came true that October when there was one fatality.

In summer 1871, there was a severe outbreak of fever which resulted in three deaths. Bayley reported in July that the number of cases, which had averaged about two annually from 1855 until 1869, had since increased to four in 1870 and 1871; altogether there had been twenty-two cases during these years, of which five had proved fatal. He thought it impossible for the fever to have been brought in from outside. He had consulted Dr Francis of the Northampton Infirmary and they had both agreed that water was not the cause, having had all sources available to the Asylum analysed. He did not think the drainage was to blame, but it was possible that there were old cesspools under the female side where most of the cases occurred; the deposits beneath the male side had previously been removed and the floors relaid. Certainly the floors on the female side were old and thoroughy saturated.

Bayley considered the most suspect source was the Northampton Sewage Works close by to the south-west of the Asylum. This was the direction from which the prevailing winds blew, bringing with them an abominable smell about which there had been many complaints, and probably the germs of the disease as well. Dr Francis thought that this line of investigation might be followed up, once all other likely sources had been investigated. Bayley asked for more workmen to hasten the removal of the old stone floors and the soil underneath, plus the installation of improved closets, the work to be completed within two years instead of being spread over several. At the same time, a proper building for isolation cases was needed, as the old one was no longer fit for use.

The Asylum's system for utilizing its sewage, which was also to come under suspicion, was given in detail in the 1871 Annual Report. As a result,

166½ tons of Italian Rye Grass, 30 tons of Mangel-wurzel, 6 tons of Cow Cabbage, 4 tons of House Cabbage, 30 bushels of Onions, 15 cwt Parsnips, 15 cwt Carrots have been grown in the previous year upon 4½ acres of land.

In July 1872 there was another case of typhoid fever, but the disease did not spread and the victim recovered. In his report for that month, Bayley could give no other reason for its re-occurrence except that previously advanced, and stated that the improvement of the sanitary conditions of the Asylum was progressing steadily. Two further cases occurred in

October 1873 and on this occasion the Northampton Medical Office of Health, Dr Haviland, inspected the Asylum and analysed the different sources of water supply. The Committee, unhappy about his report, had the water supply analysed again and the Superintendent was instructed to find out the cost of installing separate pipes for drinking water and for water used for other purposes, also the comparative expense of using the Water Board's water and that pumped from the Asylum ground. If necessary, a geologist or engineer was to be consulted. In the following month, the analysis of the water showed that the Water Company's was good, but that from the Asylum's well was unsuitable for drinking.

In August 1874, the Superintendent complained that they had been much troubled by the stench from the sewage works and announced several cases of diarrhoea and dysentry and one of typhoid. He was instructed to send this part of the report to the Northampton Improvement Commissioners and to Dr Haviland, who attended the December Management meeting, when he said he was going to recommend that the sewage works be removed as they were 'no more nor less than so many square yards of open cesspool'; it was a damning report. He thought the smells could well be the cause of the diarrhoea, about which there had also been complaints from private householders. It was agreed to make an urgent representation about the situation to the Urban Sanitary Authority.

In a letter to Dr Bayley, dated 1 January 1875, Dr Haviland introduced a new dimension to this problem by pointing to the Asylum's own sewage works as a possible source of danger to the patients. It was accordingly decided to discontinue using the sewage for irrigation purposes and the Urban Sanitary Authority was invited in January 1875 to inspect the Asylum's drainage system and to make recommendations. By now the Improvements Commissioners had become upset at the charge made about the local sewage works and asked that it be retracted, but this the Management Committee refused to do, especially as Dr Haviland had, as promised, sent in his own recommendation. Apparently the local authorities took no action.

The worst outbreak of typhoid took place in September 1875, with sixteen cases on the female side – although none on the male – and, in addition, much diarrhoea and three cases of scarlet fever. Bayley reported that he had again consulted Dr Francis of the Infirmary, who had visited the Asylum and recommended applying to the Medical Officer of the Local Government Board. While still thinking that the smells from the sewage works were probably the cause of these outbreaks, he admitted that it was just possible that the fault lay in the Asylum. He hoped the authorities in London would help.

By the end of September, the epidemic had twenty-nine victims, all but two of them female; sixteen of them were nurses and servants. Bayley reported that Dr Buchanan, a Medical Inspector of the Local Government Board, had spent two days examining the Asylum, but had been unable to detect anything wrong; he intended however to make a further inspection. The Superintendent took this occasion to emphasise the importance of having a detached hospital for infectious diseases. The laundry arrangements, which the Management Committee was now assessing, also needed to be improved. The presence of typhoid in the hospital was not mentioned either in the Management Committee's or the Superintendent's report for that year.

In February 1876, the Commissioners in Lunacy filled in the picture about the further action being taken to eradicate the source of the fever; this was also not included in that year's Annual Report. Dr Buchanan 'formed the opinion that it was due to defects in the old drains which run under some of the wards. That these drains are defective has since been actually ascertained. Such temporary remedy as was possible was immediately provided, but we are glad to learn that the Committee have decided that a new set of drains shall be constructed externally to the building, and instructions have been given for the works to be carried out under the direction of a competent sanitary engineer'. It was some time before these plans were submitted to the Committee and it was not until August that a Special Court formally approved them at a cost of £2,500; this involved, among other works, taking up and relaying timber and tile floors, removing old drains, searching for and destroying rat runs and installing new closets where absolutely necessary. The Commissioners in Lunacy in their report, dated 24 February 1877, deplored the fact that prompter action regarding the drains had not been taken.

In August 1876, Bayley reported that twenty-five persons, both staff and patients, were afflicted with the fever. Two further cases appeared in September, one of them being one of the Superintendent's own children. None of them was fatal. In October he told the Committee that 'the epidemic of typhoid fever may now, I think, be looked upon as ended'.

Cases of fever, however, continued to occur from time to time – there was one in November and two the following January – and diarrhoea remained a problem. In April 1877 there was a fresh outbreak of fever on the male side and seven attendants, including the Chief Attendant, fell sick; one attendant and a patient died. It was decided to pay the wages of the stricken attendants in full. In their Annual Report, the Management Committee referred to the large expenditure on drains, over £4,900 in that year alone.

In autumn 1878, a further four cases were reported; on this occasion the fault was found to be the Asylum's water. As the local Water Company could not supply all the Asylum's requirements, filters were placed on the pipes in every ward. By 1880, the fever had been virtually stamped out; from then onwards only the very occasional case of typhoid occurred, originating almost certainly from outside.

The other disease with which Bayley had to cope in the early years of his superintendency was smallpox. Reference has already been made to an outbreak in January 1865. Smallpox was widespread in Northampton at the time, so it was almost inevitable that cases should arise in the Asylum. Several were reported in April 1866; those affected were sent to the isolation ward on the farm. There was a fresh outbreak in 1871, as a result of which Bayley recommended that all officers, staff and patients be vaccinated, especially, according to his February Report, 'as it is notorious that there has been great neglect in this town with regard to carrying out the compulsory vaccination act'.

By December 1871, the smallpox epidemic was so widespread that the Directors agreed that no pauper patient be received from the borough while it prevailed. The Superintendent also reported that he had refused entry to all visitors from the affected districts, except in cases of emergency. The importance of vaccination was illustrated by the fate of a nurse, who had not been so treated; having fallen ill, she was removed to the Smallpox Hospital in Northampton, of which Dr Barr was the Chief Medical Officer, where she died. The question arose about workmen from the town who refused to be vaccinated. The Directors decided that they and their families should submit to the precaution and it was up to the Superintendent to see that this was done. Bayley was able to report in January 1872 that all had been vaccinated and that there had been no new cases of the disease; here was undoubted proof of his ability to cope with emergencies in a sensible and energetic way.

The Commissioners in Lunacy in July 1872, when commenting on the Asylum's refusal to admit unvaccinated paupers, asked if they could be received if vaccinated a week to ten days previously. The Superintendent at first agreed but later, when a further case of smallpox was reported in the Northampton Union in August, decided against this. It was afterwards resolved by the Management Committee in September that no pauper patients would be allowed entry until a certificate could be produced that there had been no case of smallpox in the borough Union for a month.

At the October Management Committee meeting, a deputation asked the Asylum to admit Union pauper lunatics as a month had now passed without a fresh case. This was agreed to on condition that all coming into the Asylum were re-vaccinated. From this time onwards, smallpox ceased to be a problem. The Superintendent took this opportunity to stress that as many pauper patients as possible would be received on condition that harmless chronic cases in the Asylum's care were handed over in exchange for acute cases. This last condition had been made legal by Section 43 of the Poor Law Amendment Act, 1868, which enabled workhouse guardians with the consent of the Poor Law Board and the Commissioners in Lunacy to take into a workhouse any chronic lunatic who was certified as harmless and in good health on terms as agreed between the guardians and the Asylum; as long as such a lunatic stayed in the workhouse, he was to remain a patient on the books of the asylum from which he came.

There were several staff changes during these years. Dr J. T. Hingston, who had been appointed House Surgeon in November 1865, resigned in January 1868 on being appointed Superintendent of the Isle of Man Asylum. He was replaced that February by Charles Berrell, aged twenty-five, who had served for eighteen months in the Warwick Asylum. He did not serve long as in the December of the following year he died of typhoid fever. In January 1870, John H. Bell, MD, Edinburgh, was appointed in his place. Bell had been an Assistant Medical Officer at Bethlem for six months and had acted temporarily in that capacity at the Asylum. He was to remain in this position until January 1877, when Mr de Denne was elected to succeed him.

Haines, the Chaplain, was granted six months' leave in 1868, on condition he provided a substitute in his absence. A previous request for a month's leave and payment for his substitute had been turned down as there was no precedent for this. Haines was obviously suffering from a nervous breakdown. In his letter making this request, he wrote: 'I am under great obligations to Mr Bayley and Mr Hingston for their kind treatment which has for the time being done me good but I have always fallen back again into my previous state. Cheerfulness is so essential to the performance of my duties that it is worthwhile trying every means to bring it back.' He finally resigned in November; his place was taken by the Rev. R. B. Woodward, late of Great Houghton, who had acted as Chaplain during Haines's absence.

Haines had worked with great devotion. In addition to two full services and sermons on Sundays and daily prayers on weekdays, he had performed during the year forty-three extra full services and given twenty-five sermons on Saints' Days, according to a resolution of the Management Committee. He had also been comparatively successful in teaching patients to read and write, according to his report for 1867, in which he also referred to the need for additions to the library.

Woodward, Haines's successor, served the Asylum until his death in 1875. His Annual Reports are among the shortest on record, that of 1871 being slightly longer only because of his reference to the extreme coldness of the chapel, which was subsequently rectified. His salary with no emoluments remained at £250. In 1872, the Management Committee recommended a £50 increase, in response to a request from him, but no final decision had been taken by the Court at the time of his death two years later. A gratuity of £100 was voted for his widow.

In May 1875, the Management Committee had difficulty in finding a temporary Chaplain and it was decided to investigate the duties and salaries of chaplains in other asylums; subject to this enquiry, it was thought that the post of Chaplain should be advertised at £400. In October, after the results of the enquiries were to hand, Lord Alwyne Compton recommended this sum but he was overruled by an amendment made by Lord Charles FitzRoy that the Chaplain's salary should remain at £250; it was at the same time decided that he should undertake no duties outside the Asylum, nor take pupils. In January 1876, the Rev. John Cunningham was appointed.

At the January 1872 Court, Bayley's salary was increased after much discussion from £800 to £900, while in the following year the Assistant Medical Officer's salary was raised from £150 to £200. By the end of the period under review, the Superintendent was earning £1,000, the Matron £175 – an increase of £25 – and the Secretary-Steward £350. All these officers received considerable additional emoluments such as unfurnished accommodation, free heating and service. The Chaplain's salary however remained at £250 with no extras. At the same Court it was proposed by the Duke of Grafton, seconded by the Rev. H. J. Barton, now a Canon, and unanimously resolved that the Finance Committee should work out a pension scheme for the staff. Barton was obviously the prime mover in this scheme, strongly supported by Lord Alwyne Compton. Barton was somewhat apprehensive about the future finances of the Institution; he considered it might have been sensible to wait a little longer to see how the future of the Asylum shaped before taking on this extra commitment. Perhaps he was influenced by the views of his old friend and colleague, Mr Collins who, when retiring in the previous October because of his advanced age and broken health, had written to express the greatest forebodings about the Asylum's financial future after the paupers had been withdrawn. Bayley, in thanking the Court for his salary increase, made it clear that he did not harbour the same fears as many about the Institution's financial position.

In August 1874, however, there appeared the following entry in the

Minutes regarding pensions: 'The Committee have considered Dr Bayley's letter and are quite satisfied that this Asylum cannot agree to any regular scale of Pensions, and wish to abide by the present Rule 12 which gives the power of increasing Salaries and granting Pensions, and therefore decide upon the following system already laid down of paying such liberal salaries as the Income of the Institution shall allow.' In practice, the staff at all levels continued to be given increases in wages, sick pay and pensions at what were accepted levels at that time, although occasionally the demands on them seem severe. The engine driver's wage was increased from 22s.6d. to 25s. weekly on condition that his hours were to be from 5 a.m. to 6.30 p.m., except on Saturdays when they were to be extended until 8 p.m. with attendance every alternate Sunday. He was also required to attend any emergency in connection with his normal work beyond those hours; overtime was to be allowed in certain circumstances.

In June 1875, Bayley himself asked for an increase in salary. At the July meeting, the Directors were not unwilling to entertain the request but decided first to appoint a Sub-Committee to examine the question of salaries and perquisites for all the officers. The Committee reported back that November and the next Quarterly Court confirmed its recommendation that the Superintendent's salary be increased by £100 and that '£100 a year be invested for his benefit, the whole sum so invested to be given to the Superintendent when he retires or to his representatives on his death'.

In the meanwhile, the routine of managing the Asylum went on. From March 1866 onwards, a Sub-Committee was appointed each spring 'to examine and report upon all financial details both as regards the current and also any proposed additional expenditure, that this Committee supervise all building arrangements and Farm expenditure and cultivation and also attend to any other business referred to it by the Committee of Management. Not less than two Members shall transact the ordinary routine business but one Member may check Bills and Invoices and examine cash accounts previous to their being submitted to the Committee of Management'. At the end of 1871, a Building Committee was also formed and its membership given in subsequent Annual Reports. The statutes and rules were revised from time to time, having first been shown to the officers in case there were objections, and sent to the Secretary of State, Home Department, for his approval.

In 1870, Barton emphasised his concern about the increased expenditure to which Bayley replied. The Committee begged 'to record their full appreciation of the services rendered to the Institution by both gentlemen in their several positions, and while giving their thanks to Mr Barton beg to record their full confidence in their Superintendent'. It was then resolved that in future the Finance Committee compare the cost, item by item, of each quarter compared with the previous one.

In 1873, the duties of the Secretary-Steward were re-organised in order to give the Superintendent complete control over the ordering and disposal of goods. The Secretary, who was to be solely responsible for the accuracy of the figures, was to examine all accounts and then pass them to the Superintendent for his initials. The Secretary was to carry out all the instructions of the Superintendent, but new ones were to be given in writing. Godfrey, the Secretary-Steward, had been seriously ill in 1868, involving a lengthy absence; in January 1869 the Management Committee agreed to allow him £60 towards his expenses of £90 while at Bournemouth to recuperate. He was apparently not completely well for sometime afterwards; this may have accounted for some lessening in the efficiency of the administration.

In 1875 there occurred a series of thefts by one Whiting, an attendant, and his wife, for which they were prosecuted. A Sub-Committee, chaired by Lord Charles FitzRoy, carried out a detailed investigation into how these could have happened. In their report, no blame was attached to anyone, 'but that (as often happens) from a long continuance of exemption from any occurrence, such as the recent robberies, the system has been allowed to get a little out of order and by degrees many duties which should have been performed by one person have been performed by another, thus causing some to be overworked or absent from their proper duties'. There was no system which would enable the Superintendent to see at once if anything was going wrong. The Sub-Committee was confident that it was capable of re-organising the routines within the framework of the existing rules.

A tight rein had to be kept on the attendants and junior staff. Those who proved incompetent or who ill-treated the patients were sacked and, in extreme cases, sent in front of the magistrates to be fined as well as dismissed. One attendant was discharged for wearing the patients' clothes and another for carelessness in leaving knives around. There were occasional quarrels to be sorted out. The bandmaster, an attendant, was warned not to use improper language to his Chief Attendant, who was his superior. Mention of such cases are scattered throughout the Minutes as all such details were reported to the Management Committee.

Staff also had on occasion to be protected and supported. In October, a pauper patient died through suffocation in a fit of epilepsy and the coroner accused the Matron of great neglect. The Directors examined this case and unanimously agreed that the woman had not been left uncared for intentionally. The Superintendent also reported on the vulnerability of attendants when sleeping in the patients' dormitories; one female attendant had in fact been attacked at night. He urged that they should have separate bedrooms overlooking each ward. On another occasion, as a result of a violent attack on a nurse, Bayley recommended the installation of alarm bells.

There were also problems with patients. They escaped from time to time, but nearly all of them were recaptured. On occasion, they were aided by friends. Bayley thought it odd that, while the laws provided severe punishment for any asylum official or employee who connived at or assisted a patient to get away, others could do so with impunity. Suicides, a constant source of worry because they took place when least expected, occasionally occurred and were both reported and rigorously investigated; the same applied to accidents. Cases in which restraint was used were regularly reported on by the Superintendent and by the Commissioners in Lunacy. Bayley was strongly opposed to restraint except when patients refused to allow surgical treatment to be carried out.

Amusements and entertainments continued to form an important part of the treatment. The Asylum Amateur Dramatic Company, consisting chiefly of nurses and attendants, flourished. In addition, a string band, considered more suitable for indoor entertainment than the brass band which played outdoors during the summer, was formed as well as a glee class. In 1868 there was both a Patients' Annual Ball and a Private Patients' Ball in addition to theatricals, concerts, a cricket match and an outdoor fête. The custom of a selected group of patients spending some weeks at the seaside became a regular feature in the calendar from then onwards.

Bayley insisted that all patients capable of working be employed. This was not difficult to arrange with pauper patients who usually took up their normal occupation as tradesman or labourer; private patients were more difficult, for it was quite the exception to find one capable of following any employment. He stressed the need for a suitable recreation hall where patients of both sexes could meet for musical parties and entertainments in order to break up the monotony of the long winter evenings.

It was during these years that a major project – namely the founding of a school for idiot children – was taken up with great enthusiasm, and received the unanimous support of the Annual General Court of 1865. The Rev. H. J. Barton, supported by the Rev. Chancellor Wales, considered this a subject 'well worthy of the attention of the Directors, both in a financial and moral point of view'. It was proposed in the first instance to provide places for 25 boys and 25 girls, as the census of 1861 showed that in Northampton there were 201 pauper idiots over the age of sixteen; this meant that there were probably an equal number either under sixteen or belonging to the class above pauperism. Money subscribed was to be considered as given to the Lunatic Asylum.

The proposed appeal outlined the case clearly, if somewhat emotionally:

If it be admitted
'That all the true delights of man
Should spring from sympathy',
this appeal will not be made in vain. For in what can the thoughtful mind and the tender heart find cause for deeper sympathy than the sorrows and sufferings of the Class for whom it pleads.

Outcasts from Society, often neglected, sometimes cruelly treated, these unhappy beings drag on a miserable existence without hope and without enjoyment.

The Law has mercifully provided an Asylum for the Insane: but hitherto the case of the poor Idiot has been neglected and what ought to have been regarded as a public duty has been left to private benevolence.

One great Institution there is, and one only, of this kind in the Kingdom – the Asylum for Idiots at Earlswood – which reflects the highest honour upon the individuals who founded and upon those who continue to support it. But there is no such thing as a County Idiot Asylum in existence. And yet the want of such an Institution is distressingly proved by the fact that in this County alone there can be no less than 350 of these unhappy beings but no united effort to improve their mental state or mitigate their bodily sufferings. Idiocy is not without remedy and therefore should not be left without help.

The reports from Earlswood testify that numbers have been transformed from wild, mischievous, filthy, spiteful and disobedient into the very reverse of these deplorable qualities. Many who would have been entirely unable to earn a livelihood have learnt useful trades which have enabled them either wholly or in part to maintain themselves, instead of being a permanent burden on their respective parishes . . . and it is a remarkable and most gratifying fact that a large proportion are more capable of religious than of any other instruction . . .

It remains therefore for the County of Northampton in this case as in many other instances to take the lead and by thus setting a noble example of Christian Philanthropy to induce other counties to do the same (and as in the case of Insanity cause the Legislature to take up the subject).

It was hoped that liberal contributions would be made 'from one end of the county to the other'.

A Special meeting in June 1865 received the Idiot School Sub-Committee's Report. It first emphasised that the school should work under the Lunacy Acts which empowered magistrates to send idiots to a lunatic asylum unless they could be properly cared for at home, which was usually unlikely. In this case, the expenses of the pauper children would be paid for by the parishes.

The proposed building would cost about £3,000. It would include workshops, where boys could acquire a useful trade, and a wash-house and kitchen where girls could learn to wash and cook. A playground and kitchen garden should also be included. As no convenient ground was available on the Asylum's estate, the Corporation of Northampton should be asked to provide land which they owned adjoining the Asylum.

From a purely economic point of view the School should be a great success. 'At the present time there are 200 Adult Idiots chargeable to the Union rates at a probable cost of from £2,000 to £3,000 per annum; but if the children of this class could be systematically taught useful and good habits in the manner contemplated, there are abundant reasons to hope that the Adult Pauper Idiots might be, if not entirely eradicated, reduced to a very low number indeed'.

This scheme however never came to fruition. There were no further meetings until 1868. In January of that year it was decided to ask if the Commissioners in Lunacy would vote a sum of money for the proposed building, while leaving the management of the proposed school to the Directors of the Asylum. In the meanwhile, according to that year's Annual Report, an experiment took place in the separate and systematic treatment of idiot children then in the Asylum. It had previously been the custom to treat idiot children as ordinary patients. Now seven children were placed in a large room, fitted up as a nursery, under the charge of a nurse. In each case, a great improvement in behaviour, including cleanliness, was soon achieved.

The scheme had to be abandoned in 1869 because the room was needed for other purposes and the children reverted to their former behaviour. Finally, according to the Management Committee's 1874 Report, 'the Directors took the matter into mature consideration and came to the conclusion that an institution of that kind would be most detrimental if formed in close contiguity with lunatics and therefore decided not to take part in any arrangements for such amalgamation'. Those who had subscribed were asked what they wished done with their donation; as a result £700 was invested to establish, when funds warranted it, a quite

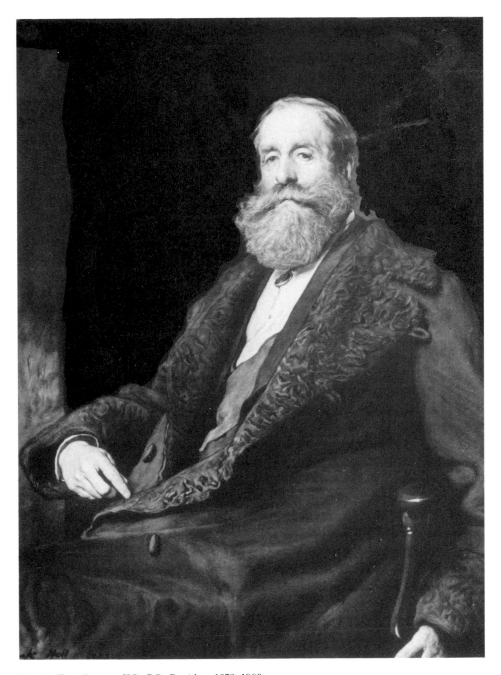

The 5th Earl Spencer, KG, PC, President 1872–1908.

separate Idiot Institution, divorced from the Asylum.

The Sub-Committee is recorded as having met on two further occasions. In May 1889 it was decided to defer the question of the Idiot School Fund, valued at £947.7s.9d. for the time being. The last meeting was held in March 1920 when it was decided to transfer this fund – then worth approximately £2,315 – temporarily to the Hospital's Reserve and Endowment Fund.

Chapter Nine

JOSEPH BAYLEY (1876–1912)

ST ANDREW'S FIRMLY ESTABLISHED

The remaining thirty-six years of Joseph Bayley's superintendency, after the departure of the last pauper lunatics in September 1876, saw both expansion and consolidation – expansion in accommodation for the patients and consolidation in the standards of care and comfort provided. Throughout this period, Dr Bayley remained in benign but complete control. Only on one occasion was his authority seriously challenged. In January 1885, a Special Meeting was called in accordance with Rule 25 at the Superintendent's request 'to inquire into circumstances which affected the discipline of the Hospital'. Bayley then explained that Godfrey, the Secretary, had informed him that the Housekeeper, Ann Collier, had called his attention to allegations reflecting on the Superintendent's conduct, a matter of the greatest importance both to the Hospital and himself.

The Committee, consisting of the Revs Wales, G. S. Howard Vyse, H. Crawley and of Dr Barr with the Rev Maze W. Gregory in the chair, spent over four hours in examining the case in detail. At the end of their investigation, they unanimously concluded that the female side of the Hospital was in a very unsatisfactory state, owing to quarrellings and jealousy among the staff, and that this situation stemmed from the conduct of the Housekeeper and her sister, both of whom had been frequently reprimanded by the Superintendent for dereliction of duty. They found that Ann Collier had stirred up dissension and raked up charges with the avowed intention of getting rid of the Superintendent. Accordingly, both women were dismissed with a month's wages in lieu of notice.

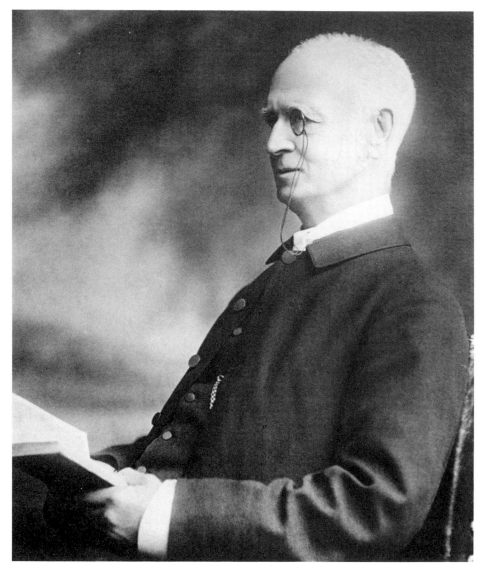

The Rev. Maze W. Gregory, Vice-Chairman 1879–93.

In 1878, now that only private patients were being catered for, two notable decisions were taken. The first was to change the name of the Institution from that of the Northampton General Lunatic Asylum to St Andrew's Hospital for Mental Diseases, the new name to become operative from the beginning of 1879; this was to avoid confusion with the new Northampton County Lunatic Asylum, now established at Berry Wood.

The second, taken in October, was to purchase the Moulton Park Estate, some two miles to the north of the Hospital, consisting altogether of 453 acres, including a farm of 410 acres, together with a modest-sized country house.

A Sub-Committee on Investment, which had met in mid September with the Duke of Grafton in the chair, asked for a Special Court after the next committee meeting 'to consider the propriety of purchasing land'. At this Special Court on 26 September with the Duke of Grafton again presiding, it was decided by four votes to three to bid up to £30,000 for the estate; it was acquired for this sum, plus £600 for timber and fixtures. A reason for this purchase was to provide the Hospital with a suitable site should it ever become necessary to move St Andrew's from the Billing Road; it might also be the place for a convalescent home or an isolation ward. Lord Charles FitzRoy, later the 7th Duke of Grafton, was one of those who voted against this proposition and later withdrew from membership of the Moulton Park Committee; he had favoured the suggestion that part of the new estate should be sold so that the Hospital's charitable funds should not be drawn upon nor the Institution saddled with a heavy debt.

Lord Charles FitzRoy's sentiments were shared by other members of the Management Committee. At a Special Court, held in January 1879, the Rev. Maze Gregory, who served as a very active Vice-Chairman from then until 1893, proposed that the estate be resold. In this he was supported by the 5th Earl Spencer, Lord-Lieutenant of the County, who was to serve in Gladstone's second, third and fourth administrations; he thought £30,000 a very large outlay for a possible convalescent home if there was no immediate plan for removing St Andrew's from its current site. This motion was lost by six votes to five.

The debate on how best to utilize the Moulton Park Estate continued through most of 1879. It was decided in March to consult a land agent both on the advisability or otherwise of selling some 150 acres and to arrive at a fair rent for the farm. The agent, Mr Edward K. Fisher, reported back a week later that:

> The Estate has features, which for the purpose of a large institution, it would be difficult to equal. It is in a ring fence and it is so compact as to be complete in itself – it has also the advantage of being a Parish in itself, which is an important consideration, situated as this property is with a perfect independence as to water supply and drainage. It is also a situation as to which privacy is combined with a convenient proximity to Northampton . . . I should strongly advise the Committee to hold the Estate as purchased, and by judicious planting to prepare it for the

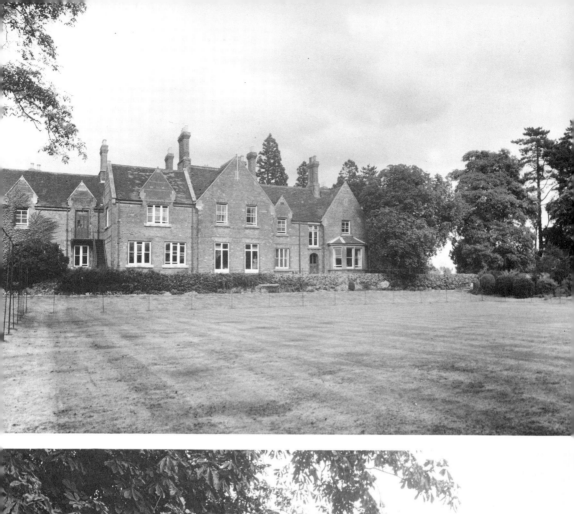

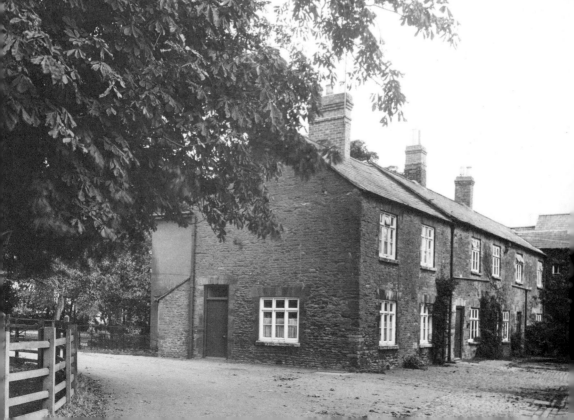

purposes they have eventually in view and for which there is within my knowledge no situation to equal it in the County.

As for rent, the Committee was advised, in view of then current agricultural depression, to meet Mr Hill, the tenant, 'in a somewhat liberal spirit' and to offer him the farm for £710 per annum; the rent was finally fixed at £650 with a lease for two years.

It was accordingly decided to sell no part of the estate for the time being and to ask the Superintendent to submit a report on how best the house could be utilized, supported by facts and figures, after consulting the Commissioners in Lunacy on using it as a convalescent home. In April, it was resolved on a proposal by Lord Spencer, seconded by Lord Charles FitzRoy, that the Committee should take no measures about adapting the estate for hospital purposes, beyond utilizing the farm, until the necessary funds became available.

At the October 1879 monthly meeting, the Superintendent recommended that a few chronic patients be moved from St Andrew's to Moulton Park House to make more room at the former for acute cases, several of which he had recently been compelled to turn away for lack of space. In the previous August, he had informed the Committee that a large proportion of the cases in the Hospital were incurable but at the same time not fit to be out of an asylum. Many might be kept in a hospital for chronic cases with a much smaller and less experienced staff, if such an institution existed. He was, therefore, asked to prepare and have printed for circulation to the Directors a detailed proposal showing how Moulton Park House could be used and what would be involved financially. This was done and considered by a Special Court held in the following month.

Patients were now divided into two classes, according to what they could afford. The plan showed that eighteen quiet and chronic cases of the second class could be given good accommodation at Moulton Park together with beds for five attendants. There would also be room for a first-class patient in the gardener's cottage. It was therefore decided to spend up to £600 on furnishings for the house up to second-class standard. The Superintendent recommended that the post of Housekeeper and Ladies' Companion at Moulton Park be offered to Mrs Grant, the Matron, who had been ill since that July and who had written to say that she very much doubted whether she would be able to fulfil 'the excessive duties which have devolved upon

ABOVE LEFT: *The ladies' house, Moulton Park Farm.*

LEFT: *The Lodge, Moulton Park Farm.*

me for the last few years'. As a result, the post of Matron at St Andrew's was replaced by a Housekeeper, responsible for supervising the kitchen and the laundry, and by a Ladies' Companion for the second-class female patients in addition to the Companion for the first-class female patients already appointed.

By 1880, the debt on the Moulton Park Estate had been completely paid off and a start made on adapting the buildings for hospital use. Eighteen 'chronic ladies' were installed in the house and the Commissioners in Lunacy, who now regularly visited the estate as part of the Hospital, reported on 31 May that 'we saw the ladies at Moulton Park for the most part sitting in the garden watching a cricket match between the Officers of the Militia and listening to the Band'.

In 1882, it was decided to convert the Moulton Park farmhouse into a residence for second-class male patients, who could help in the farm work. A further house was fitted up in 1884 as a residence for four male patients in the care of a married couple and an attendant. An important addition, made in 1886, was the erection of a building for patients with infectious diseases, should any arise in the Hospital. In 1891, however, this was turned over to patients working on the farm and the isolation ward transferred to the house on the forty acres of land to the east of St Andrew's, acquired in 1887 from Lord Wantage, of which Mr Perkins had been the tenant for many years. A high price of £400 per acre was paid, plus £1,200 for the house, excluding the glass-houses, but the Committee was confident that the debt would quickly be paid off. There was a danger that these forty acres would otherwise be used for building development.

By 1895, further additions and improvements had been carried out at Moulton Park. In March of that year, seventeen and half acres of land were purchased from Lord Wantage to join the farm buildings to the Kettering Road and a new villa for up to six male patients built on the road to Boughton Green. There were further additions between 1897 and 1911 when a chapel was erected.

The farm was tackled with similar vigour. In 1881 it was taken over by the Directors from the tenant and a farm bailiff appointed. Considerable expense was involved in renovating the farm buildings and in stocking the farm. By 1882, shelter had been erected for some fifty cows, together with a new dairy, a dairyman's cottage and extensive piggeries. A large orchard and a kitchen-garden of nearly twenty acres were also laid out, as a result of which the land at St Andrew's, previously used as farm and garden, was put down to grass for use not only as grazing land but also for football and cricket. In 1883, Dr Bayley reported that the Moulton Park kitchen-garden was able to supply all the vegetables and fruit required by the Hospital.

The profitability of the Moulton Park Farm was largely held back by the nationwide agricultural depression. Its losses would have been considerably greater but for the free labour provided by the male patients. In 1892, a Sub-Committee appointed in the previous year, decided 'that it would be a great advantage for the Sub-Committee to have the assistance of a practical farmer'. There were two meetings at Moulton Park that October with a Mr Richard Britten, presumably a practical farmer, and various recommendations made; it was also decided that the primary object of the farm was to provide the Hospital with milk.

It is difficult to assess the effectiveness of the Farm Sub-Committee's efforts as no further reports of its meetings were included in the Minutes after 1893, except that, after a poor year in 1895, the farm finally moved into profit in 1896. A small loss was reported in 1899 but in the following years up to and including 1914, the accounts invariably showed a favourable balance in spite of the failure of the fruit crops in 1903 and 1907. The greatest attention was paid to all aspects of the farm, including the regular inspection of the livestock by a veterinary surgeon.

Great attention was also paid to the development of the main hospital buildings and grounds adjoining the Billing Road. Scarcely a year went by during the last two decades of the nineteenth century without further acquisitions or improvements. The 6th Duke of Grafton announced in 1875 that St Andrew's was the largest hospital of its kind in the country; its steadily increasing income, a proportion of which always went to patients who needed help with fees, on average about 20 per cent of the total, was constantly used to extend its facilities and comforts.

In 1881 work was started on a new kitchen and a storeroom for the Steward. In addition, two good houses and some property in the Cliftonville Avenue area adjoining the Hospital were purchased to provide privacy and additional accommodation. This was also the year in which the elegant stone steps from the carriage drive in front of the main entrance into the Hospital down to the lawns were constructed to the Superintendent's design. The building of the long-desired recreation hall and the new offices for the Secretary were started in 1882. These works were completed by 1885, together with a new entrance to the grounds from the Billing Road. The Superintendent was then able to report that the centre or administrative block of the Hospital had been virtually rebuilt; that the new arrangements of offices, kitchen and stores had added much to the comfort and convenience of the staff and that the recreation hall, in use throughout the previous winter, had been much appreciated by the patients. Great attention was paid to fire precautions.

Utility alone was not the only consideration. Much attention was given to making the accommodation decoratively attractive. Funds were granted in 1885 for providing suitable chimney-pieces, grates and hearth tiles in the Central Drawing Room. Double doors, instead of a single one, were inserted in the main entrance. In 1886, ten stained-glass windows were placed in the new recreational hall.

Queen Victoria's Jubilee in 1887 was commemorated by the embellishment of the chapel under the guidance of J. Oldred Scott, the architect responsible, among other works, for the Greek Orthodox Cathedral in Moscow Road, London. His suggestions aroused the greatest interest. Part of the plan was for a chancel screen and the addition of a stained-glass window at the east end, designed by Messrs Burlison and Grylls. The 4th Marquess of Northampton, who had succeeded the Duke of Grafton as Chairman of the Management Committee after the latter's death in 1882, was invited to take away this design and 'to be good enough to make suggestions thereon which he might deem advisable'. He accordingly consulted, among others, his younger brother, Lord Alwyne Compton, by then Bishop of Ely, and reported back that it was generally thought satisfactory but that Messrs Burlison and Grylls 'should have their attention called to the design representing the casting out of the evil spirits into the swine with the view of substituting some other subject not connected with demoniacal possession'.

It was also unanimously agreed at the 1887 Annual General Court:

> that the Hospital having now been erected fifty years, and having in that time had such success in its beneficent efforts to alleviate Mental Disease that it ranks as the largest Institution of its kind in England; and this year also being the Jubilee Year of the Reign of Her Majesty the Queen: this Annual Court resolves that a humble address be presented to Her Majesty praying Her permission that the Hospital may be in future called and known by the name and style of the 'Royal Hospital of St Andrew Northampton'. And this Court further resolves that their Chairman, the Most Noble the Marquess of Northampton K.G., be requested to present the address through the proper quarter and use his influence in securing the object in view.

No further reference to this matter appears in the records available.

More progress was reported in 1888. New buildings at the Hospital included a detached steam laundry, a new slaughter-house and farm stables. Electric light was introduced into the centre buildings, kitchen, the recreation hall and the offices. A new lodge was built at the Bedford Road entrance to the Estate and the old laundry buildings converted into an

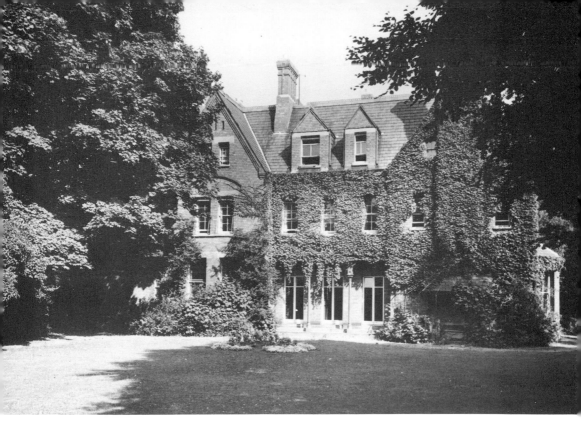

Fernside, a villa in the Hospital grounds, c.1900.

infirmary for females with dormitories above, which provided between forty and fifty more beds plus quiet and comfortable sitting-rooms for the feeble and sick.

Another house, Fernside, adjoining the Hospital, was purchased in 1892 and incorporated into the estate; five male patients were accommodated therein. The Commissioners in Lunacy had for several years been pressing for improved and increased space for male patients and the Management Committee at last felt in a position to respond, not only by this purchase, but by the extensive alterations to the male side which were started in 1893. In spite of a strike by bricklayers' labourers, two-thirds of the work had been completed by the end of 1895, which also saw the erection of the workshops, authorised some years previously, for carpenters, painters and upholsterers, together with buildings for washing, cleaning and drying the horsehair with which the hospital beds were stuffed. The building of an organ chamber in the chapel for the new organ was also carried out.

The alterations and additions to the male side of the Hospital were only completed in 1900; the work had been much delayed by strikes in a period when trade unionism was developing its muscle. By this time, a new boiler-house had been built in which the machinery, boilers and electric light plant were installed, the old engine and boiler-house having been converted into grocery and linen stores for the Steward. The Cedars, a villa on the hospital grounds close to Fernside, had also been converted for the use of patients. A reserve water tank, capable of holding 200,000 gallons of water and connected with a smaller tank in which the suction-pipe of the fire-engine was placed, had been installed by 1896 and proved its worth three years later when a fire broke out in the kitchen.

In 1903, the Committee discussed in detail how to bring the female side up to the same standards as the recently completed male side and, in July of that year, sanctioned the expenditure of £25,700 on building work and £3,588 on heating. In 1907, Bayley was able to state 'the extensive alterations and additions, which have been carried out for many years past to bring this Hospital up to the standard of more modern buildings and to make it suitable for the present requirements for the treatment of the insane, have been completed. The whole of the interior of the Hospital has been altered and re-modelled, and many new buildings have been added to it.' Gone were such prison-like features as iron bars and bare brick walls, the patients' comfort had been greatly increased and the appearance of the grounds much improved, all of which had been paid for out of income. During the remaining years under review, there were only minor alterations and additions at St. Andrews's. A cricket pavilion was erected in 1908 and a garage in 1909. There were slight alterations to the offices to give extra staff room in 1910, while in 1912 the temperature in the engine-house was reduced to enable the engineers to work more efficiently.

As more accommodation became available, the number of patients grew. In 1878, there were 286 patients; by 1912, this figure had reached 430. As already stated, there were two classes: first-class patients paid a minimum of 42s. a week throughout this period, a few very much more, and second-class patients were charged 25s. until 1902 when the payment was increased to 31s.6d.

From 1880 onwards, the Directors were consistently able to report a healthy financial situation. The charitable purposes of the foundation, moreover, were never forgotten. In 1881, the number of patients who received charitable assistance was 84 out of a total of 312; in 1912, the comparable figures were 103 out of 430. These figures varied slightly from year to year but on average those who received help in varying degrees were between 20 and 25 per cent of all patients at any one time. The amount laid out by the Directors for charitable assistance naturally also varied. In 1896, for example, £3,500 was allocated for this purpose, while in 1901 the sum dropped to £2,813, rising to £3,235 in 1906 and £4,302 in

1912. At every monthly meeting, requests for charity were objectively examined, care always being taken to ensure that relief was given where it was most needed.

The Management Committee explained their approach to helping patients financially by quoting, in their 1896 Annual Report, the principles followed by the Governors of the Gloucester Lunatic Asylum:

Patients who are admitted at reduced rates must satisfy three requirements:

1.   They must possess so much education or refinement as would cause them to feel the loss of comfortable surrounds.

2.   They must, from want of means, be unable to pay the ordinary rate.

3.   Their mental condition must be such as to show a reasonable prospect of their recovery.

[The report continued]: It is obvious that (3) is a very necessary precaution in order to prevent the Hospital from becoming blocked with chronic cases, which would not only be a constant drain on the finances, but would also bar the way to the admission of a much larger number of curable cases. In selecting patients paying at reduced rates, preference, all else being equal, is always given to persons connected by birth, residence or otherwise with the County of Northamptonshire, but cases are admitted from all parts of the country.

The devoted attention given by the Management Committee to making St Andrew's as comfortable as possible was rewarded by the increasing number of patients entrusted to their care. In Bayley, they had a Superintendent who translated their benevolence into a practical regime which gained the confidence of both guardians and trustees. From the first, as reported in the previous chapter, he based his hopes for achieving cures on providing his patients with occupations. It proved an uphill struggle. Nevertheless, he persevered with reasonably successful results.

By 1885, there were seventy-nine male patients employed in various pursuits. Sixty-one of these laboured out of doors. In his report for that year, Bayley wrote: 'Eighteen of them live at Moulton Park Farm and are all employed there under the charge of the attendants with whom they live and under the supervision of the Farm Bailiff. The experiment of establishing the small colony of working patients at the farm, which was commenced about two years since, has proved a great success. The patients like the work and always appear to be happy and contented.' Others were occupied in the ornamental gardens at St Andrew's, while a few worked at carpentry, upholstery, printing and similar crafts.

In the following year, he referred to a paper, 'Outdoor work as a Remedial Agent in Insanity', written by Dr Lloyd Francis, the Senior Assistant Medical Officer, in which the system developed was described and in which the atmosphere of the Asylum comes alive. This system

[was] carried out on a more extensive scale in this hospital than in any other of the same type with a completeness indeed which frequently elicits expressions of interest and astonishment from visitors both lay and medical and has more than once been favourably commented upon and held up for imitation by the Lunacy Commissioners.

Putting aside its proved remedial value in the treatment of recent insanity, its effect in raising the standard of physical health, in combating excitement, turbulence and disorder, and lessening the discomforts and annoyance of an asylum patient's life, would fully compensate for the trouble and expense in carrying it out. Nothing illustrates the fact more clearly than the behaviour of the working patients on a week-day and on Sunday; a contrast highly unfavourable to the Day of Rest. Missing the accustomed round of work, incapable of intellectual occupation of any kind, they become restless, noisy, mischievous, destructive, quarrelsome, turning the ward into a bear garden and sorely trying the patience and temper of the attendants.

Still more marked is the difference of the male and female wards of the same class; the inmates of the latter being noisier, more excitable and difficult to manage, to a degree far greater than can be accounted for by the mere difference of sex. At meals, for instance, the male dining-halls are generally a marvel of order and quietude, the female often quite the reverse.

The Commissioners in Lunacy in their June 1885 report made very similar comments.

It is interesting to note that, in the year after the report, Dr Francis's salary was increased from £200 to £250. In January 1892 his request for a further increment was turned down. In 1893 he resigned on being appointed Superintendent of the Earlswood Asylum, Surrey, originally founded for idiots which by 1881 had over 560 inmates.

Dr Bayley always emphasised that, in his opinion, exercise and amusement came next in priority after occupations. The increase in land at

St Andrew's and at Moulton Park made possible the provision of football and cricket pitches, tennis courts and crocquet lawns for patients and staff; archery also became an option. According, however, to the May 1881 report of the Commissioners in Lunacy, not more than twenty male and twelve female patients were able to take part in these exercises. Three carriages were acquired to take patients for drives and, in 1886, Bayley introduced a pack of beagles, costing £20, which were followed on foot by ten to twelve patients; in 1891, the beagles were out on thirty-four occasions but were soon afterwards given up because of the scarcity of hares. Reference was also made to 'hunting parties' up to 1896 and 'to parties to hunt meetings' up to 1901. A few patients actually rode to hounds. Boating, fishing, hockey, skating and swimming are also mentioned on occasion. Walks within the grounds were a normal feature of daily life for those capable of so doing, and a few trusted patients ventured on parole into the town.

Amusements included visits to theatres, concerts, agricultural and horticultural shows and to places of interest in the vicinity. The monotony of the long winter evenings was relieved by theatricals, dances, smoking concerts and such indoor games as snooker. Details of these events were a regular feature of Bayley's Annual Reports. He also re-established in 1879 the custom of selected first-class patients dining regularly with the Hospital Officers. In 1901 he was allowed to hire amateur dramatic societies once a month and was granted £100 to cover railway fares and hotel rooms.

Dr Wing had been the first Superintendent to introduce the annual expedition to various seaside resorts, starting with the visit to Llandudno in 1862. There had been a break in this practice due to Wing's illness and death, but Bayley re-instated these annual excursions in 1868 when a party spent a month at Lowestoft. The Directors, as previously, made a contribution of £150 as they were to do in each subsequent year, in order to help those patients whom the Superintendent considered would benefit from the sea air but who could not afford the holiday unaided. Other resorts visited included Eastbourne and Scarborough. Then in 1887 began the long association of St Andrew's with the North Wales coast when Benarth Hall near Conway was rented. In 1889, the lease on Benarth was renewed for a three-year period and an additional house, Tan-y-Foel, taken. Benarth came to be occupied throughout the year.

So successful was the North Wales enterprise that it was decided in 1896 to give up Benarth Hall and instead to rent the much larger Deudraeth Castle near Portmadoc for five years, as from February 1897. The Commissioners in Lunacy, who visited it in May 1897, described it as 'a handsome modern mansion, in castellated style, pleasantly situated in the midst of beautiful scenery and near the sea. The grounds are very charming, and the house itself is roomy, comfortable and well furnished . . . The lighting is by mineral oil lamps, which are . . . of the safety form, and are extinguished if upset.' There was also a smaller house, Plas Penrhyn, occupied according to the Commissioners by six ladies 'of the more demented class'.

In November 1898, the Management Committee, conscious that the lease on Deudraeth was due to end early in 1902, resolved that a seaside property be purchased when the right opportunity presented itself. This came in 1900 when Bryn-y-Neuadd Hall, with some 180 acres situated close to the railway station at Llanfairfechan, North Wales, came on the market. Standing in its own park with its private entrance close to the

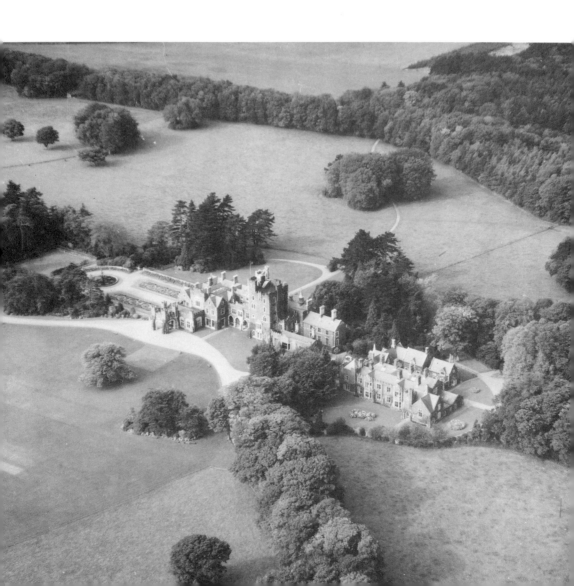

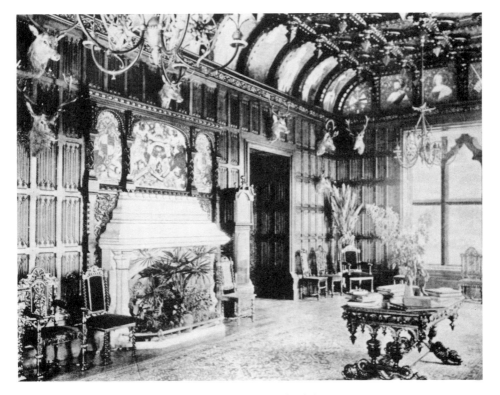

LEFT: *Bryn-y-Neuadd, the Hospital's holiday home near Llanfairfechan.*

ABOVE: *Interior, Bryn-y-Neuadd.*

station, so that patients did not have to be driven through the town, the house contained five large reception rooms, two entrance halls, a billiards room and some thirty bedrooms, with excellent sanitary arrangements and drainage and some central heating. There were, in addition, two lodges and three other small houses in the park, suitable for those requiring special accommodation. Altogether the property was capable of providing room for some forty invalids. A Sub-Committee visited the property and decided to offer up to £40,000. It was acquired for £37,500.

As usual, every attention was given to ensure that the buildings and the estate at Bryn-y-Neuadd were maintained to the highest standards. Electricity, produced in the words of a Lunacy Commissioner 'by pressure of water from the adjacent mountain', was installed in 1904, additional accommodation and a sea-wall built, and in 1907 a Resident Medical

Officer appointed. The sea-wall was extended in 1908 to provide a splendid mile-long promenade. The Annual Report for 1910 noted the construction of twelve additional bedrooms while in 1912 the stables were pulled down and additional accommodation built on the site for the male patients who resided there permanently.

The Commissioners in Lunacy continued to keep a close watch on developments at St Andrew's, Moulton Park and the accommodation in North Wales. The Northampton establishments were regularly visited twice a year by two of their number, one a medical practitioner and the other a barrister, and their findings were published in the Hospital's Annual Report. There was also an annual visit by one of the Commissioners to North Wales, whose report was also reproduced. These reports had to be laid every six months before the Lord Chancellor who also appointed Chancery visitors to examine patients classified as lunatic by inquisition, on occasions when the safe-keeping of an estate was involved. From 1903 onwards, extracts from past reports, in addition to those made in the year under review, were included for promotional purposes at the end of each Annual Report.

The 1890 Lunacy Act had tightened up the procedures leading to the admission of patients. The documents required now included the petition to a judicial authority, two accompanying medical certificates and the order given by the judicial authority. If the case was considered to be one of great emergency, the patient could be received with one medical certificate but the additional papers had to follow within seven days if the patient was to be retained. The purpose of this Act, partly the result of keen public concern originally stirred up by the Alleged Lunatics' Friends Society, that sane people might wrongly be detained as lunatics, was to ensure that every reasonable precaution was taken to avoid this. A disadvantage, foreseen by Lord Shaftesbury, who had died in 1885 while the state of the lunacy laws was being debated, was that delays in obtaining legal sanction to commit someone afflicted with insanity to an asylum could endanger recovery.

Newly admitted patients were always examined by two Directors, who were also magistrates, to decide whether they were being rightly detained. The new Lunacy Act made one minor change in the procedures of the Management Committee. Before 1890, it had been customary for letters from patients to persons in authority to be vetted at the monthly meetings and not sent if they were likely to cause a nuisance. It was not unknown for a patient to write several letters a day to some well-known personality such as the Prime Minister. From 1890 onwards, such letters were no longer read at committee meetings but forwarded unopened. The Commissioners had powers to direct that notices explaining this situation should be placed in asylums.

The reports of the Lunacy Commissioners were scarcely altered, if at all, by the requirements of the 1890 Lunacy Act. They continued to record the numbers admitted, discharged and died, plus the payments actually made by patients; in 1880 they reported three who were admitted free and, at the other end of the scale, four who paid £350 per annum, one £500 and one £1,000. They discussed the numbers and adequacy of the staff, the illnesses and accidents of the patients together with details, when they occurred, of suicides, restraint, seclusion and on one occasion (1888) wet-packing. Suicides were rare although, in their April 1894 report, they noted that seventeen patients were believed to have a suicidal disposition and pointed out that the instructions in writing for the constant supervision of these cases could be improved; action was duly taken. Restraint by instruments and appliances was only used, as laid down by the Act, to allow for medical or surgical treatment or to prevent self-inflicted injuries.

Bayley explained in his 1895 report that restraint had to have his sanction and that a special atttendant was put on duty to watch the patient concerned at all times. The methods used were the fastening of hands behind the back with padded straps; if in bed, the patient was fastened to the bedstead with bandages while allowing the body some movement. He quoted cases when restraint had been necessary. Two patients had tried to put out their eyes with their fingers. Another, who had received a scalp wound, persisted in tearing off the bandages. A fourth had attempted suicide by stabbing himself in the abdomen with the steel spring of his truss. Because he persisted in tearing off the bandages, he was restrained in bed until the wound had healed, a period of 614 hours.

The Commissioners also commented upon the appearance of the patients, whether they were calm or excited, whether or not there had been any illnesses and the quality of the food. In 1883, for example, they considered the dinner service to be 'substantially good, but the tables might be made more ornamental by the introduction of flowers'. In 1896, they suggested 'a better supply of books and periodicals for No. 3 Female Ward and greater attention to the table appointments and service of meals in the dining hall'. They were eager to point out when improvements in furnishings, decorations, lighting and heating might contribute to the greater comfort of the patients. In 1904, for example, some electric light bulbs were considered too weak. In 1907, they suggested that the pads in one of the padded rooms were too hard and should be replaced by some of a more modern style. They also recommended that garments of exceptionally strong material be provided for two female patients in seclusion who insisted on tearing off their clothes. Perhaps more important, in 1909 they considered that the system of dividing the patients into two classes, depending upon payment, was objectionable and recommended classification by disorders only.

The Commissioners constantly warned the Hospital during this period against the dangers of retaining too many chronic patients whose life-span must often have been extended by its good food and kindly environment. Bayley himself was always conscious of this danger. As early as 1881, when arguing the case for transferring chronic patients to Moulton Park, he pointed out that St Andrew's might 'soon become an Asylum for chronic lunatics, instead of a Hospital for the reception and treatment of acute and curable cases of brain disease'.

Overall, adverse criticism by the Commissioners was rare and they frequently congratulated the Directors on the consistently high standards of their Institution and the efficiency of their Superintendent and staff. They were enthusiastic about the care provided for the upper and middle classes and especially about the charitable help, occasionally suggesting that this help might be increased. They obviously approved of the additions to the buildings as they occurred and encouraged the Directors to make further improvements. In 1897 they reported the large number of patients who expressed gratitude at the treatment they received. They were alert to the need for an efficient fire-precaution service. They took great interest in the occupational and recreational side of the Hospital's activities, applauded the Hospital's efforts to stimulate recovery, and were always ready to offer advice of a helpful nature. When in 1895 they found that one of the Lord Chancellor's visitors had seen an inmate, who was not a Chancery patient, and had suggested to his friends that he be removed elsewhere, they were quick to point out that this patient was quite unfit to leave the Hospital and that they did not think it would be to his advantage to leave the comfortable quarters in which he found himself.

Who, after the departure of the paupers, were the patients of St Andrew's? Throughout these years and for many afterwards, it was customary to include in the Annual Report a table showing 'the previous Position or Occupation of the Admissions' during the year under review. Table *xi* for 1901, which is typical, gave the following details:

MALES

Army Officers	3	Brass Founder	1
Art Decorator	1	Brewery Pupil	1
Barrister	1	Brewery Agent	1

Builder	1	*FEMALES*	
Civil Engineer	1		
Clergyman	1	Army Officer's daughter	1
Clerk (Gov.)	1	Auctioneer's wife	1
Clicker	1	Book-Keeper	1
Corn Merchant	1	Builder's daughter	1
Drapers	2	Commission Agent's wife	1
Electric Engineer	1	Cook	1
Farmers	6	Earl's daughter	1
Gentlemen	6	Farmer's wives	3
Graduate	1	Gardener's wife	1
Grazier	1	Governesses	2
Grocer	1	Manufacturer's wife	1
Journalist	1	Minister's wife	1
Land Agent	1	Nurses	3
Manager (Textile)	1	Tradesmen's wives	2
Medical Practitioner	1	Tradesmen's daughters	4
Paper Factor	1	Travellers' wives	2
Restaurant Keeper	1		
Solicitor	1	*VARIOUS*	
Student	1		
Telegraph Engineer (Gov.)	1	Married	7
		Single	24
Persons	41	Widowed	5
		Persons	62

No doubt such lists gave confidence to relatives that mental illness was an affliction suffered by all social groups and that those committed to St Andrew's would be likely to find some patients with broadly simiar backgrounds. This table was omitted from the Annual Reports after 1939.

Another table, Table X, showed 'the probable cause, apparent or assigned, of the disease in the admissions, discharges and deaths'. This was included in the Annual Reports up to 1907; from 1908 until 1940, it was given a more elaborate form and headed 'Aetiological', but did not include discharges and deaths. During the earlier period, causes were differentiated under the headings 'Moral' and 'Physical'. Amongst the causes given under the first heading were 'anxiety, trouble, disappointment in love, fright, jealousy, pecuniary difficulties, religion, novel-reading and spiritualism'; those listed under the second heading included 'apoplexy, brain disease, change of life, drink, fall from horse, heart disease, hereditary, injury to head, masturbation, old age, over-study, over-work, self-indulgence, sunstroke, syphilis and unknown'. This table, like Table XI, may have been included to indicate the wide range of conditions with which the hospital was able to deal.

A broad indication of the percentage of cures achieved during Bayley's superintendency may be gathered from the following table:

Year	Total number of patients under treatment	No. of admissions in year	No. of patients recovered	% of admissions cured	% cured of all those under treatment
1878	394	112	55	48	14
1888	379	48	19	38	5
1898	448	86	26	33	6
1908	485	70	23	53	5

These figures are not intended to show a trend nor are they a reflection on the efficiency of the Hospital. The basic treatment was to provide a comfortable, relaxed atmosphere, involving employment, exercise, entertainment and good food with the hope that patients would recover in these friendly, helpful surroundings. What is perhaps significant is that those who recovered were almost invariably patients who had been admitted to the Hospital within the year.

That it was considered that more could not be done is perhaps indicated by the size of the medical staff. In 1878, Dr Bayley had one Assistant Medical Officer. In 1886 a Clinical Assistant was appointed, his title being changed to that of Junior Assistant Medical Officer in the following year. In 1889, the Commissioners gave their opinion that 'if more patients are received here, we think that another Assistant Medical Officer is absolutely needed'. A third Assistant Medical Officer was not however appointed, presumably on the Superintendent's recommendation, until 1904, by which time the total number of patients under treatment had increased from 381 to 482. There was no criticism at any time by the Commissioners that there was an insufficiency of nurses or attendants.

The continuing complaint by the Commissioners that the Hospital housed too many chronic patients resulted in many of these, whose condition had deteriorated to such an extent that they were barely aware of their surroundings, being discharged. Nevertheless, the Hospital was in practice, far more a home for incurables than a place for cures. It is argued by some that the role of the mental hospital became one of acting as a warehouse for the useless, the intolerable and potentially troublesome, especially when earlier hopes that the newly established asylums and mental hospitals would be effective in curing the majority of the mentally ill had been proved misplaced. That the Commissioners became progressively less optimistic, may be seen from the tenor of their reports. There were times when they seemed surprised to find patients who were apparently on their way back to sanity. In their second report for 1910, for example, they found that 'two gentlemen and three ladies show signs of mental improvement'. Nevertheless, the Hospital must have helped restore the mental balance of some patients by taking them away from family backgrounds in which their presence had caused intolerable strains.

There were on occasion changes of policy regarding the types of afflicted taken in by the Hospital. In 1882, the Commissioners noted that epileptics were no longer accepted. Ten years later, however, four patients were reported as epileptics and epilepsy was classified in the Aetiological Table as one of the diseases of the nervous system.

Dr Lloyd Francis's paper, mentioned above, advocated outdoor work to help treat patients with violent, noisy temperaments. There is no indication in the Superintendent's reports of how these were kept under control if unresponsive to occupation, exercise and amusement. In their reports for November 1887, February 1891 and July 1892, the Commissioners referred to sedatives being taken by patients; it is to be assumed that their use was standard practice.

Seclusion was employed throughout Dr Bayley's superintendency. From the details noted by the Commissioners, the number of patients subjected to this treatment appears to have increased during the first decade of this century, but this may merely reflect the steady growth in the number of inmates. With so small a medical staff, not much individual attention could have been given to the widely varying afflictions of the inmates, many of which were apparently physical as distinct from moral or psychological.

Another factor which must have influenced the number of cures achieved, was the calibre of the attendants. There was a considerable turnover of staff, due partly, perhaps, to the low wages generally paid to this type of employee and partly to lack of training. While staff had occasionally served in similar institutions, the majority appear to have had no previous experience, nor is there any indication of staff-training schemes; a significant proportion of staff must therefore have proved unsuitable. Discipline was strict. Any attendant found in any way ill-treating a patient was immediately suspended and almost invariably dismissed when his case was reviewed by the Management Committee. The attendant could also be prosecuted in the Magistrates' Court and fined. By contrast, in 1888, an attendant and his wife, discharged from Moulton Park, brought an action in court against the Superintendent for wrongful dismissal but were unsuccessful.

If an attendant was found to have been negligent when a patient escaped, he would be made to pay part of the sum involved in apprehending and returning the patient to the Hospital. The 1890 Lunacy Act laid down that, if an escaping patient was not recaptured within fourteen days, he could not be brought back unless fresh proceedings for certification were completed. On the rare occasions when this happened, the Management Committee usually allowed the case to lapse.

Up to and including 1906, a return of the number of officers, attendants and servants, with their salaries, wages and emoluments was published in the Annual Report. From a comparison of the table for 1878 with that for 1906, it can be seen that, with the possible exception of the Chaplain, the senior staff and those with specialist skills gained considerably. The Medical Superintendent's salary rose from £1,000 to £2,000 and that of the Assistant Medical Officer, later the most senior of three, from £200 to £500. At one stage, in 1898, it was discovered that the salaries of the Assistant Medical Officers were below average and they were accordingly adjusted upwards. The Chaplain's salary however was only £310 in 1906 as compared with £280 in 1878.

The wages of the lower grades of male staff however showed little change. Those of the most senior attendants remained constant at £45 per annum, while the lowest paid received £24 in the earlier and £25 in the later year, when there were also four junior attendants at £16 per annum. Nurses did rather better: the Chief Nurse earned £40 in 1878 and £70 in 1906, while the highest paid ordinary nurse received £22 in the earlier year and £40 in the later. Throughout, a firm hand was evident. A servant receiving a gratuity or commission from a tradesman was liable to instant dismissal.

In 1889, the Coachman's wages were increased from 22s. to 25s. a week 'but he must strictly understand that he will be entitled to no provision in case of incapacity to follow his duties'. Employees were expected to take out insurance against sickness; on that condition, the wages of attendants who were ill were made up to the full amount, part of the money coming from their 'club'. In 1899, all staff and their families had to be vaccinated; seven refused to comply and were forced to resign. In 1912, Mr Stops, the solicitor, was instructed to find out the position of the Hospital's employees under the National Health Insurance Act, as the benefits they were

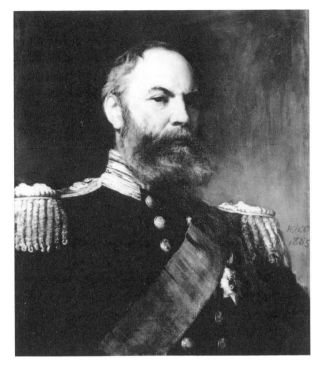

Admiral The 4th Marquess of Northampton KG, Chairman 1882–97.

receiving during sickness were thought to be greater than those proposed by the Act.

Pensions or payments on leaving the Hospital's employment were not automatically given. A house carpenter, leaving presumably on retirement after twenty years' service, asked for a gratuity and received £10. A mason received a pension of 15s. a week in 1893 after forty years' service. Overall the impression gained is that the Directors, always guided by the Superintendent, treated the staff fairly according to the standards of the day. In 1897, a Miss Chapman, aged forty, Chief Nurse at St Andrew's for fifteen years was granted a pension of £100 a year when forced to retire through ill health, as a result of having been kicked by a patient. In July 1899, the Chief Attendant was forced to resign after twenty-one years' service as a result of alleged grave misconduct – details unknown – while on holiday; in the following month the Committee accepted the Superintendent's recommendation that the man be appointed the official in charge of Deudraeth Castle at £100 a year, a reduction of £25. Widows of long-serving attendants were often granted a small weekly payment for one year; an attendant's wife, widowed by her husband's death in the South African War in 1900, was granted 3s. a week for five months. On one occasion, in 1909, an attendant at Bryn-y-Neuadd, who had undergone an operation for a rupture which arose while working in the Hospital, was refused compensation and took the Hospital to court when he was awarded £50 damages plus costs – perhaps a unique occurrence.

During these years there were inevitably changes in the membership of the Management Committee. The 6th Duke of Grafton, who succeeded William Smyth as Chairman in 1870, regularly attended meetings until 1882, when he died in harness. His widow donated £1,000 to the Hospital in his memory. His successor was the 4th Marquis of Northampton, then aged sixty-three. His attendance at meetings was infrequent, and his place was usually taken by the Rev. Maze W. Gregory, the Vice-Chairman, who held this office until 1893 when he felt compelled to resign and was made a Vice-President; he nevertheless continued to attend Management committee meetings almost up to his death in 1905. He was succeeded as Vice-Chairman by Mr Christopher Smyth who in turn became Chairman in 1897 on the death of Lord Northampton; he was to hold this position until 1932. Lieutenant-Colonel J. Rawlins was at the same time elected Vice-Chairman and remained so until 1917.

The main reason for Gregory's resignation as Vice-Chairman was the reawakening of the vexed question of linking St Andrew's with the county asylum. In 1894 the Visiting Committee of Berry Wood Asylum actually instructed solicitors to prepare and lay a case before Counsel. The Commissioners in Lunacy did not approve of this.

> We hear that the County Council [they reported in October 1894], has renewed efforts to wrest the Hospital from the governing body, and to combine its management with that of the County Asylum. Success on part of the Council would, we believe, be disastrous to the prosperity of the charity . . . It must not be forgotten that this Hospital, though founded for lunatics of all classes, was founded when there was no compulsory legal provision for paupers; and that the ratepayers should not be the objects of this charity, but those for whom there is no sufficient provision in this country, viz, the lunatic class, just above pauperism.

This was a very different attitude to that adopted a quarter of a century earlier.

The Management Committee appeared unwilling to meet the Berry

Wood Committee, but a Sub-Committee was eventually appointed for this purpose after a letter had been received from Lord Spencer, the Lord-Lieutenant, who wrote: 'I desire very strongly that some arrangement should be voluntarily made with the County Council for co-operation in regard to County or Borough Patients who come under the supervision of the County Lunatic Asylum and who would be fit objects for treatment and consideration at St Andrew's'.

It emerged at a meeting in December 1896, that there were some twenty inmates at Berry Wood, some private, some pauper, who would be better placed at St Andrew's, which should be asked to accept them *en masse* and on lower terms than the minimum rate. The impossibility of doing this was explained, partly because it would be against the provisions of the 1890 Lunacy Act, partly because some of these patients were chronic and their acceptance by St Andrew's therefore against the recommendations of the Lunacy Commissioners, and partly because there were not the vacancies.

It was eventually resolved, 'That the Visitors of Berry Wood be invited to send in, through the relatives, applications for the admission to St Andrew's Hospital of Patients now at Berry Wood: and that the cases be considered on their merits; and those which the Committee are able to accept shall be received at rates below the present minimum charges as vacancies occur'. This resolution was accepted in 1897 and a letter sent that July to the relatives concerned from Northampton County Hall, telling them that they could apply to St Andrew's if they wished. There the matter ended.

In April 1906, John Godfrey, who had been appointed Secretary and House Steward in April 1858, tendered his resignation after over forty-eight years' continuous service. He was then in his seventy-fifth year. His letter to the Chairman ended: 'I venture to add that at the time of my appointment, the income of the Hospital was £13,019.2s.6d. and it is now £66,929.8s.3d., whilst the capital account has increased in the same period from £44,493.2s.7d. to £373,573.0s.8d.; thus showing the wonderful progress of this great hospital'. He was voted the maximum pension of £466.13s.4d. per annum but died within three months: the law regarding pensions did not allow a continuing payment to his widow.

As a result of a recommendation by the Superintendent, it was decided that the Secretary's work should in future be undertaken by two officials; one was to be termed 'Medical Superintendent's Clerk and Clerk for Statutory Work' and the other 'Financial Clerk and Accountant', titles subsequently abbreviated to Clerk and Accountant respectively. In July 1906, E. E. Caesar received the former appointment at a starting salary of £250 and J. Walker became Accountant at £350. William Arkell, the

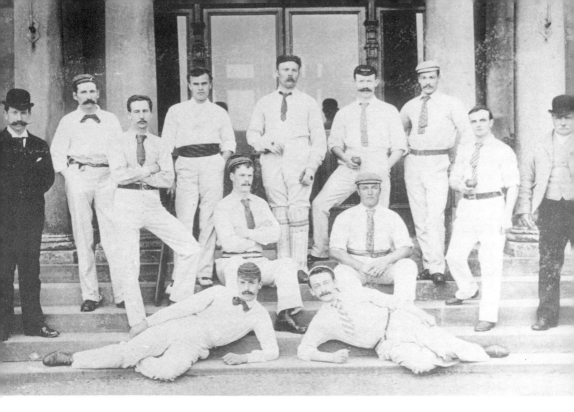

St Andrew's cricket team, 1894.

Steward, who had served the Institution for just on forty years, also retired that spring and was replaced by H. W. Clarke at a salary of £250. The Rev. John Cunningham, Chaplain since 1875, retired on maximum pension in 1911 and was succeeded by the Rev. E. J. Whittall with a salary of £310.

There were various changes in the way the Management Committee organised its work. In 1886, all matters, previously discussed separately by the various committees, were now covered by the monthly Management Committee meetings. By this time, the following method of decision taking had been adopted. The Committee made its recommendation to the next Court, still held four times a year. If the Court approved, it remained for the succeeding Court to confirm the decision. Except when a Special Court was held for the purpose, it normally took at least three months before a recommendation by the Management Committee could be put into action.

By now the original way of becoming a Governor, which was by subscribing £20 or more to the Hospital, had been replaced by election. This gave the Court the opportunity of doing honour to a prominent or popular personality by inviting him to become a Governor, the number of whom was not to exceed seventy.

The last thirty years of Bayley's superintendency were calm compared with his early years and those of his predecessors. Only an occasional cloud shadowed the Institution. In 1883, the Surveyor of Taxes, on behalf of Somerset House, asked for copies of the Hospital's rules, the Committee's reports for the previous four years and details of any interest payable annually by the Committee. The Secretary was instructed to reply that, in the Committee's opinion, the Hospital was not liable for income tax. For this reason, they could not furnish copies of the Annual Reports, but were glad to send a copy of the rules as this showed the principles on which the Hospital was supported and managed. The only interest paid was on bank overdrafts. This did not satisfy the tax authorities and Mr Hensman, the Hospital's legal adviser, was briefed to fight the Hospital's case.

In their second report for 1885, the Commissioners in Lunacy supported St Andrew's:

We learn [they reported], that this Hospital, which is clearly a charitable Institution, receiving as it does many patients gratuitously, and many more at less than their cost, has recently been called upon to pay Income Tax. As the question is about to be argued, it would be out of place to say more than that we shall regret extremely if the building operations be hindered, the comforts of the patients curtailed, or the recipients of the charity lessened, by any diminution of the money hitherto available for the Hospital expenses.

The tax authorities won and in 1887 the judicial decision of the Institution's liability to pay Schedule D income tax was finally accepted.

For several years in the 1890s a stream, known as the Brook which ran through the Hospital's grounds from an adjoining meadow, was foully polluted in the wet season from, it was thought, the local sewage works. The water was unfit for cattle. The Governors complained and the matter was placed in the hands of Messrs Becke and Green, solicitors. The pollution came and went and came again. In October 1898, it was discovered by the borough engineer that the culprit was not the sewage farm but the gut-scraping works of a Mr Bates. Not only was the discharge into the Brook stopped immediately but action taken to remove Mr Bates's activities from the vicinity.

The Hospital gave generously to charities both in the county and borough of Northampton and, after the acquisition of Bryn-y-Neuadd, in Llanfairfechan and neighbourhood. In 1900, handsome donations were made to various funds for those serving in the South African War. At the end of the war, £500 was given, but only after much debate, to the Northamptonshire Imperial Yeomanry. In 1905, £105 was devoted to a new church in Abington and there were many smaller gifts over the years such as an annual £5.5s.0d. to the Llanfairfechan District Nurses' Association. The Hospital's inmates also benefited when, on the Coronation Day of King Edward VII in May 1902, first-class patients received a glass of champagne and those of the second-class a glass of port.

The Hospital took advantage of advancing technology. A telephone connected the Hospital and the Superintendent's house as early as 1881; further connections were added both at St Andrew's and on the Moulton Park Estate. By 1909, the Superintendent reported that the service between St Andrew's and Moulton Park had been adversely affected by the new electric trams in Northampton and asked permission to rent a 'second wire' to improve it. A duplicate electric plant was installed in 1898 for use in the event of a breakdown. In 1899, a male shorthand typist was appointed in the Clerk's office. The latest fire-fighting equipment was acquired in 1903. In 1912 a new hydraulic lift to connect the bakehouse and the kitchen was installed.

In 1909 the building of a 'motor house' was sanctioned. This followed the decision to purchase a motor vehicle; the model chosen was a Beeston Humber 20 hp, whose cost, including all accessories, was not to exceed £600. This necessitated the employment of a mechanic to act as chauffeur; a wage of about 30s. a week was offered on the understanding that, when not engaged in his own work, he assisted the engineer. The motor was found so useful that a second machine was acquired in May 1912, this time a 30 hp Standard; its price, including accessories, was £750. As a result of its first purchase, the Hospital recorded receiving in January 1911 'An Appeal to every owner of a motor vehicle in Northamptonshire' from the Northamptonshire Territorial Force Association. Its purpose was to try and establish a Civilian Motor Vehicle Organisation in the county 'to aid in case of urgent Military necessity – in defence of the County, as regards transport and supply', as it was 'both the duty and privilege of everyone to help in the defence of the country'. The Hospital replied that it would be willing to lend a motor for one day each year.

One innovation, reported upon at length by the Superintendent in 1904, was the introduction of machinery to make the most economic use of coal. An investigation in 1902 had revealed a great wastage of steam and hot water. Messrs Ashwell and Nesbit Ltd., specialists in this type of engineering, were called in and, as a result, great savings in coal achieved as well as improved heating and ventilation. The role of the Senior

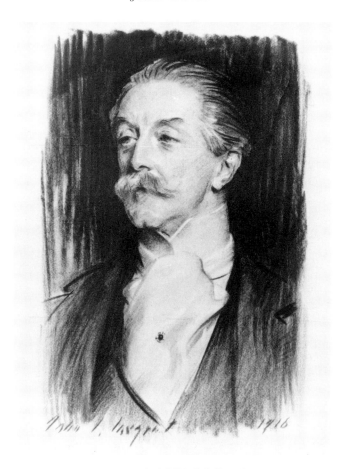

The 6th Earl Spencer, KG, GCVO, PC, President 1908–22.

Assistant Medical Officer was particularly mentioned in this connection. This official was Dr J. H. Bayley, the eldest of the Superintendent's six sons, three of whom died young; there were also four daughters, one of whom was married to Dr Archdall, the Resident Medical Officer at Bryn-y-Neaudd. J. H. Bayley had joined the staff as Second Assistant Medical Officer in September 1892 on the recommendation of the Superintendent, without, apparently, a competitive election. He had been short-listed for the position of Senior Assistant Medical Officer when Dr Lloyd Francis resigned in 1893 but Dr C. W. Ensor had then been chosen. Ensor resigned on account of ill health in 1894, whereupon Bayley succeeded to the post, holding it throughout his father's superintendency. He was to leave the Hospital's service in mysterious circumstances in 1913, perhaps suffering from a severe nervous breakdown. The Superintendent had, on a previous occasion in 1881, successfully recommended his brother as a Gentleman's Companion but he had resigned in the following year through ill health.

Bayley's career as Superintendent of St Andrew's for over forty-seven years from 1865 to 1912 was altogether a remarkable one. The Hospital's high reputation must then have been largely due to his skills as administrator and to his pleasing personality, especially towards those in authority. He seems to have been indefatigable in carrying out his duties. New regulations were produced on his initiative when they seemed necessary, new forms designed, diet tables prepared, plans drawn up for the development of newly acquired buildings and land. No detail was too small for his attention.

His standing with the Lord Chancellor's Visitors and the Commissioners was always excellent. In 1881, according to the Minutes of the March monthly meeting, 'the Medical Superintendent mentioned that one of the Lord Chancellor's Visitors had requested him to take his duties for the month of July and that, with the sanction of the Committee, he proposed to take his holiday in this way, stating that as the tour would be through the North of England he should find it a pleasant change. This was sanctioned'. He was called into discussions in 1886 on the Lunacy Acts Amendment Bill which became the Lunacy Act, 1890. Throughout, he appears to have acted wisely, speedily and decisively.

In August 1906, the monthly Minutes record the unanimous thanks of the Committee to Bayley 'for the handsome additions he has made to the Hospital Chapel: they consist of an altar frontal, jewelled brass cross and flower vases, and were placed in the Chapel in memory of Dr Bayley's three sons who had died young'. In July 1908, he was given a gratuity of £10,000 'in recognition of his invaluable services to the Hospital'. He was then seventy-three.

Bayley continued in the Hospital's service for another four years, paying close attention to all that took place. Every year the reports of the Management Committee praised him warmly and those of the Commissioners noted the efficiency and good order of the three establishments. The Commissioners knew that he would give early attention to any criticism, however unimportant.

It was at Bryn-y-Neuadd that Bayley, then seventy-seven, was taken ill late in 1912 when on a visit of inspection; here he remained until his death on 19 January 1913. The dismay was universal. The Secretary of the Commissioners wrote:

I am directed by the Commissioners in Lunacy to express their very deep regret at the death of Mr Bayley, of whose valuable services to St Andrew's Hospital for so many years they have such a warm appreciation. At their numerous visits to the Hospital they were invariably impressed by the accuracy and extent of his knowledge of the patients and of all the details of administration of the Hospital, and it is unnecessary to say that they have always fully recognised the enormous extent to which its progress and development and present high position are mainly due.

The local press was equally complimentary. Both the *Herald* and the *Mercury* praised his keen, far-sighted perception, his shrewdness, great practical organising abilities and decisiveness; both also noted his strictness as a disciplinarian while at the same time rewarding faithful service. The *Herald* commented that 'he may have seemed sometimes a little quick-tempered but at heart he was the best of men'. The *Mercury* reported that under his rule 'from being rather a grim and comfortless building, St Andrew's had grown into a lordly mansion, set in the midst of one of the prettiest parts of the Midlands. Its extensive grounds have been likened to those of Warwick Castle', and often used for local sporting contests. With none of these observations would Dr Bayley have been likely to have disagreed.

Chapter Ten

DR DANIEL RAMBAUT (1913–1937):

NEW HORIZONS, NEW HOPE

D r Bayley died in harness at the age of seventy-seven. To say that
his death was timely is in no way to detract from his outstanding
achievements. He left St Andrew's as one of the largest and most
respected of the thirteen Registered Hospitals of England organised on a
charitable basis. His last years, however, saw an increasing tempo of
change.

The legislation introduced by Asquith's first Cabinet (1908-14) reflected
the need to improve the standards of living and the working conditions of
the labouring classes against a background of rising inflation and the
growing strength of the Trade Unions, which did not leave the Hospital's
staff unaffected. The Trade Boards Act of 1909 was carried by Churchill,
when Home Secretary, to suppress sweated labour, and the National
Insurance Bill of 1911 passed to help protect the working population
against sickness. These years also saw the emergence, especially in Europe,
of much new knowledge about the causes and treatment of insanity, which
a man of Dr Bayley's age might not have been expected to pursue with the
vigour required. In any case, the First World War with all its diversity of
problems was only eighteen months away. The opportunity of appointing a
new Medical Superintendent came at the right time.

Dr Daniel Frederick Rambaut was forty-seven when he was elected to
succeed Dr Bayley in February 1913 at a salary of £1,200 together with
unfurnished residence, free coal, electric light, vegetables and washing.
Descended from a Huguenot family, which had escaped to Dublin early in
the eighteenth century, the new Superintendent was the fifth son of the

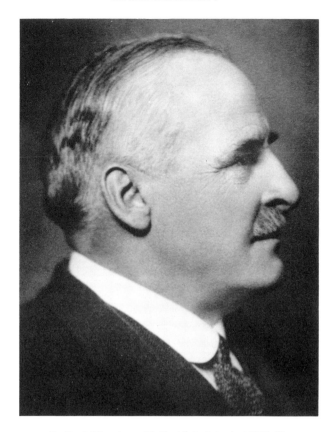

Dr Daniel Rambaut, Medical Superintendent 1913–37.

Rev. Edmund Rambaut, the incumbent of Carysfoot Church, Blackrock, near Dublin. He was educated at the Royal School, Armagh, at Trinity College, Dublin, and at Vienna University. At Trinity, he achieved honours and prizes in logic and mathematics and came first in his final medical examination. He was a rugby international, playing for Ireland in 1887 and 1888. He was also a champion hurdler and a fine cricketer. At the age of fifty-two during the 1914–18 war years, he took up hockey and played in the Hospital's team.

On qualifying, he became Assistant Medical Officer and Pathologist, Bacteriologist and Radiologist at the Grangegorman Mental Hospital, Dublin, where he introduced weaving looms for the purpose of occupational therapy. In 1902 he was appointed Medical Superintendent of the Salop and Montgomeryshire Mental Hospital at Shrewsbury, the post he, like Dr Bayley before him, held when he was elected Superintendent of St Andrew's.

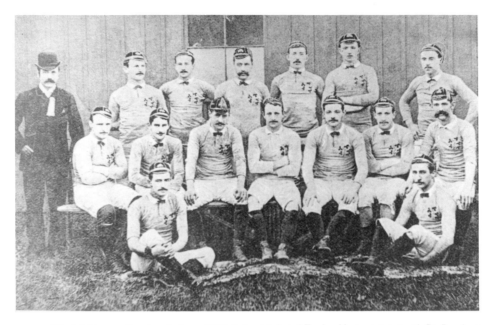

ABOVE: *The Irish international rugby team, 1887. Ireland defeated England by ten points to nil, Dr Rambaut (seated at far left) scoring two conversions.*
TOP RIGHT: *The Hospital cricket team, c.1920, of which Dr Rambaut was an active member.*
BOTTOM RIGHT: *The Hospital hockey team, c. Dr Rambaut, bare-headed, is seated in the front row in both photographs.*

When Rambaut took over, he had Dr S. E. Martin as Senior Assistant Medical Officer and Dr N. R. Phillips as second Assistant Medical Officer, the former earning £600 per annum and the latter £350; both received emoluments in addition. There was later a third Assistant Medical Officer who left the Hospital's service before the end of 1914 and was not replaced.

The first problem facing the new Superintendent was to apply the provisions of the National Health Insurance Act to the staff of the Hospital. Having discussed the matter with the other Registered Hospitals, he recommended that it would be advisable for the Committee to contract out and for the Resident Medical Officers to form an 'Institutional Panel' to treat all staff members living in the Hospital. He advised the Committee 'to undertake to pay full wages until insurance benefit accrues, whereupon a deduction from wages shall be made equal to the money benefit received under the Act, the result being that a sum equal to the full amount of wages will be received in addition to board, lodging, allowances and medical attendance by the Hospital staff. I would suggest that the amount received

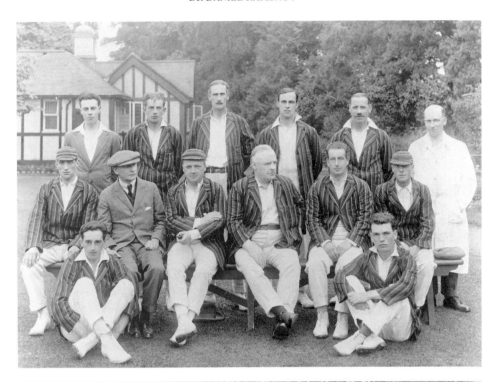

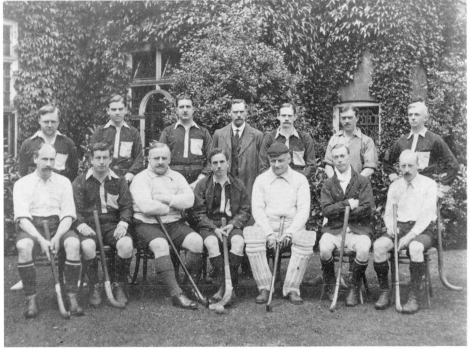

in payment should be divided among the resident medical staff after deducting the cost of drugs and appliances'. Those living outside the Hospital should make their own arrangements with their own doctors, the Coommittee deducting from their wages an amount equal to the money benefit received under the Act. No comment from the National Health Insurance Commission is recorded in the Minutes, so presumably this recommendation was implemented.

More pressing than the question of insurance was the demand for increased wages. At nearly every meeting of the Management Committee in 1913, requests were received for improved pay, many of which were granted by small increments but others 'not entertained', as in the case of the chapel organist. Dr Rambaut obviously gained the Committee's confidence from the start. The artisans employed by the Hospital had asked that March for a weekly half-holiday and the Committee decided to await the new Superintendent's decision, which was given in their favour at his first monthly meeting; their work was to end at 1 p.m. on Saturdays. In the following month, he authorised the reduction of the printing workers' hours to fifty-two weekly. One suspects that many requests might not have been made if Dr Bayley had still been in command.

These requests for improved pay and working conditions culminated in an approach by the attendants to the Management Committee in November 1913, which resulted in a thorough examination of the whole situation by Rambaut. His findings were submitted to the Management Committee in January 1914 in which he stated:

> I have made out a table showing the conditions in seventy-eight other Mental Hospitals and Asylums in England. From this it will be seen that the number of hours of duty at St Andrew's are more than those in any other Mental Hospital or Asylum in England, while their wages are the second lowest. As a result I find it difficult to obtain suitable applicants, and several newly appointed Attendants have left suddenly after a few days' service.

He then made the following recommendations, which throw an interesting light on working conditions before the start of the First World War:

> By an alteration of the hours of the various breakfasts, by the alteration of the hours of Night Attendants and the assisting artizans, and the addition of a few Attendants, I can arrange to give Attendants one additional half day's leave each week, one additional half day's leave each month, and the whole of every third Sunday off duty instead of

every second Sunday half day; Senior Attendants an additional half
day's leave each month and the whole of every third Sunday instead of
every second Sunday half day. I think the Night Attendants, should
have two nights off a month instead of at present one night a month.

Rambaut's recommendations on salaries, spelt out in detail, were aimed at
encouraging attendants to aspire to more responsible posts. He had already
introduced courses of lectures, run by the senior medical staff, on mental
nursing, as sponsored by the Royal Medico-Psychological Association;
these were not interrupted by the Great War. 'To encourage this most
necessary change', he wrote, 'I would ask you to authorise me to give an
annual increase of £1 to those who pass the Preliminary Examination and
£2 to those who obtain Certificates in Mental Nursing in both Male and
Female Departments'. In his 1928 report, Rambaut referred back to this
event: 'It is interesting to see the wonderful change that this training brings
about in the Mental Nurse. The knowledge of anatomy, physiology, and
mental illness and its treatment properly implanted, changed the prison
warder, drill sergeant and policeman type of attendant into the
sympathetic long-suffering skilled and tactful modern Hospital Nurse.'
From 1916 onwards the names of those who had passed the Association's
final examination were given in the Annual Reports. In 1916 there were 16;
in 1937 there were 132.

He did not approve of the system, complained about by the Attendants,
under which many of them slept in the same wards and rooms as the
patients. 'It is dangerous for the patients and unfair to the Attendants who
have been on duty all day. I believe that it should be gradually altered.' He
suggested that a recreation room should be provided for the male nursing
staff. 'Almost all Mental Hospitals and Asylums now have a Recreation
Room for the Attendants. The female staff already have such a room.
When possible a separate Mess Room should be given to the charge
attendants.'

He recommended that the beer allowance to attendants, nurses and
maids be stopped. 'In most English Asylums this allowance has been
discontinued for some time, and compensation in money has been given to
the staff in lieu of beer . . . Many of the young Attendants and Nurses who
come to the Hospital have not been in the habit of drinking beer. I have not
seen any of the staff intoxicated, but I have found several Attendants asleep
and fuddled in the middle of the day, and actively homicidal and suicidal
patients grossly neglected.' His report was adopted *in toto*, the salary
increases taking effect from the beginning of that year. Not all the requests
of the junior staff, however, were accepted. A plea by unmarried attendants

to be paid monthly instead of quarterly was turned down. Discipline, moreover, remained as strict as ever; two attendants, for example, were dismissed in July 1914 for drunkenness and neglect of duty.

So well had Rambaut established himself with the Governors of St Andrew's that his salary was raised in October 1914, only eighteen months after joining the staff, from £1,200 to £1,500, backdated to 1 May. It was further increased to £2,000 in August 1917. The visiting Commissioners of the Board of Control to which, under the Mental Deficiency Act, 1913, the duties of the Commissioners in Lunacy had been transferred, were equally pleased with his appointment and, in the report of their second visit to St Andrew's that year, referred to the 'judicious and thoughtful administration under the superintendence of Dr Rambaut'.

Then came the outbreak of war in August 1914 which was to affect considerably the balance between male and female staff. Rambaut reported late in August that thirteen attendants who were reservists, had been called to the colours. In December, he announced that a further nineteen had volunteered, one of whom had been killed in action. The Committee decided in September to allow those attendants, who had been in its employment before August, 5s. per week while serving with the colours and to guarantee their re-employment if they returned in good health at the end of hostilities. Then, at the end of that year, they resolved that all junior staff called up should be paid their full wages, less their army allowances. This measure was re-affirmed in October 1915.

Senior as well as junior staff were affected by the war, especially Dr S. E. Martin, Senior Assistant Medical Officer, whose salary was raised in January 1915 from £600 to £700 with annual increases of £25 per annum up to a ceiling of £800. That April, he was given permission to take a temporary commission in the RAMC for one year. In May 1916, he was recalled to St Andrew's. In April 1917, the Board of Control requested that both Martin and Phillips, the second Assistant Medical Officer, be allowed to join the RAMC; the Committee decided that Dr Phillips, whose salary was now £400 per annum, could be released from St Andrew's but not Dr Martin. Phillips however was found to be fit only for home service. The names of Martin and Phillips continued to appear as Assistant Medical Officers in the Annual Reports but, in spite of objections by St Andrew's, it appears that in 1918 Martin was again in the RAMC and was demobilised in January 1919 to return to the Hospital. Phillips, who had been granted permission to marry in 1915, was not called up after all.

By 1916, 116 members of the Hospital's staff were serving in the Forces and there were increasing difficulties in getting suitable replacements. That January, compulsory military service had been introduced for single men between eighteen and forty-one: this was extended to married men as well in the following April and the Management Committee drew up its list of those for whom it sought exemption. Female attendants, at the suggestion of the Board of Control, were now being increasingly employed in male wards, thus reviving a practice introduced in 1861 by Dr Wing but later apparently allowed to lapse. In August, the Board of Control was informed that no nurses could be spared to work in Asylum war hospitals.

A letter, dated 29 September 1917, from the Board of Control, which revealed something of the tragedy of war, was considered in October. In it the Board outlined a scheme whereby 'Service patients', those non-commissioned officers and men discharged from war service through being afflicted with insanity, were to be maintained in asylums classified as Private Patients. ' "Service Patients" are maintained by the Ministry of Pensions at a rate but slightly exceeding the current pauper rate in each institution. Those who are dealt with under the scheme are thus relieved of the so-called stigma of pauperism which would have been attached to them had they continued on the footing of pauper patients.'

The letter went on to explain that the Minister of Pensions was now concerned with making arrangements, in many cases permanent, for the care and treatment of officers in more or less straitened circumstances who had been discharged from the services 'on account of insanity, arising from War conditions to which they have been subjected'. The Board of Control hoped that the Registered Hospitals would here be able to help. The Management Committee was accordingly asked to state the maximum number of such patients they would be willing to receive on the understanding that the Minister might be prepared to pay up to £2.2s.0d. a week for the maintenance of each patient. The average weekly cost per patient that year was £3.0s.11d.

The Committee decided to take in ten commissioned officers at two guineas a week, but excluding clothing, wines and spirits, tobacco, washing or a special attendant. They also reserved to themselves the power of having an officer removed, should he become unmanageable, and to consider annually whether or not to retain an officer who did not recover.

Quite apart from staff difficulties, the war inevitably imposed extra work in carrying out the instructions of various wartime officials, such as the Food Controller and the Live Stock Commissioner. Wages rose considerably in line with the cost of supplies, some of which became increasingly difficult to find. The Northamptonshire War Workers' Committee appealed to the Hospital in 1916 for dripping; as none could be spared, a cheque for £5 was sent instead. In March 1917, the Board of Control pressed for the utilization of all available land for growing

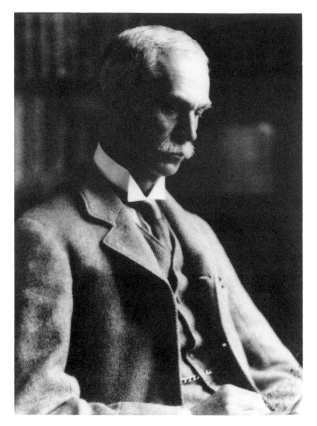

Christopher Smyth, Esq., Vice-Chairman 1893–7, Chairman 1897–1932.

vegetables, to which the Hospital responded by employing over 25 per cent of its male patients for this purpose. The Board's Commissioner after his visit in November 1917, reported that 'the Food Controller's requirements as to bread, meat and sugar are being strictly observed in the amounts issued to the officers, attendants and patients, except so far as the diets for the sick are concerned'; this included the use of potatoes in making bread. In his 1918 report, the Superintendent wrote that 'the restrictions in diet have been borne by both the patients and the staff in a praiseworthy and most patriotic manner'.

Altogether 135 members of the male staff joined the Armed Forces during the war, of whom 13 were killed in action, 3 died of wounds and 2 of illness. A list of their names was included in the 1918 Annual Report. In March 1919, it was agreed in principle that a war memorial in some form should be set up; £20 was also given to the Llanfairfechan war memorial. That May, it was decided that war service should count for staff pensions, including increases made during those years. Twenty-five war savings certificates were also given to each of the 34 who had been members of the staff before 4 August 1914 and who had returned to the Hospital.

Inevitably there were changes on the Management Committee. In February 1917, Colonel Rawlins, who died in the following year, resigned as Vice-Chairman and the Rev. H. H. Crawley was elected in his place. In 1918, Colonel Hill, who had served on the Management Committee from 1907, also died. A patient asked that a letter of condolence be sent on behalf of the patients to his widow. The Duchess of Grafton gave £2,500 five per cent War Stock to the Hospital to maintain a personal friend, to be used afterwards to maintain some poor gentleman.

In spite of wartime difficulties, the new Superintendent did not allow conditions to deteriorate. He strove, supported by the Board of Control, to provide the nursing staff with better accommodation. In 1915, he introduced a scheme whereby patients were encouraged to hire small plots of land on the estate, grow their own produce and sell it to the Hospital at a profit; this proved a great success and was continued for many years. He reported in 1917 that, 'Employment in gardening has had a marked curative effect'. An annual Arts and Crafts Exhibition became a regular feature in the Hospital's calendar. Two qualified masseuses were added to the staff. An improved scale of wages was introduced for the nurses, taking into account their varying responsibilities, and other groups of employees were also given increases as the cost of living rose. When the Berry Wood County Asylum was taken over by the War Office in October 1915, St Andrew's offered to accommodate several private patients at the rates they were then paying, which were considerably below the weekly average cost at the Hospital.

The good relations established by Rambaut with the Commissioners became firmly cemented. In July 1916, the visiting Commissioner reported: 'I feel satisfied that Dr Rambaut and his somewhat depleted staff are exercising all their energies to render the patients comfortable and content'. Like his predecessors, he took seriously any criticism or suggestion the Commissioners might make and was usually successful in following their lead.

Of particular significance for the future of St Andrew's was a statement made in April 1915 by A. H. Trevor, the visiting Commissioner on that occasion. 'I should be glad', he reported, 'to see better facilities provided for the nursing and treatment of recent and acute cases; the absence of verandahs and other means of nursing suitable for patients in the open air, such as are now generally adopted with good results, must add very considerably to the difficulties of the medical and nursing staff . . . I agree with my colleagues as to the desirability of providing better sleeping accommodation for the nurses.'

This report gave Rambaut, who already enjoyed a reputation for using new methods in the treatment of mental illness, the opportunity he had been seeking. In October 1915, he submitted a preliminary paper to the Management Committee on 'the Provision of Improved Infirmary Accommodation and Better Sleeping Accommodation for the Nursing Staff', in which he divided the insane needing care into three classes.

These were:

1.
Those requiring constant care, supervision and the best possible medical treatment, either because (a) they are in an acute stage of mental disease and are violent and dangerous to themselves or their fellow men or (b) they are in an incipient and presumably curable stage of insanity and required special and immediate attention in order that their chances for recovery may be materially increased.

2.
Those requiring less constant care and supervision, but who are suffering from chronic forms of insanity and are fitted only for institutional life.

3.
Those who, although not capable of taking care of themselves, are able to live in villas in the grounds or farms of the Hospital.

He considered that the last two classes were well provided for at St Andrew's.

To cure all recoverable cases, which meant taking them in hand at the earliest possible moment, first-class facilities were still needed. Only a few hospitals in Britain had been built with this problem in mind, and he hoped to visit them with the Hospital's architect: the best of such establishments were to be found in Germany and America. To achieve this end more beds were required. Many sufferers from acute insanity, he explained, did far better when confined to bed until the acute symptoms had passed. Treatment in bed was also essential in dealing with melancholia and the acute attacks which occur during the course of chronic

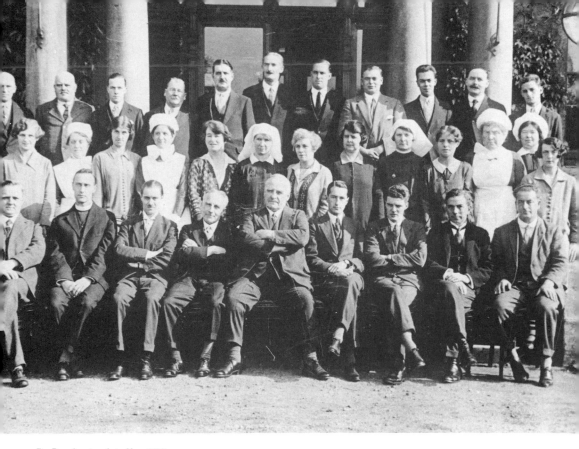

Dr Rambaut and staff, c.1927.

insanity. During the previous ten years, a great advance had been made by treating new cases of insanity in bed in the open air. Open-air verandas connected to the Infirmary on to which beds could be rapidly and easily wheeled were therefore most important.

The continuous warm-bath treatment had been found to be one of the most reliable means of quietening excitement in the insane and in calming patients suffering from acute mania. Rambaut himself had recently succeeded in curing two acute cases by this means, but the present equipment in the Hospital was inadequate. The lavage of the intestines and stomach in acute melancholia had proved highly effective but special apparatus was needed for this. 'In addition', he wrote, 'the rain, needle douch, sitz and hot air or Turkish baths are invaluable in the treatment of the different varieties of insanity. In addition to hydrotherapeutic equipment, there should be apparatus for electrical treatment'. This was not electroconvulsive therapy.

Before carrying out any changes, he reiterated the need to consult the experts who were responsible for the finest mental hospitals in Britain.

Then, as a first step, he considered it desirable to build a separate acute hospital for twelve patients of each sex. Even before this was done, he recommended that the existing infirmary wards should be enlarged, the number of beds and of single rooms increased, hydrotherapy apparatus added plus verandas for open-air treatment. The erection of a separate building for a nurses' home, also recommended by the Commissioners, would give more room on the female side of the Hospital. A large number of county asylums had already built separate nurses' homes at a reasonable cost. War conditions, however, made the implementation of these recommendations impossible.

The period between the end of the war and 1927 was one of adjustment as well as development. According to the Superintendent's report, 1919 was 'in many ways as difficult and anxious as the years of War. Problems of wages, hours of work, the price of food, fuel and commodities have followed one after another without intermission'. Prices rose steeply at first but afterwards steadied at slightly below the peak. In 1913, the average weekly cost per patient had been £2.12s.9¾d.; by 1919 it had risen to £3.5s.0d. and by 1921 to £5.0s.3d. after which the figure fell to £4.14s. 8¾d. in 1925 and by 1927 was £4.16s.1.1½d.

The Hospital continued to help patients in straitened circumstances. In 1913, £4,250 was set aside for this purpose, in 1919 the figure was £3,521, while in 1921, 1925 and 1927, it was £3,307, £3,037 and £3,325 respectively. The average daily number of patients had fluctuated between 464 and 473 during the war years; it fell to 423 in 1921 and 1922, and rose again to 473 in 1927, 3 more than in 1914. From 1928 onwards, the number varied between 503 and 518 and was 510 in 1937, when Rambaut died.

Salaries and wages increased modestly over the years, while working hours were no doubt modified from time to time in line with the national trends. At the same time, war allowances were progressively reduced. Little information on these matters is given in the Board of Control Commissioners' reports but in 1919 the working week for the nursing staff was one of sixty hours, exclusive of meal times. The male attendants had one and a half days off each week and one evening from 6 p.m. to 9 p.m. in addition to every alternate Sunday, while the nurses had one day off in the week, two hours every day, and all day every other Sunday. Senior attendants and nurses were allowed three weeks' annual leave, while the rest of the junior staff received two weeks. While pay and working conditions may compare unfavourably with those of the 1980s, Rambaut

TOP RIGHT: *Nursing staff in the grounds, c.1920.*
RIGHT: *Nursing staff in one of the female wards, c.1920.*

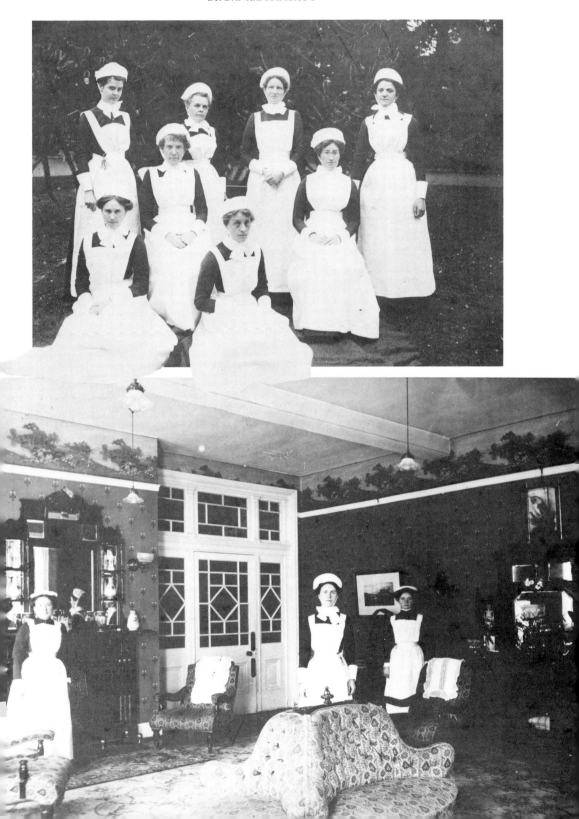

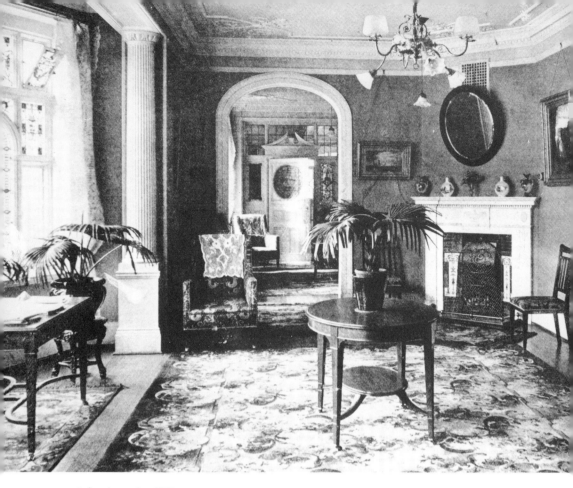

A female ward, c.1920.

was able to report in 1919 that 'all members of the staff who joined the colours and who have survived have now been demobilised and have returned to the Hospital'; conditions at St Andrew's must therefore have been reasonable. He added that, being fit young men, they brought a new lease of life to the recreational and sporting activities of the patients.

Between 1919 and 1927 the patients' activities and entertainments were increased to such an extent that there was at least one event daily; these attracted some 50 per cent of the patients while Divine Service on Sundays was usually attended by between 25 to 30 per cent. Fresh forms of entertainment were acquired as they became available. In 1919, Mr Gervase Elwes, of Billing Hall, Northampton, the distinguished tenor who had joined the Management Committee in 1916, was invited to enquire into the purchase of two gramophones. In 1922, the golf-course was improved by Len Holland, a well-known professional. Later that year, a piano and gramophone were sent to Bryn-y-Neuadd and in December the Superintendent was authorised to purchase cinema equipment for up to £105.

Throughout this period, Rambaut's prestige was rising. In 1919, he was authorised to attend the Annual Meeting of the Mental Hospitals' Association. In the following year, he was elected a member of the Educational Committee of the Royal Medico-Psychological Association, of which he became the Registrar in 1924. In July 1922, his recommendation that a consulting room in Harley Street should be rented, where he could meet the relatives of patients and prospective patients, was accepted. He was also empowered to invite the Medical Superintendents of the Registered Hospitals to meet at St Andrew's later that year. Such was his work load that, in January 1924, the Management Committee considered the advisability of providing him with a Personal Assistant. He turned this down because he considered that it would be more helpful to have an additional Assistant Medical Officer and a Junior Clerk in the Steward's office.

Senior medical staff at first posed something of a problem. In October 1920, Rambaut submitted a report on Dr Martin's relationship with himself and the Institution; Martin was then invited to resign, which he did. The matter did not end there. In November the solicitors to the Medical Defence Union threatened proceedings on Martin's behalf against the Hospital.

Martin issued a writ in January 1921 which was considered at a Special Meeting of the Management Committee. Mr J. F. Stops of Messrs Becke, Green & Stops, solicitors to the Hospital, suggested that a basis for settlement would be the withdrawal of the writ and agreement to a request by Martin for a voluntary grant in view of his fourteen years' service with the Hospital, together with a reasonable reference. The Committee, after considerable discussion, instructed Stops to proceed along these lines, indicating that a grant of 500 guineas would be made, 'that being a sum', according to the Minutes, 'which the Committee had always had in their minds as a reasonable sum, prior to the Action having been commenced'. Martin accepted this sum and the matter was closed, but not before the Chief Attendant, the Chief Nurse and the Front Lodge Keeper were dismissed with six months' salary and allowances 'on account of their conduct in connection with the circumstances arising out of Dr Martin's resignation'. Correspondence from the Professional Union of Trained Nurses was acknowledged but no action taken.

Dr N. R. Phillips had in the meanwhile been appointed Senior Assistant Medical Officer in Martin's place at a salary of £750, rising annually by

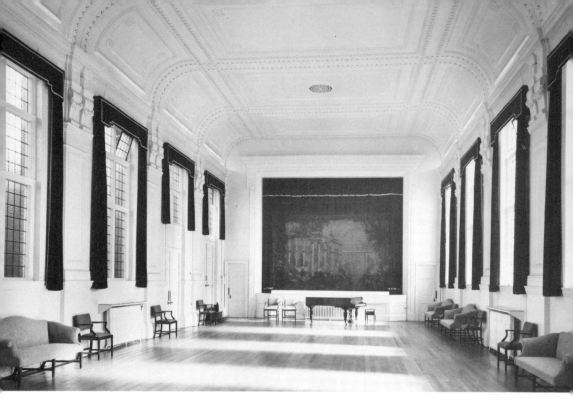

The Great Hall at St Andrew's, c.1930.

£50 to a ceiling of £900. A Second Assistant Medical Officer was not appointed until October 1922 when Dr G. W. J. Mackay took up this position at £400 per annum, rising annually by £25 to £450. As he was then found to have a serious heart condition, he was told he could only be considered as temporary. Two years later, having been passed fit, he was given a permanent post which he retained until 1928 when he resigned on being appointed Deputy Superintendent to the Nottingham City Mental Hospital. By this time, Rambaut's salary was £2,600.

In June 1922, Dr Archdall, who had been Resident Medical Officer at Bryn-y-Neuadd since 1907, retired. Although a pension of £600 was at first proposed, it was scaled down at the following Quarterly Court to £400. The Management Committee however asked that the matter be re-considered, as a result of which his pension was finally agreed at £600. His place at Bryn was taken by Dr Sidney Hillier, starting at £500 per annum. A third Assistant Medical Officer, who stated his wish to marry, was appointed in November 1925, only to be rejected three weeks later when it was discovered that he already had a wife. There were other changes in the senior staff. Mr Walker, the Accountant, retired in 1923 after fifty-five years service: he was granted an annual pension of £433, plus a gratuity of

£300 and a piece of plate. He was succeeded by Cyril Baker, his assistant for sixteen years. Each had received a gratuity in 1922 for recovering £6,774 income tax for the years 1920-22. In 1925, the Rev. E. J. Whittall, the Chaplain, died. The election of a successor had to be deferred because the salary of £400 then offered proved insufficient. The Rev. J. T. Stevens accepted the post at £465 per annum.

In September 1922, a Sub-Committee to study the question of pensions was formed under the chairmanship of Christopher Smyth, to whom the Superintendent in November submitted a scheme; this was agreed in principle. In the following March, it was decided that the Hospital should guarantee pensions on the basis of a 3 per cent contribution by the staff.

In 1919, the 8th Duke of Grafton announced that he could no longer attend meetings as he was leaving the district and could not be persuaded to allow his name to remain as a member. In 1920, the Rev. H. H. Crawley, who had succeeded Colonel Rawlins as Vice-Chairman, died, to be

The Billard Room at St Andrew's, c.1930.

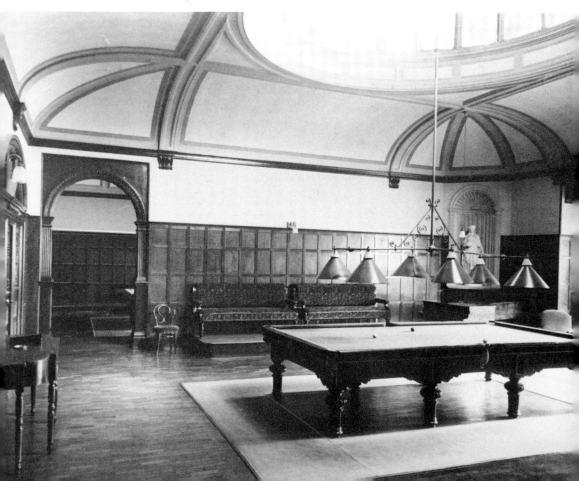

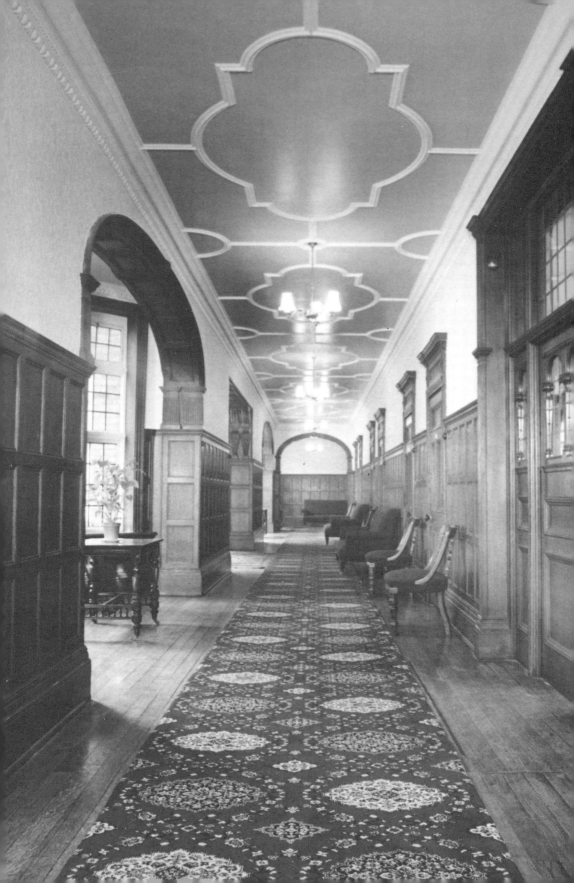

followed in this position by Sir Charles Gunning, 7th Bt. It was also decided to appoint the 7th Lord Vaux of Harrowden, a member of the Committee since 1913, together with Sir Frederick V. L. Robinson, 10th Bt., a member since 1920, to succeed Crawley as Trustees of the Superintendent's Superannuation Fund. Colonel (later Major-General) Sir Hereward Wake, 13th Bt., whose family had been associated with the Institution from the start, and Lieutenant Colonel H. G. Sotheby joined the Committee in 1922. That year, the 6th Earl Spencer, Lord-Lieutenant of Northamptonshire and in that capacity president of St Andrew's, died; he was succeeded in both positions by the 5th Marquis of Exeter.

The Board of Control Commissioners, which in 1920 was placed under the Ministry of Health and thus finally divorced from the Local Government Board and its associations with the Old Poor Law Board, continued to report favourably on the Hospital. They encouraged the Management Committee to keep pace with new ideas and their few criticisms were mainly about the need for redecoration. On several occasions, they reported the gratitude felt by patients about conditions in the Hospital and were increasingly impressed by the personality, methods and aims of Dr Rambaut.

Cures however were achieved by only a small percentage of the patients, nearly all of them direct entries of less than a year's sojourn. In 1919, for example, 74 patients, excluding those transferred from elsewhere, were received into St Andrew's, 39 of whom were discharged recovered; this represented under 8 per cent of the total number of patients under treatment which was 520. In 1922, the number of certified patients was 483, only 28 of whom were released as recovered, or under 6 per cent of the total. These results reflected the influence of the 1890 Lunacy Act which made certification dependent upon mental illness being recognised as such by a lay authority, namely the Justice of the Peace. Because this made it very difficult for hospitals to deal with early cases, they became increasingly homes for the incurable. Under the act, Superintendents had also to deal with an enormous amount of paper work in notifying the Board of Control about the state of each certified individual.

As a Registered Hospital, unrestricted by public expenditure controls, St Andrew's was encouraged by the Commissioners to take the initiative in new ways of dealing with mental illness. They were well aware of Rambaut's ambitions to introduce the most up-to-date methods and equipment, as evidenced by his paper of October 1915. In 1920, they

A male ward, c.1930.

Can you do "Squigglies"? See page 14

Daily Mirror

THE DAILY PICTURE NEWSPAPER WITH THE LARGEST NET SALE

FIVE WOMEN ON INQUIRY INTO STREET OFFENCES

LORD CHANCELLOR OPENS £68,000 EXTENSION TO NORTHAMPTON MENTAL HOSPITAL

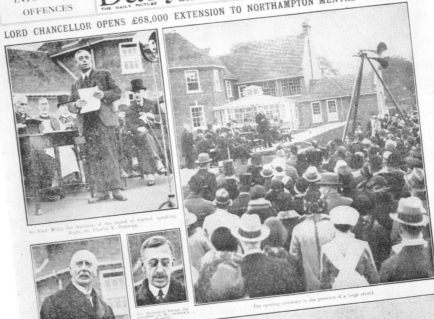

Sir Fred. Willis, the chairman of the board of control, speaking. Right, Sir Charles V. Gunning.

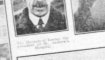

The Marquis of Exeter, the President of St. Andrew's Hospital.

The opening ceremony in the presence of a large crowd.

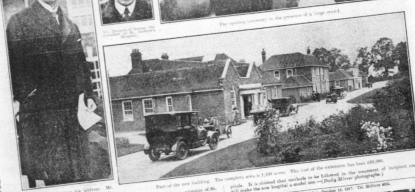

Lord Cave delivering his address. Mr. Christopher Smyth was the chairman.

Part of the new building. The complete area is 1,100 acres. The cost of the extension has been £68,000. It is claimed that methods to be followed in the treatment of incipient cases will make the new hospital a model one.—(Daily Mirror photographs.)

The Lord Chancellor, Lord Cave, yesterday opened at Northampton an extension of St. Andrew's Mental Hospital, which is said to be the largest of the thirteen registered hospitals.

Printed and Published by The Daily Mirror Newspapers, Ltd., at Geraldine House, Rolls Bldgs., Fetter-lane, London, E.C.4.—Saturday, October 15, 1927. Tel. Holborn 4321.

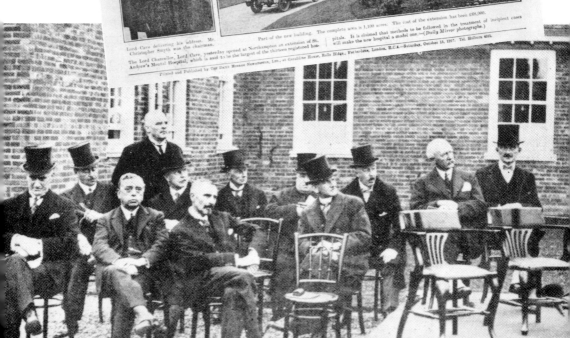

reported that, 'he is clearly anxious that this important Hospital should take its full share in the development of special means for the treatment, on modern lines, of early cases of mental illness'. Again, in 1921, they urged the Management Committee not to overlook certain medical facilities to enable the Hospital to carry out modern treatment, and to purchase additional equipment for the laboratory to enable routine laboratory work to form part of its daily clinical work. Rambaut in his report for that year had hoped that expenditure would soon be sanctioned for a complete installation of hydrotherapy apparatus.

While 1919 and 1920 had been difficult administratively, the revenue had been satisfactory; in the following three years it grew considerably and enabled the Management Committee to spend £6,000 on enlarging and re-equipping the kitchens at St Andrew's, buying thirty-six acres of the Western Favell Estate and sixty-four acres of Moulton Lodge Farm, both adjoining the Moulton Park Farm, and renovating the farm buildings. Then, in 1922, Rambaut disclosed the Committee's decision to erect a special Hospital where patients could receive 'the most modern treatment in the early stages of their illness in a building separated from the main institution, without coming into contact with the chronic insane... They propose that detached houses be built for convalescent patients. A Sub-Committee has been formed and has visited several of the more recently built Hospitals recommended by ... a commissioner of the Board of Control'. His 1915 scheme was about to be implemented.

During 1923, the Sub-Committee, consisting of Sir Charles Gunning, Sir Thomas Fermor-Hesketh, 8th Bt., later 1st Baron Hesketh, and Major

The opening of Wantage House in October 1927 by the Viscount Cave, Lord Chancellor (by kind permission of The Daily Mirror*).*

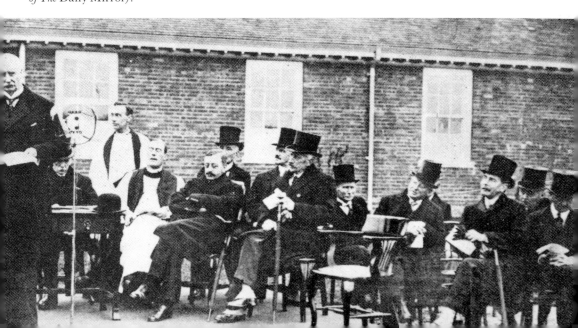

Leslie Renton, accompanied by Rambaut and Sidney Harris, the Hospital's architect, visited a group of mental hospitals, not only in Britain but in Amsterdam, Utrecht and Brussels as well, to study the latest methods and equipment in use there. Up to £50,000 was to be spent in providing accommodation for sixteen patients of each sex, together with rooms for all forms of hydrotherapy, including the prolonged warm bath, the Plombières treatment, Turkish and vapour baths and douches. There were also to be rooms for electrical, X-ray, dental and ophthalmic treatment, psychotherapy and treatment by massage, together with pathological laboratories and a medical library. Harris was responsible for the plans in consulation with the Board of Control and other hospitals. In March 1924, Messrs Henry Martin, who did much construction work for St Andrew's, gained the contract for building the new Hospital for £49,800 with completion promised within eighteen months.

It was originally hoped that the laying of the foundation stone, fixed for 27 June 1924, would be carried out by Lord Exeter, the Lord-Lieutenant, or, failing him, by Colonel S. G. Stopford Sackville, then the senior Vice-President. As neither was available, the ceremony was performed by the Chairman, Mr Christopher Smyth. Those who attended, in addition to Governors of the Hospital, the Management Committee, and senior members of the staff, included Sir Frederick Willis, Chairman of the Board of Control; Miss Margaret Bondfield, Member of Parliament for Northampton, who later became Minister of Labour in Ramsay MacDonald's second Labour Cabinet in 1929, the first woman to achieve such rank; and the Mayor of Northampton.

The new Hospital, known as Wantage House, was not formally opened until 1927, two years behind schedule. England was then passing through a period of industrial unrest which culminated in 1926 in the Coal Strike and the General Strike. There was also said to be a lack of skilled artisans, especially plasterers, according to Rambaut who that year for the first time opened his annual address with the words 'My Lords, *Ladies* and Gentlemen' as several ladies had now been elected Governors of the Hospital.

Work on Wantage House did not bring all other activities to an end. In 1924, a new staff dining room was provided for the charge sisters. In 1925, a separate home for nurses received consideration as Rambaut declared it unpleasant for them, when off duty, to be conscious of disagreeable sounds and scenes. In 1926, the male infirmary was enlarged and a new bathroom with facilities for the prolonged warm immersion bath treatment and other forms of hydrotherapy installed. A verandah for six beds was also erected there. All other activities continued normally, including the training of nursing staff as laid down by the Royal Medico-Psychological Association. In October 1926, after the death of Colonel Stopford-Sackville, Sir Hereward Wake, the 4th Lord Annaly, Sir Frederick Robinson and Sir Thomas Fermor-Hesketh were appointed Trustees.

In January 1927, with Wantage House nearing completion, it was agreed to approach Lord Exeter, the Hospital's President, to try and persuade King George V to perform the opening ceremony any time after 1 June, 'pointing out that the new Hospital shows a marked advance on any Mental Hospital in the British Isles, and is, in many ways, unique'. Neither the King nor the Prince of Wales was available and it was therefore decided to invite the Lord Chancellor, Viscount Cave, or, failing him, Neville Chamberlain, the Minister of Health. Lord Cave accepted and the date of the ceremony was fixed for Friday 14 October.

That April, Dr W. H. Ford Robertson, who had been temporarily Superintendent of the Laboratories of the Scottish Asylums, was appointed Assistant Medical Officer, Pathologist and Bacteriologist at a salary of £750 per annum, a position he held until his appointment in 1932 as Director of the West of Scotland Neuro-Psychiatric Research Institute, when Rambaut paid tribute to his extraordinary zeal, industry and scientific skill. In October 1926, £10,000 was allowed for purchasing furniture and scientific equipment for the new hospital, while £2,000 was earmarked for X-ray and electromedical equipment with a further allocation of £500 that September. By this time, two entrance lodges had been built together with a separate drive leading to Wantage House, which stood apart from the main Hospital in its own gardens and recreation grounds.

At the opening ceremony, Lord Exeter invited Christopher Smyth to take the chair as a compliment to his long services as Chairman of the Management Committee. Smyth's brief introductory speech, which gave full credit to Rambaut's role in the project, was followed by one from Sir Frederick Willis, Chairman of the Board of Control, in which he placed in perspective St Andrew's very great achievement in being the first Registered Hospital to build a fully-equipped admission unit. He first said:

> It is interesting to learn from the history of the Hospital that there are so many descendants of the first Board of Governors ninety years ago on the present list. [He then pointed out that] the scientific atmosphere is pervading our mental hospitals today as it never did before, and this new hospital is fully equipped for the treatment of patients according to the most modern methods which science has taught us . . . I am particularly glad to observe that research will have a prominent place in your

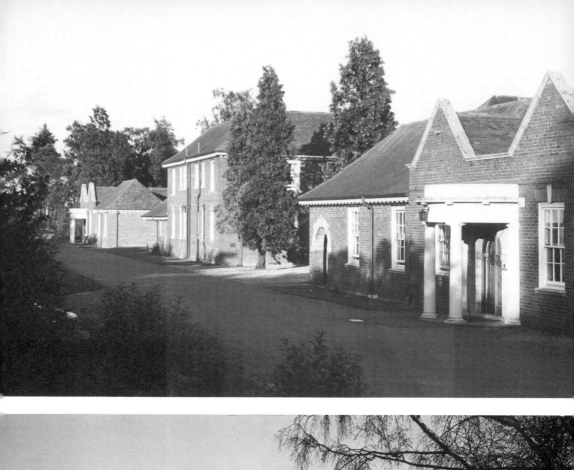

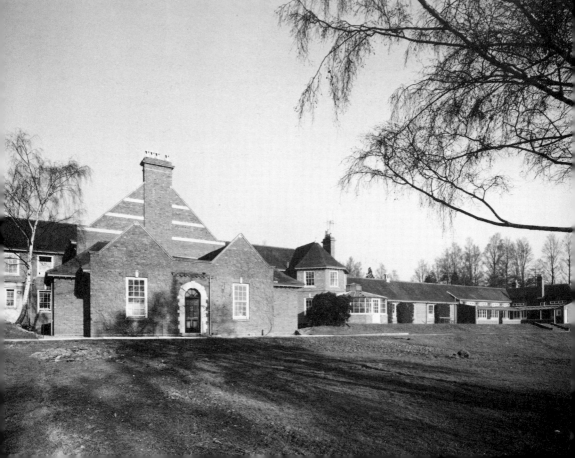

work . . . The public health of the country has immensely improved during the last fifty years. The same cannot be said of public mental health, notwithstanding the great improvements which have been made in the treatment of the insane. The recovery rate shows no material improvement and the prevention of insanity has made little or no headway. There is obviously a great field to be worked.

One thing I am sure the Government will realise, and that is that a well-equipped scientific institution of this kind must, for the successful prosecution of its objects, be provided with competent scientific workers. You are fortunate in possessing a distinguished and progressive Medical Superintendent, but Dr Rambaut would be the first to admit that he cannot cope unaided with all the scientific work which is to be undertaken here.

My hope is that work such as you are doing and proposing to do in Northampton will lead to a big diminution in the numbers of those patients whose illness goes on until they are placed in that pathetic class – the chronic insane. It is impossible to over-estimate the importance of well-equipped admission units in every institution devoted to the treatment of mental disorders, and I can only hope that other registered hospitals will follow the lead given by St Andrew's.

Lord Cave, in declaring the building open, said:

Today it was recognised as essential to keep recent and presumably recoverable cases away from contact with those whose cure had been found beyond hope, to put them, so to speak, in a special atmosphere, an atmosphere of hope, and in a place where every facility was found for examination and for curative treatment. This system has many advantages. Among others it encourages persons who know – for many of them do know that they stand in danger of mental aberration – to submit to a voluntary course of treatment without the distasteful process of certification under the law. That is a good thing, and I have every hope that the system of voluntary submission to treatment may be extended before long to the other hospitals, the county hospitals, by legislation on the lines of the Royal Commission, whose report I know to be under active consideration.

ABOVE LEFT: *Wantage House from the front.*

LEFT: *Wantage House from the Bedford Road end.*

Lord Cave was here referring to the Royal Commission on Lunacy and Mental Disorder set up in 1924 under the Labour Government because of the uneasiness aroused in the public mind by a number of charges, somewhat recklessly made, to the effect that large numbers of sane persons were being detained as insane; that the whole system of lunacy admission was wrong; and that widespread cruelty existed in our public mental hospitals. The Commission produced some highly constructive recommendations. That regarding admission to mental hospitals stated: 'the lunacy code should be recast with a view to securing that the treatment of mental disorder should approximate as nearly to the treatment of physical ailments as is consistent with the special safeguards which are indispensable when the liberty of the subject is infringed'. Treatment should be the priority and certification used only as a last resort. Voluntary patients should be allowed to enter mental hospitals without legal formality and to discharge themselves after notifying the authorities. The Mental Treatment Act of 1930 was to legalise this recommendation.

In this connection, St Andrew's had been receiving voluntary patients as boarders for many years. During Dr Bayley's superintendence, there were rarely more than one or two, but in 1914, Dr Rambaut's second year, the number climbed from 3 to 23 and in 1926 reached 70, diminishing to 40 in the following year, then climbing back in 1937 to 74. The 1930 Mental Treatment Act was also to introduce a third classification, namely temporary patients. These were defined as patients 'suffering from mental illness and likely to benefit from temporary treatment, but for the time being incapable of expressing [themselves] as willing or unwilling to receive such treatment'. The intention was to help in cases where the affliction might have a physical cause, such as childbirth or alcoholism. A Temporary Order, which lasted for six months with two extensions, each of three months, could be granted on a petition from a near relative plus two medical certificates made out not more than fourteen days before reception into hospital. In 1931, the average daily number of temporary patients at St Andrew's was two and in 1937 five.

Wantage House undoubtedly placed St Andrew's in the forefront of mental hospitals. The Board of Control wrote in 1928 that:

we know of no line of treatment for mental illness which is not available in this unit; and it is with the greatest satisfaction that we have seen that full use is being made of those medical sources available, both in the various treatment rooms and in the well-equipped Laboratories. It has also been apparent to us – and this we regard as very important – that the value of this reception unit is by no means confined to the forty-one patients we saw under treatment there, but that it is having a stimulating influence throughout the whole of the Hospital.

Visitors came from abroad as well as from elsewhere in Britain. In 1929, Rambaut was authorised to entertain the Superintendents of the Dutch Psychiatry Society at St Andrew's in 'a fitting manner'. A letter of 23 November 1930 to Rambaut from Dr M. A. Bliss, Mental Specialist and Governor of the St Louis and Missouri State Board of Mental Hospitals, enshrined in the Minutes, reads:

Dear Dr Rambaut.
    First I want to thank you. Second I want to express my most sincere admiration for the beautiful spirit which your genius has brought into the care and treatment of mental sufferers at St Andrew's, and, third I want to express my admiration for the Hospital itself – especially of Wantage House and its splendid equipment for a kindly and scientific reception service – something more than money is necessary to produce a St Andrew's. Lastly I hope you may take seriously the suggestion of coming to America. You can do us good, and we will not be slow in showing our appreciation.
    Sincerely,
    [signed]
    M. A. Bliss

From 1928 onwards, the Superintendent expanded his Annual Report considerably, describing the various treatments at Wantage House in some detail, while continuing to give facts and figures about the rest of the St Andrew's group, supported by the usual tables of statistics which remained little changed throughout his superintendency.

Progress at Wantage House was keenly watched by the Board of Control who, in 1929, was encouraged to learn of the good results obtained there with some longstanding and protracted cases and that two houses, 'Merchiston' and 'The Rowans' on the Billing Road, acquired that year by the Hospital, were to be used for convalescent patients who wished to continue with treatment. Demand for admissions already exceeded accommodation. In November of the following year, however, they noticed that several cases of long duration were resident there and went on to express the hope that such cases would not be allowed to occupy beds which could be much better used for recent and acute cases. They continued to comment favourably on the clinical and laboratory work.

Dr Ford Robertson contributed considerably to the success of Wantage

House and Rambaut generously referred in his 1930 report to a thesis, then shortly to be published, entitled: 'A Study of the Pathogenesis of the Anaerobic Corynebacterium Diptheriae, Anaerobic Diptheroid and Anaerobic Leptothrix Infections in relation to the Psychoses, Neuroses and Neurotoxic States, compared with 260 cases of Symptomatic Physical Disorder'. When Robertson resigned, his clinical and pathological responsibilities were separated. Dr D. J. O'Connell, the second Assistant Medical Officer, was put in charge of the former department at a salary of £500 while the latter became the responsibility of Dr Ruby Stern, the first woman doctor to be employed at St Andrew's. Dr Stern remained at Wantage House until January 1936 when she gained the Sebag Montefiore Fellowship in Morbid Anatomy and Histology at the Hospital for Sick Children, Great Ormond Street.

Rambaut's next most important building achievement was the erection of a separate nurses' home in the Hospital grounds. The Management Committee's decision was taken in October 1927, only two weeks after the opening of Wantage House. Twenty-six thousand pounds was allocated for this purpose, to be the responsibility of a Sub-Committee with Sir Charles Gunning as Chairman supported by Sir Thomas Fermor-Hesketh, Major Renton, Mr H. M. Stockdale of Mears Ashby Hall and Major Thurburn. The Sub-Committee decided, after finding the originally proposed site too low, to convert Rose Cottage with extensive additions into sleeping accommodation for sixty-seven nurses, later further expanded, together with a dining-room for forty, a recreation room, sitting-room, a room for study and lectures and a three-bed sick bay. It was first thought appropriate to invite Northampton architects to submit plans competitively but this proved expensive and, instead, Sidney Harris was invited to undertake the work. The contract was given in November 1928 to Messrs E. Green & Son, whose tender was £24,478. Completion was to be in eighteen months, which was successfully achieved. Three thousand pounds was allowed for furnishing the house and it was occupied that September by seventy-five nurses and eight staff.

The Board of Control Commissioners were evidently pleased with the result. 'The bedrooms, supplied with hot and cold water, are most comfortable, and the sitting-rooms are attractive in their decorations and supplied with everything to make them suitable for rest and recreation. This home is a great addition to the amenities of the Hospital, and supplies a much needed want'. There was a separate wing for the night staff.

The Superintendent remained responsible for the maintenance of the Hospital's buildings. His Annual Report listed year by year the continuing round of repairs, redecoration, alterations and additions. The building

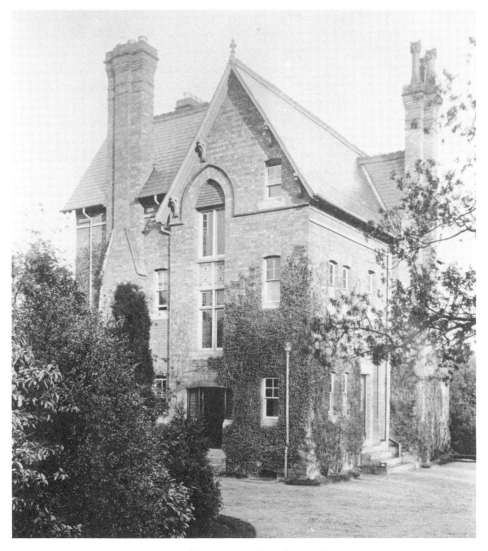

Rose Cottage, which formed the nucleus of the new nurses' home built in 1930.

work carried out during the final years of his superintendency revealed the Committee's intention of keeping all accommodation up-to-date. Four additional fully-equipped clinical rooms were added to the main Hospital between 1929 and 1931; the nurses' former quarters in the Hospital converted into two female infirmaries in 1932; a mess provided for the artisans in 1933; the laundry completely renovated and brought up-to-date in 1934; separate dining-rooms provided both for the Assistant Medical Officers and the Chief Attendants, and recreation rooms for the nurses in 1936. A new central dining hall for patients was built, thus allowing the recreation hall and theatre to be used solely for its original purpose. In 1937, Rheinfelden on the Billing Road, purchased for £3,000, was opened as a home for those nurses who could not be accommodated in the main house. Other additions that year included a consulting room for the Deputy Superintendent, a flat for the Matron and a sitting-room for the Assistant Matron; to enable these improvements to be carried out, a new female block was added.

Rambaut was usually, but not always, successful in obtaining whatever he considered important. In 1935, for example, he pointed out that the X-ray plant then in use in Wantage House had been superseded by more modern equipment; by the following year the latest apparatus had been installed. In his 1931 report, he hoped that special occupational rooms for both male and female patients would be erected and an expert Occupation Officer engaged to teach handicrafts, a recommendation made by the Commissioners in 1928. He referred to this need again in 1932, quoting Galen who wrote 'Employment is Nature's best physician'. In 1933 both he and the Commissioners were pleased to report that a carpentry workshop had been made available for the gentlemen and that new handicrafts rooms for both sexes would be constructed as soon as circumstances permitted, but these hopes had not been fulfilled by 1937.

There was a switch from horse-drawn to petrol-driven vehicles during these years In 1933 it was decided to dispense with horses altogether; as a result, the coachhouse was given over to coal and a large garage erected on the former coal store. A special Locomotion Sub-Committee was appointed to examine the whole question of transport under the chairmanship of Mr A. H. Sartoris, the other members being Sir Charles Frederick, Major Renton and Colonel N. V. Stopford Sackville. The Hospital then owned four motors, the largest and oldest being an eleven-year-old 30 hp Daimler, and two Morris vans. It was decided to dispose of the worn-out Daimler, and replace it with a second-hand car, preferably a 40–50 hp Rolls Royce, costing up to £1,500. In future the Hospital's motor vehicles were inspected annually.

The Management Committee found it increasingly difficult to cope with the growing complexity of running an organisation which cared for over 500 patients at any one time and employed a staff of over 300. Accordingly, it was decided to delegate greater responsibility to Sub-Committees. In January 1929, an Expenditure Sub-Committee was established to scrutinise all monthly and quarterly bills and other expenditure in order to

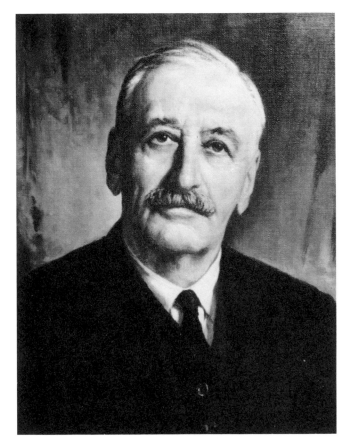

The 5th Marquess of Exeter, KG, CMG, TD, President 1922–51.

advise the main Committee, whose Vice-Chairman, Sir Charles Gunning, was nominated Chairman. One of the new Sub-Committee's first recommendations was the setting up of a Farms and Grounds Sub-Committee under Major Maunsell; its other members were Major Geoffrey Elwes and Sir Frederick Robinson. Both Committees met immediately before the monthly Management Committee meeting, occasionally at other times as well.

From 1931 onwards, the names of these Committee members were shown in the Annual Report. The work they carried out was extensive. In 1932, for example, the Committee of Management had 12 meetings, the Expenditure Committee met 13 times and the Farm and Grounds

Committee 10. Another important Sub-Committee was formed in March 1930, first to deal with the furnishing of the nurses' home and then of 'Merchiston' and 'The Rowans'; all matters regarding furnishing and decoration were subsequently allocated to it. Its chair was taken by Miss Mary Bouverie, the granddaughter of Edward Bouverie, who had played so vital a role in bringing the Institution into being; other Committee members were Major Elwes, Colonel Stopford Sackville and Lieutenant Colonel H. G. Sotheby, later to be joined by Mrs St. John Mildmay and Mrs Wentworth Watson. Sub-Committees were appointed to deal with insurance and investments, meeting when required, and others for *ad hoc* purposes such as short-listing candidates for a senior hospital post. Because of these pressures it was decided to alter the rule concerning the size of the Committee's membership from fifteen to 'not less than fifteen'.

Important changes in the composition of the Management Committee took place during the 1930s. In 1932, Christopher Smyth retired after thirty-five years as Chairman, having served on the Committee since 1879. During those years, he had rarely missed a meeting and his outstanding services were widely acknowledged. He and his family served St Andrew's devotedly. His uncle, William Smyth, had been Chairman of the Committee from 1865 to 1870 and his father, the Rev. Christopher Smyth, had for many years been a member of the Committee on which both father and son sat from 1879 until 1894 when the latter became Vice-Chairman. Christopher Smyth's great friend and partner in local affairs and for long a member of the Committee was Sir George Gunning, 5th Bt., whose daughter he married. Sir George died in 1903 and his younger son, Sir Charles Gunning, 7th Bt., served as Smyth's Vice-Chairman from 1920 to 1932. Smyth died in 1934.

Sir Charles Gunning became Chairman in 1932 with Major A. H. Thurburn as Vice-Chairman. In 1937 he indicated his wish to retire; he had joined the Committee on succeeding to the baronetcy in 1906, taking the place of his elder brother who had died that year. Sir Charles was persuaded to remain in office for one final year while the Committee decided on his successor. The choice fell on the Rt. Hon. Sir George Stanley, the sixth son of the 16th Earl of Derby; he had held posts in both the Bonar Law and Baldwin administrations, had been Governor of Madras, 1929–34, and was briefly Viceroy of India in the latter year. He had become a Governor of the Hospital as recently as 1936 and elected to the Committee in 1937. Sir Kenneth Murchison, for many years a Member of Parliament and a colleague of Stanley in the Ministry of Pensions, was elected Vice-President at Stanley's recommendation. Mr Stephen Schilizzi joined the Committee in 1928, having been a Governor since 1921. In 1932,

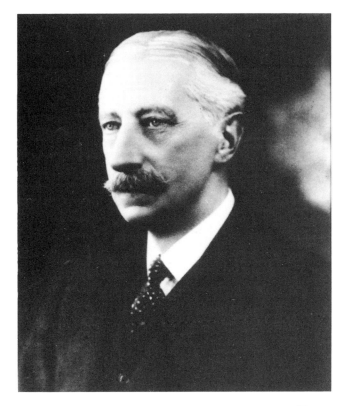

Sir Charles V. Gunning, 7th Bt., CB, CMG, Vice-Chairman 1920-32, Chairman 1932–8.

Sir Charles Knightley, Bt., later Lord Knightley, died after forty years' service as did the 7th Lord Vaux of Harrowden, another attentive long-serving Committee member and a Vice-President, in 1933; Major-Gen. Sir Hereward Wake became a Trustee of the Superannuation Fund in his place. Mr Hugh Sartoris, who had been a Committee member for thirty-two years and a Vice-President, died in 1937.

Sir Charles Gunning's tenure of office, first as Chairman of the Expenditure and then of the Management Committee, had not been easy. In October 1929, the crash on Wall Street and the inability of the United States to buy British goods resulted in a great economic depression in Britain. By December 1930 there were over two and a half million unemployed. There were fears of a large budget deficit and increased taxation unless government expenditure was reduced. A general lack of confidence in the economy did not leave St Andrew's unaffected.

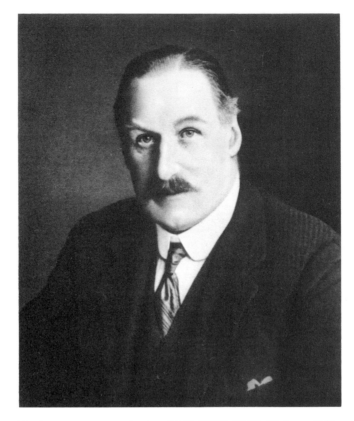

The Rt. Hon. Sir George Stanley, GCSI, GCIE, CMG, Chairman 1938.

On 7 September 1931, Sir Charles asked the Superintendent to call a Special Meeting of the Expenditure Committee as:

'important matters connected with patients' fees and salaries and wages of staff and general expenditure will be before the Committee for consideration . . . The Accountant will submit the usual financial statement and a statement of the work in hand, etc. In addition to this I should like him to prepare a statement showing what a reduction in patients' fees would be of five per cent all round, also another statement of a ten per cent cut in salaries of £500 and over, and a five per cent cut in all salaries and wages of under £500 and over £150. This is in view of the serious financial situation which I fear may become worse, before it's better.

Rambaut, agreeing to these arrangements, wrote:

I see clearly that it is the duty of all patriots to make sacrifice in times of
danger to the State, but I do not agree that the more highly skilled and
hardest working of the Staff on whose scientific knowledge and energy
the success of the Hospital depends, should have a higher percentage of
cut in their salaries than their inferiors. If a cut is really necessary, with
much deference I venture to think that it should be the same percentage
for all, unless Socialist or Communist principles are to influence us. The
Government no doubt may be trusted to see that none of us escapes our
fair share of extra taxation.

At the Special Meeting, held on 22 September, the Superintendent
submitted a paper on the Hospital's financial situation. He did not
recommend a reduction in patients' fees. He had already dealt with those
few relatives who were in financial difficulties; a reduction merely meant
that the great majority who had not asked for a reduction would benefit. As
for wages, there were fifty employees earning between £150 and £500; of
those twenty-one would receive less than £150 if a cut of 5 per cent were
made and so would be on a lower wage level than those who originally
received less.

I would like to point out [he continued], that when the cost of living was
over 100 per cent above that of July 1914, the Officers received no
addition to their salaries, and it was not until 1920 that a thirty per cent
increase was granted when the cost was 125 per cent above that of July
1914. The increase to 50 per cent was only granted in 1929.
    The Officers will pay considerably more Income Tax under the
Economy Budget, and they have also contributed three per cent of their
salaries since 1st January 1924 under the Hospital Superannuation
scheme.
    In the year 1912, the receipts from the patients were £63,600 and in
1930 they were £148,800 – an increase of 133 per cent. This increase was
due to the reputation which the Hospital had gained; this reputation was
in a great measure created and maintained by the skill, assiduity, and
painstaking attention to detail of our Officers.
    Patients do not arrive in this Hospital automatically as they do in a
General Hospital. Before a patient is admitted there is considerable
correspondence, many interviews at the Hospital and in London take
place, and relatives are shown over the Hospital. If this work were left to
subordinates, and the special personal element were not always in

evidence, the number of admissions (especially of the better-paying patients) would soon decrease.

I have communicated with the other Registered Hospitals, and I find that none of them has made a general reduction in the rates of patients' payments or has reduced salaries and wages.

He ended by recommending that further improvements, except for the completion of contracts in hand, be postponed for six months. The logic of Rambaut's argument was accepted, and no reductions were made. That year, it should be noted, the medical staff, in addition to the Superintendent, consisted only of Dr Phillips, the Deputy Superintendent; Dr O'Connell, the second Assistant Medical Officer; Dr Dorothea Tudor, temporary Assistant Medical Officer; Dr Ford Robertson at Wantage House, and Dr W. Starkey, Assistant Medical Officer at Bryn-y-Neuadd. In July 1934, the Royal Medico-Psychological Association, of which Rambaut had been a member since 1894, held its ninety-third annual conference in Northampton. This was a compliment both to St Andrew's and to its Superintendent's achievements in his profession, including his work for the Association. This was recognised by his investiture as the Association's President for 1934–5. The Management Committee showed its appreciation by granting £250 towards entertaining the visitors, because 'it was felt that the presence of so many mental specialists will be a great asset to St Andrew's Hospital'. The Conference was a great success and Rambaut was able to inform the Management Committee at its July meeting that he had received many letters of congratulation.

In 1934 the Annual Report of the Board of Control made the following references to St Andrew's:

Good progress continues to be made in the provision of separate admission hospitals with their ancilliary convalescent villas. As we have pointed out in previous Reports, an adequately equipped admission unit and treatment centre is an essential part of a complete mental hospital and the operation of the Mental Treatment Act (1930) has emphasised the necessity for these units . . . Where the admission hospital is situated, as it should be, well away from the main building with entirely separate access, there is much to be said for the practice which has already been adopted in a few cases, e.g. at Wantage House, St Andrew's, of giving the admission hospital a name of its own. There are those who say that this is a mere concession to prejudice, a distinction without a difference. We do not share this view, and experience convinces us that it will help to attract voluntary patients and encourage earlier admissions if the patients and, perhaps an even more important point, their relations feel that treatment is being offered to them without the necessity of having to enter institutions still unfortunately too often associated in the public mind with permanent mental disorder . . . From the point of view of complete examination of patients, clinical laboratory tests, and of treatment, Dr Rambaut emphasizes the value of the Reception Hospital [Wantage House] at St Andrew's.

Rambaut noted in 1935 that, of the sixty-one new patients admitted to Wantage House, thirty-five were voluntary. 'This number of voluntary patients in proportion to the total number of admissions is highly satisfactory, as it bears witness to the fact that public opinion is now beginning to regard mental illness in its true light and appreciates the advantages of early treatment before recourse to certification becomes imperative'. This trend continued.

The years 1936 and 1937 were uneventful. There was a further request in 1936 from the Ministry of Pensions for a reduction in payment for their patients. Rambaut, after consulting other Superintendents, recommended that no further reductions for these cases be made. The Soke of Peterborough, having asked whether St Andrew's would accept voluntary patients chargeable to the County Council, was told that rate-aided patients were not received. In June 1937, the Annual Reunion of the Superintendents of Registered Hospitals was held at St Andrew's.

In October, Rambaut raised the question of providing adequate shelter for patients and staff in the event of gas attacks during air raids. A month later, he was reported to be so ill that it was decided to form a Committee under Sir George Stanley, the Chairman elect, 'to deal with matters how and when necessary'. On 30 November, four days later, Dr Rambaut died. He was seventy-two.

His death was greatly lamented. The Committee of Management recorded in their Annual Report for 1937 that the Hospital's 'high state of efficiency is in no small measure due to his administrative abilities, his strong personality, and his great charm. Those of us who met him so frequently at our monthly meetings will miss him greatly, and he will be remembered by all with affection and respect'. The Committee voted a gratuity of £7,000 personally to Mrs Rambaut in recognition of his exceptional services and advanced her £4,000 out of his pension fund of £23,000 to help pay estate duty. The Commissioners, in their first report for 1938, observed that 'his views with regard to the need for occupying patients and his recognition that physical treatment often had an important bearing upon the recovery of certain cases of mental disorder had an influence far beyond his Hospital. It was in 1927 that Wantage House, which he had designed for the treatment of early and recoverable cases, was opened. Its value as a treatment and research centre was soon recognised and it became a model for Admission Hospitals not only in Great Britain, but in many parts of the Empire.'

A long obituary in *The Times* of 1 December ended on a more personal note. 'During his time at St Andrew's Hospital, Dr Rambaut treated numbers of poor patients in Northampton and the county from whom he took no fee. He was generous in lending the beautiful grounds of the hospital to local organisations. He was beloved by the patients and by every member of staff.' In addition to his widow, he left two sons, one of them, a Flight Lieutenant in the RAF, and a daughter, who was married to a son of Sir Kenneth Murchison, a future Chairman of the Management Committee.

Chapter Eleven

DR THOMAS TENNENT (1938–1962):

NEW TREATMENTS,

NEW LEGISLATION

D r Thomas Tennent was Deputy Superintendent of the Maudsley Hospital, London, when he was elected to succeed Dr Rambaut early in 1938 at a salary of £2,000 per annum, plus generous emoluments. Born in 1900, Tennent, a Lowland Scot, was educated at Lenzie Academy and at the Universities of Glasgow, London and John Hopkins, Baltimore, USA. He had held posts as Assistant Medical Officer at the Dykebar Mental Hospital, Paisley, 1924–6, and at the Maudsley, 1926–31. In 1927–8 he was Rockefeller Medical Fellow at the Phipps' Psychiatric Clinic of the John Hopkins Hospital, Baltimore. While Deputy Medical Director at the Maudsley, 1931–8, he had also been Assistant Physician in Psychological Medicine at King's College Hospital, London. On his appointment, he was allowed to retain his position as Lecturer in Psychological Medicine at London University. He was married with a son and two daughters. On paper, Tennent could not have had better qualifications and the Governors of St Andrew's were to have every reason for congratulating both him and themselves on the soundness of their judgement in choosing him.

There were many similarities between the careers at St Andrew's of Dr Tennent and his predecessor. Both served the Hospital for twenty-four years, both died in harness, and both enhanced its already prestigious reputation by ensuring that the latest and most advanced techniques were successfully adopted. Both were faced with guiding the Hospital through a World War, which they successfully achieved, within some eighteen months of taking up their appointments. Both successfully initiated a new venture, in Rambaut's case the creation of Wantage House and in Tennent's the introduction of a School for Occupational Therapy. Both gained universal respect.

The Board of Control were delighted with Tennent's appointment and in their second report for 1939 spoke of 'his high attainments and considerable clinical and administrative experience at the Maudsley and other Hospitals'. There was also local approval. The Northampton General Hospital offered him the appointment, which he accepted, of Honorary Physician in Psychological Medicine; Dr O'Connell, St Andrew's Senior Assistant Medical Officer, was at the same time invited to become the Assistant Honorary Physician. By now, Dr Phillips, the Deputy Superintendent at St Andrew's since 1929, was approaching retirement which he took in 1939, to be succeeded by Dr O'Connell.

This year, 1938, also saw the election of a new Chairman and Vice-Chairman of the Management Committee. Sir George Stanley in his few months as Chairman had gained the respect and affection of Governors and staff alike, but he died that July after a short illness. His successor was Sir Kenneth Murchison who, when a young man, had been on the Asylums Committee of the London County Council. His proposal that the 6th Baron Braye of Stanford Park, near Rugby, should become Vice-Chairman, which also made him Chairman of the Expenditure Sub-Committee, was accepted; both attended meetings assiduously, Sir Kenneth until his retirement in 1949 and Lord Braye until 1951, and both died in 1952. Captain G. E. Bellville was now Chairman of the Farms and Grounds Sub-Committee and Miss Bouverie continued as chairman of the Furnishing and Decoration Sub-Committee.

Tennent was immediately concerned with improving two aspects of the Hospital's work, the research being done at Wantage House and the occupational therapy facilities, in both cases planning to build on the foundations laid by Rambaut. In his first Annual Report, he pointed out that the facilities at Wantage House for investigating the physiological and psychological factors of nervous and mental illness were outstandingly good. 'Nevertheless', he continued, 'I am somewhat perturbed in mind as to whether or not this unit is achieving all that was visualised by those responsible for its creation. My interpretation of their intentions is that its function should be threefold, for the treatment of acute and recoverable patients, for investigations that may become necessary in the patients in other parts of the Hospital, and for research work on nervous and mental disorders. I cannot feel that our position with regard to the third of these is at present worthy of our status and high traditions.'

Like Rambaut before him, Tennent believed fervently in the value of

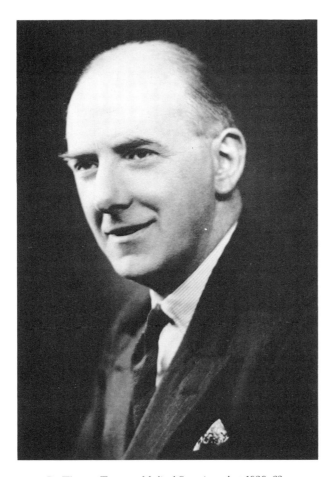

Dr Thomas Tennent, Medical Superintendent 1938–62.

occupational therapy. He acknowledged in 1938 the excellent progress already made by the Hospital, especially in gardening work, but was anxious to see even greater emphasis on this form of therapy. He was glad to report the appointment of an occupational therapist for the female patients and, as the demand for male occupational therapists appeared to exceed the supply, sent a male nursing attendant, who was afterwards likewise employed on the male side, for instruction in this field to the Maudsley. He, like Rambaut, hoped that an adequate occupational therapy department would be created. In this he was supported by the Board of Control.

In March, 1940, he emphasised to the Management Committee the need

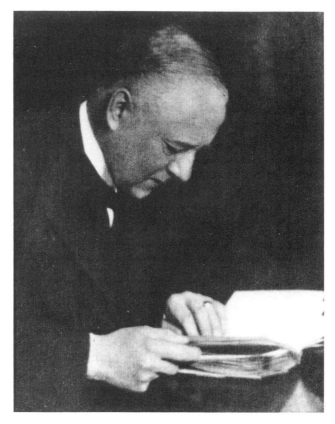

Sir Kenneth Murchison, Chairman 1938–49.

for indoor occupational and recreational therapeutic facilities and better library arrangements. Had it not been for the war, he would have asked for this project to be provided immediately, estimating the cost at about £15,000. He suggested that a fund be opened for this purpose. These proposals met with the Management Committee's unanimous approval but it was not until well after the war that action was possible.

Immediate steps were taken, nevertheless, to increase the supply of professionally trained occupational therapists. By 1941, Tennent had obtained official recognition of a School of Occupational Therapy at St Andrew's with three students already undergoing instruction. Theoretical and practical training in the arts and crafts was carried out at the Northampton School of Art, whose Principal, Mr F. E. Courtney, and Miss Burrows, its teacher of needlework, judged the patients' entries at the

Hospital's annual Arts and Crafts Exhibition. By 1943, there were seven students engaged on the two-year course under Miss Mabel Thompson and in the following year Mrs Joyce Hombersley was appointed Director of Training.

Great strides were also made in methods of treatment, especially of schizophrenia. In 1938, Dr Tennent introduced the use of cardiazol and insulin with encouraging results. The insulin technique was a complicated one and arrangements were made for a Dr Gross to come from Switzerland to train the Hospital's staff involved. In 1941, however, the use of cardiazol was replaced by electrically induced convulsive therapy which was far less unpleasant for the patient. The pre-frontal leucotomy operation was also introduced, although the Superintendent pointed out that there had been neither a sufficient number of treatments nor a long enough period of observation for conclusions about its efficacy to be reached.

These new methods had a dramatic effect upon the number of patients who were discharged as recovered between 1938 and 1947 as shown in the following table:

Year	Average daily number of patients	Number discharged as recovered
1938	504	40
1939	500	49
1940	515	56
1941	496	76
1942	483	90
1943	509	131
1944	530	137
1945	563	182
1946	570	191
1947	558	205

From then onwards up to and including 1955, the average daily number of patients varied between 524 and 547 and those cured between 152 and 209, the peak figure in both cases being achieved in 1955. The greater the number of patients cured, the greater the number of patients who could be accommodated. From 1956 onwards, the numbers in both categories began to decline and in Tennent's final year the average daily number was 416 and those cured 115.

That so much progress should have been made immediately before and

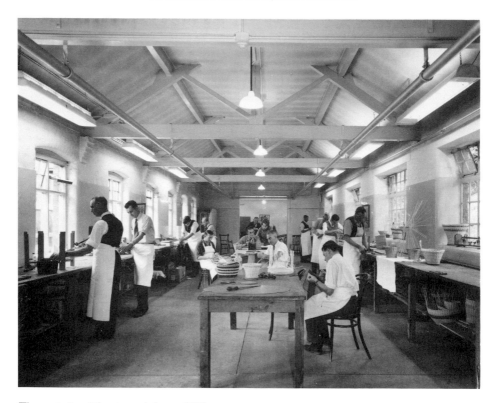

The occupational therapy workshop, c.1938.

during the Second World War speaks much both for Tennent and for the Hospital's Management Committee who accepted his initiative. The wartime conditions inevitably imposed considerable strains. There were extensive alterations to convert underground rooms and passages at St Andrew's into well-ventilated air-raid shelters. Staff had to be trained in anti-gas measures and in dealing with incendiary bombs. Those called up into the Services had to be replaced, arrangements made for their pay during their absence and their jobs safeguarded.

Both the X-ray equipment and the operating theatre at Wantage House needed special protection, especially as the Chief Constable hoped that they could be available for the community should the Northampton General Hospital be put out of action. Bryn-y-Neuadd was made ready to receive evacuees and fifty female patients were transferred there on the outbreak of hostilities, although others continued to be sent there for the usual holidays. Not all services could be kept going as the war years lengthened; fuel shortages put the Russian and Turkish baths out of

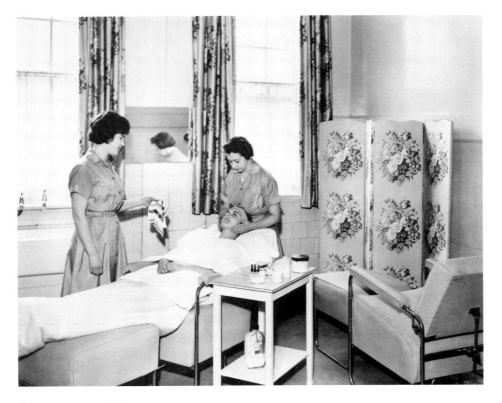

Beauty treatment, c.1935.

commission and X-ray films could only be used in essential cases. Overall, however, the Hospital functioned normally.

With the German invasion of Belgium, France and Holland in May 1940, many of the male staff retained by the Hospital were anxious to form a unit of the Local Defence Volunteers (LDV). The Management Committee agreed on condition that the Hospital had first call upon their services. The Board of Control thought differently. They pointed out in a circular letter that, in the event of enemy activity in their vicinity, the duty of the Hospital staff was to look after the patients. The LDV was part of the army and therefore could not necessarily be allocated to protect the Hospital. They therefore recommended that staff, whose absence, however brief, might prejudice the welfare of the patients should not be allowed to join. Major-General Sir Hereward Wake, a member of the Management Committee, who commanded what became the local Home Guard, hoped that any unit formed by the Hospital staff would have the protection of the Hospital as first priority. The Board of Control replied that a Home Guard volunteer unit could be called up by the War Office without consulting its employer. It was therefore decided that the Hospital's staff should not join the LDV; in any case there was need for more fire-fighting staff. In 1942, the Hospital set up its own fire-fighting unit as membership of the Auxiliary Fire Service could involve staff being sent for duty elsewhere.

St Andrew's did not survive unscathed from enemy action. On 15 January 1941, the Hospital received a direct hit from a *Luftwaffe* bomb. There were no casualities either from this or from another bomb which landed on the golf-course. In March, a claim of £23,933.12s.3d. was lodged for the damage done. The Governors recorded that they were 'very greatly impressed by the foresight, efficiency and promptitude displayed by Dr Tennent under such trying circumstances, especially for the way in which he arranged for the accommodation of the patients whose sleeping quarters had been made uninhabitable.' Various mutual arrangements were made by the Superintendent in 1940 and 1941 with other hospitals, especially

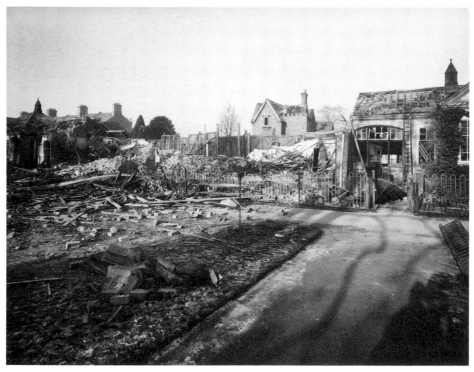

Some of the few bombs to fall on Northampton during the Second World War landed in St Andrew's, destroying one male ward and leaving a large crater in the front lawn. No one was injured.

ABOVE: *Bomb damage to the male ward.*
RIGHT: *The crater in the front lawn.*

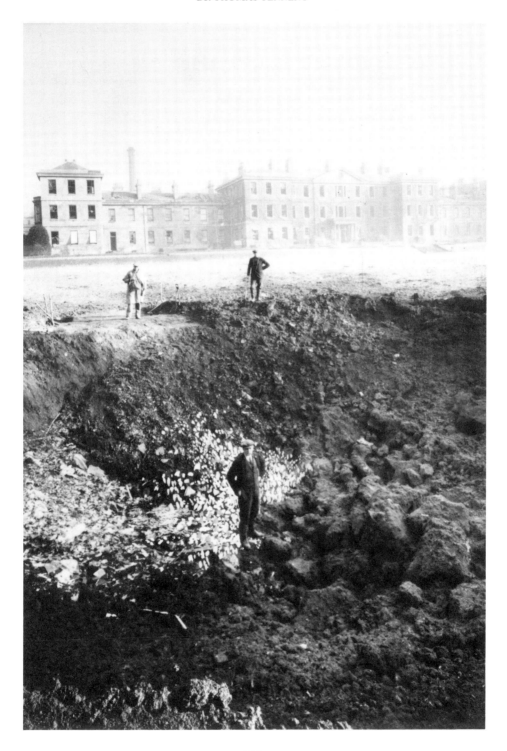

those in the Registered Hospitals Group for which St Andrew's became the central control point.

In June 1940, Tennent agreed to the Board of Control's request to receive twenty-seven officers when the Royal Naval Hospital was evacuated from Great Yarmouth. He also arranged with the War Office to establish a military hospital and take in from fifty to a hundred officers and other ranks from the Women's Services; thus temporarily Tennent became a Lieutenant-Colonel and O'Connell a Major. The work proved greater than anticipated. Insufficient staff was provided by the War Office. In October 1942, the War Office was informed that, if they did not keep to their side of the agreement by providing adequate clerical and medical staff, St Andrew's would not be able to continue with the Military Hospital. A Quartermaster-Sergeant was accordingly sent to put the office in order.

A principal wartime problem was lack of adequate nursing staff. Tennent first looked for help from the local Women's Voluntary Aid Detachment (VAD) and the Red Cross, but these did not fully meet requirements. It was therefore agreed that he be allowed to increase the hours of duty of his own nurses and give them additional pay. To this the nurses agreed. Tennent later told a Sub-Committee, convened by Lord Braye in 1941 to enquire into nurses' pay, that he was dissatisfied with the type of nurse being recruited, partly due, he considered, to their poor wages which were lower than those being paid by many comparable hospitals. The Committee of Management, anxious to maintain its charitable payments for the less fortunate, had habitually held down salaries and wages and had thus lost valuable staff to better paid jobs elsewhere.

This question of inadequate wages was not new. In October 1939, Tennent had been approached by the nursing staff through the national organiser of the Mental Hospital and Institutional Workers' Union about hours of duty, sleeping-in arrangements, ration allowances and holidays. On that occasion, he had sent a questionnaire to a wide range of hospitals about working conditions. An analysis of the replies showed that the ratio of nurses to patients was higher at St Andrew's than at any other mental hospital contacted and that salaries and wages were lower than most. The majority of the hospitals paid emoluments when the staff were on holiday, as well as when away sick, while the average hours of duty were between fifty-four and fifty-six per week. On this occasion, the Management Committee increased pay to a competitive level and reduced weekly working hours from sixty to fifty-five.

Equally difficult was the availability of doctors. At a meeting in July 1941, Tennent explained that his normal staff of six doctors had been reduced to two. Three doctors had recently been offered to him but only because they had proved unsatisfactory in their previous posts; these he could do without. Because of the shortage of male doctors he had engaged a woman: by 1943 there were two women doctors on the staff but by 1945 they had gone. He reminded the Committee of one possible source of trained medical staff which had so far been debarred. He was referring back to a meeting held in spring 1939 when he had called their attention to a number of distinguished Austrian and German psychiatrists then in England as refugees and asked if one could be employed on research work. Tennent had later added that the doctor he had in mind was both a naturalised British subject and held a British medical qualification. This proposition was, however, turned down by eight votes to six. Brigadier-General M. F. Gage, supported by Mrs Wentworth Watson, had afterwards tried to get this decision reversed, but allowed the matter to drop when the Superintendent explained that he could no longer fill the position.

In July 1941, it was agreed that the situation had completely changed and the 1939 decision was unanimously revoked. Tennent was accordingly authorised to obtain any help he considered necessary with the proviso that any doctor not of British nationality, not excluding a German, should first be approved personally by the Chairman and Vice-Chairman. No such doctor however appears to have been employed.

The Hospital's property did not remain inviolate during the war. The Ministry of Aircraft Production requisitioned a ten-acre field at Moulton Park Farm, later purchasing it outright, while the Royal Observer Corps established an observation post at Bryn-y-Neuadd and were extremely reluctant to release it after the end of hostilities. In 1942, the Air Training Corps was allowed to use the cricket field on condition that they provided petrol to enable the grass to be cut; in 1944, the US Army was given permission to play baseball there. Repairs to and redecoration of the buildings were limited to what was essential but old medical equipment was replaced by new whenever possible.

Throughout these years, the Board of Control was sympathetic towards the Hospital's problems and enthusiastic about its achievements and its exceptional facilities for treatment. Its high standards, its Commissioners noted, were not impaired by the war; the food, supplemented from the Moulton Park Farm, was generous and the buildings kept in excellent order. The visiting Commissioner in October 1944 recorded that: 'Progress continues in every direction possible in war-time. All modern methods of treatment are being employed, and this year it is believed that the turn-over of patients will reach record figures'.

The form of the Annual Reports underwent changes during Tennent's superintendency. In 1940, the reports of the Board of Control Commissioners, which had previously been placed immediately after that of the Chairman, were relegated to the back; after 1956 they were omitted altogether. At the same time, the impressive array of statistical tables was dispensed with, either because of wartime conditions or on Tennent's recommendation; the only one retained was the General Table showing the movement of the Hospital population – the total numbers of cases treated, discharged, transferred, etc., during the year under review. The names of the consulting physicians and surgeons were now shown for the first time.

With the end of hostilities, staff began returning to St Andrew's, among them male nurse Thomas Myles who had been awarded the DSM while a sergeant in Burma; the Management Committee presented him with a gold watch. Altogether seventy had served in the Armed Forces, two of whom had been killed and one seriously wounded. Two of the Assistant Medical Officers had also been called-up. Rear-Admiral Wellwood G. C. Maxwell, who had served with distinction during and after the First World War and who had been called back into the Navy from retirement in 1939, was knighted for his services in 1943. In 1945 Lt. Col. Sir Gyles Isham, 12th Bt., of Lamport Hall, having served in the Western Desert and Palestine, was elected a Governor of the Hospital. It was also in 1945 that Tennent, with the full approval of the Management Committee, was appointed Examiner to London University for the degree of Doctor of Medicine in Psychiatry and for the Diploma in Psychological Medicine.

A somewhat sad association with the past occurred in 1943. The 7th Earl Spencer, a member of the Management Committee, wrote that year as Chairman of the Northampton Yeomanry Association to Sir Kenneth Murchison, reminding him that in 1828 the Northampton Yeomanry had voted £6,000 to help erect the original Asylum and that there was an unwritten agreement that the Governors in their turn should help the Yeomanry when in need. The Hospital had in fact donated £500 to Yeomanry funds at the end of the Boer War. Help was needed again and it was agreed to give £1,000 if approved by the Charity Commissioners. Approval, however, was not forthcoming.

Consideration of the mental health services needed in the future did not cease during the war and, if anything, was given greater impetus through the publication in 1942 of the Beveridge Report on Social Insurance and Allied Services. The need for an integrated medical service, instead of the complexity of voluntary, municipal and Public Assistance hospitals, became clear. The wartime Emergency Medical Service, divided into twelve regions, was to become the framework of the National Health Service, each region under the authority of a Regional Hospital Board.

While the Minister of Health became the ultimate authority for mental health, the Board of Control remained an independent organisation with the right to visit hospitals and review individual cases.

The Registered Hospitals, whose Superintendents met for consultation from time to time, agreed in principle in 1943 that they should continue apart from the Municipal Hospitals but should join the British Hospitals Association. That year, they decided at a meeting of Chairmen and Superintendents, attended by Sir Kenneth Murchison and Tennent, to form an Association of Registered Hospitals of which Tennent was elected the first Chairman, his expenses paid by the Hospital. In 1945, Tennent stated that Sub-Committees of the Royal Medico-Psychological Association, the British Medical Association and the Royal College of Physicians had recommended in a memorandum, entitled 'The Future Organisation of the Psychiatric Services', that the Registered Hospitals should carry on as before. When the Health Services Bill was published, Murchison and Tennent had talked to Dr Hill, later Lord Hill of Luton, who was then Secretary of the British Medical Association, to Lord Moran and Sir Arthur Rucker, Deputy Secretary of the Ministry of Health, to press the case of the Registered Hospitals which were now, it had been decided, to be integrated into the National Health Service.

In September 1947, a formal letter was received from the Ministry, saying that St Andrew's, according to the Act, came under the Oxford Regional Hospital Board, which would be responsible to the Minister of Health for all hospitals in the area. The Minister, however, had power 'to disclaim any hospital, the transfer of which will not be required for the purpose of providing hospital and specialist service'. If it was desired that a particular hospital should be disclaimed, the Minister would be glad to consider any reasons put forward to support that view. The Hospital took appropriate action. In May 1948, it was announced that only four of the Registered Hospitals were to be disclaimed, namely Cheadle Royal, Barnwood House, The Retreat, York, and St Andrew's. Tennent was delighted. He reported with great satisfaction that the Hospital was to be allowed to function outside the National Health Service. 'The history and present status of Registered Hospitals show that they have been responsible for much of the pioneer work and progress in psychiatry, quite out of proportion to their relative size. We are of the opinion that this progressive outlook and approach can better be maintained by an independent management.' Nevertheless the Registered Hospitals' Association was disbanded that year.

St Andrew's, fully aware of its responsibilities, offered to place beds in the Hospital at the disposal of the National Health Service, an offer accepted by the Oxford Regional Hospital Board. During the years under review, some fifty-six to eighty beds, the number varying according to circumstances, were reserved for the Regional Board, the fees in general keeping pace with the average maintenance cost of a patient.

With the war barely ended, immediate steps were taken to improve the facilities of the School of Occupational Therapy. A hut was built in the grounds to provide extra accommodation for students, twenty of whom were now being admitted annually. In October 1945, Tennent visited hospitals and institutions in Edinburgh, Dumfries, Chester and Loughborough with a view to designing, in co-operation with the architect, a new building for the Ocupational Therapy Department. In 1946, he stated that arrangements had been made to train students for the full Diploma of the Association of Occupational Therapists, a three-year course. In the past, St Andrew's had offered training in the psychological side but had had to go elsewhere for orthopaedic training. Now, thanks to the Manfield Hospital, Northampton, which had granted orthopaedic training facilities, and to the continuing help of the Northampton School of Art, the complete curriculum could be carried out in Northampton.

Permission to build the long-contemplated Occupational and Recreation Unit, consisting of a reading room, library and physiotherapy department and to include a gymnasium, squash court and swimming pool, had the full approval of the Management Committee, but funds could not yet be made available. In the meanwhile, full-time appointments of a male and female supervisor for physical recreation were made, encouraged by the Central Council of Physical Recreation.

In 1949, it was arranged for the occupational therapy students to gain orthopaedic experience at the Hospital of St Cross, Rugby, at the Thorpe Hall Rehabilitation Centre, Peterborough, and at Creaton Sanatorium as well as at the Manfield Hospital. By 1952, further training facilities for students, whose numbers were slowly increasing, were made available at the Northampton General Hospital and at the St Edmund's, St Crispin and Danetree Hospitals. The Arts and Crafts Exhibition remained an annual fixuture in the Hospital's calendar.

Tennent pointed out in 1957 that, if St Andrew's was to remain in the forefront, the Occupational and Recreation Unit was essential, especially as Cheadle Royal had opened its own that year, but funds and rising costs were still a problem. The architect, P. R. Rees Phillips, submitted revised drawings for the unit in May 1959. In February 1960, with no decision yet reached, Tennent stated that, in view of its size and cost of nearly £70,000, he felt that a full commitment by the Committee was essential. Approval was thereupon given, an appeal launched, which by 1961 had brought in

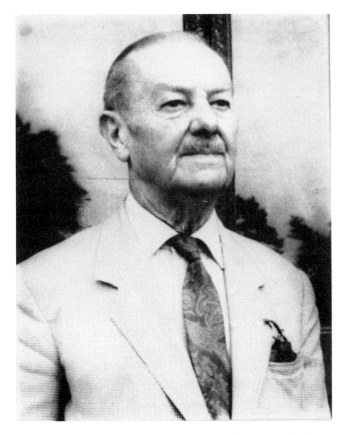

Sir Frederick V. L. Robinson, 10th Bt., MC, Chairman 1949–56.

£10,500, and the construction set in motion. It was sufficiently advanced by the end of 1961 for its official opening in May 1962 by HRH the Duchess of Gloucester (now Princess Alice, Duchess of Gloucester) to be considered.

Another important addition to the Hospital's facilities had been the opening, in spring 1950, of a Preliminary Training School for nurses; a fee of £10 was charged for the eight-week course, excluding meals. The old Turkish baths at Wantage House were converted for this purpose. The Board of Control considered it a great asset to the Hospital and an attractive way of recruiting junior nursing staff. Members of the General Nursing Council visited the Training School in 1953 and recommended the provision of extra equipment, for which £300 was allocated.

Tennent continued to emphasise the importance of research. In 1947 he had visited hospitals and clinics in North America to investigate recent developments there. He reported that all institutions, comparable in importance to St Andrew's, had research departments well-provided with funds. While, however, conscious of various shortcomings, he reported that he was gratified by the comparatively high standards maintained at St Andrew's.

In 1952 Dr T. McLardy, MBE, with a brilliant reputation in the field of neuro-pathological research, was appointed Pathologist, Biochemist and Bacteriologist at Wantage House. During his years at St Andrew's, he carried out much research and read papers at medical congresses both in Europe and North America.

The pattern of medical treatment changed considerably during the post-war period. In 1945, for example, forty-six major operations were carried out, thirty-five of which were pre-frontal leucotomies. In 1946, Dr Michael Partridge, with much experience of psychiatry in both England and the United States, had been engaged to carry out research into the merits of the pre-frontal leucotomy operation, a task completed to Tennent's satisfaction by 1949. Treatment by insulin and convulsive therapy was also then in regular use and in 1948 the Hospital was asked by the Admiralty to accept naval nurses for training in the former technique.

By 1958, while treatment by insulin and by convulsive therapy was still available, the use of the former in the treatment of schizophrenia had been diminishing through the introduction of tranquillising drugs. Caution, according to Tennent, was required when dealing with these drugs, since their side-effects had not always been fully tested; in general, however, they had proved of great benefit, particularly in psychotic forms of illness – and at times the improvement was described as dramatic. The pre-frontal leucotomy operation was less and less used as, indeed, was the operating theatre. In 1960, only five major and three minor operations were performed; only one of these was a pre-frontal leucotomy. During this period, the average daily number of patients began to decline, partly as a result of the effective use of tranquillising drugs and partly because of rising fees.

Great financial difficulties were experienced in the post-war years. At the Budget meeting in March 1948, Tennent pointed out that in 1947 wages were £11,000 more than in 1946, and this was £35,000 higher than four years previously. The Management Committee may have been slow in meeting the wage demands of organised labour but, by 1944, wage scales were being recommended by such bodies as the Rushcliff and Hetherington Committees, the former covering nursing staff and the latter domestic staff, which could not be ignored. Once these scales had been accepted, it became virtually impossible to ignore subsequently recommended increases. Consultation with other hospitals showed that all were in the same position. All sections of the hospital staff were included in these increases which reflected the generally inflationary situation. Repairs, replacements and improvements were also becoming ever more expensive. Under these circumstances, patients' fees had also to be raised and so the charitable funds inevitably decreased: nevertheless, by 1957, more than £22,000 was available to assist patients.

The Confederation of Health Service Employees, formerly the Mental Health and Institutional Workers Union, was long refused recognition by the Management Committee, in spite of consistent pressure and support by other Unions. In May 1946, the Committee was persuaded to allow a ballot to discover whether the employees favoured being represented by this Union, a condition being that the vote was counted by Sir Kenneth Murchison and Sir Wellwood Maxwell. When the vote was found to be 225 in favour and only 102 against, recognition was accorded to the Union.

Finding suitable nursing staff remained difficult. In 1952, it was agreed that Afro-Asian students could be engaged as nurses. In 1953, the Roman Catholic Chaplain, the Rev. E. M. Phillips, first appointed in 1950, stated that there were 105 Roman Catholics on the staff including Irish, French and Austrian girls. In the following year, the Superintendent announced that many of the European nurses were proving unsatisfactory, the Austrian girls tending to marry locally, and that he hoped to recruit male nurses from Nigeria, as those from Jamaica had been a success. In 1961, the Roman Catholic Chaplain reported that seven different nationalities were employed, including a number of Spanish nurses, for whom he was arranging visits by a Spanish priest. Tennent reported that he could not employ State Registered Nurses because they suffered a drop in wages if they worked for a mental hospital. Permission was accordingly given for this loss in wages to be made good.

In 1956, the Board of Control Commissioners referred to the increasing difficulties at St Andrew's in recruiting staff, without stating whether or not this problem was encountered at other hospitals. The staff, they reported, were of many nationalities, which created language difficulties, but it was remarkable in spite of the lack of qualified women how high the nursing standards remained. The staff shortage extended to domestics, although a group of some thirty mental defectives, working on license, were proving most useful. The greatest difficulty was at Moulton Park where, because of its isolation, there was only one sister and two nurses with no cook or domestic staff whatever to look after some thirty-eight patients. The cooking was done by the nurses and many of the patients helped with the housework.

Another problem was the Superannuation Fund. Admittedly it had many shortcomings. So narrow was its constitution that, for example, a nurse who after twenty-seven years service had to retire to look after her widowed and invalid father, could not receive a pension because she was only fifty-one. There was, moreover, no provision for widows nor for inflation. In other respects, also, the Hospital's pension plan did not compare favourably with the National Health Service Superannuation Scheme. It was accordingly decided in 1948 to seek the advice of actuaries on the relative merits of the two schemes and on the question of widows' pensions.

The actuaries, Messrs Bacon & Woodrow, London, reported in 1949 that the employees' contributions were inadequate. A Sub-Committee, consisting of Lord Spencer, Sir Wellwood Maxwell and Mr H. C. M. Stockdale, son of H. M. Stockdale (jnr) and a Governor since 1938, agreed in 1950 to recommend increased contributions by the staff, according to their grade, and to ask for wider investment powers to be granted to the Trustees of the Superannuation Fund; these were subsequently given by the Charity Commissioners and Messrs Robert Benson, Lonsdale were appointed investment advisers. It was however not until 1957 that a scheme, backed by the Hospital's assets, to provide benefits comparable to those granted under the National Health Service scheme, including pensions for widows, was adopted.

In spite of these financial difficulties, the Hospital's properties were kept in good repair. Modern office systems and machinery were introduced. Equipment in the operating theatre was updated as necessary. Two new houses adjoining St Andrew's were acquired in the early fifties for patients and staff. In 1954, the rebuilding of the blitzed site was completed, providing private rooms for male patients together with a dining- and sitting-room, the cost of which was far greater than War Damage Refunding. The repair and renovation of the boiler plant and heating services became necessary in the mid fifties at considerable expense. A start was made in 1955 to provide wards with built-in wardrobes, hand basins, bedside lockers and wooden bedsteads. Television was made available, through an ample provision of sets, to all who could benefit. Through the initiative of a Northampton ladies' hairdresser, a salon for hairdressing and beauty treatment, paying 15 per cent of the profits to the Hospital, was established. The golf-course was extended to nine holes and the bowling green completely returfed.

The Hospital's farm of some 600 acres at Moulton Park and the extensive vegetable gardens at St Andrew's had, for many years, provided the Hospital with milk, meat, fruit and vegetables. Profits were usually satisfactory, although there were losses in 1943 and 1945, and patients capable of gardening and working on the farm derived much benefit therefrom. Even if the return on capital employed was sometimes commercially unsatisfactory, it was more than balanced by the therapeutic advantages obtained.

Post-war conditions, however, especially the escalation of wages, made it increasingly difficult to achieve a profit. The Farm and Grounds Sub-Committee, under the successive chairmanship of Captain G. E. Bellville, Sir Gyles Isham, Lieutenant-Colonel R. L. Findlay and Lieutenant-Colonel R. A. Collins, devoted much time and effort to the problem. In 1959, it was decided that it was no longer economical to grow vegetables at St Andrew's and the kitchen gardens were put down to grass. One source of pride was the outstanding success in the immediate post-war years of S. M. Gault, the Head Gardener, in winning Royal Horticultural Society prizes for produce grown at the Hospital; between 1945 and 1949, when he joined the staff of Messrs Sutton & Sons of Reading, he gained, among other distinctions, eleven gold medals.

Consideration was given on several occasions to selling Moulton Park Farm. During the 1950s the value of building land rose rapidly, owing to the expansion of Northampton town, and various parcels of land were sold at satisfactory prices.

The Hospital was fortunate in having a strong and dedicated Management Committee during these testing years. Sir Frederick V. L. Robinson, who had seen action in the South African and First World War, became Chairman in 1949; he was the great-nephew of the Rev. Sir George Robinson, who had fought so vigorously to establish St Andrew's in its early years. Sir Frederick had at first the support as Vice-Chairman of Lord Braye, and then of Sir Wellwood Maxwell, a most capable Chairman of the Finance Sub-Committee. He and Sir Frederick retired in 1956 and were succeeded as Chairman and Vice-Chairman respectively by Sir Gyles Isham and by Admiral Sir Geoffrey Hawkins of Grafton Underwood, Kettering.

Sir Gyles, born in 1903, brought to his chairmanship, which he retained until 1973, a keen imaginative intelligence together with a great capacity for hard work. The Management Committee's Annual Report now became much longer and far more detailed; those who received copies were taken into the Committee's confidence as never before, which must have helped in raising funds for the new Occupational Therapy Unit and other projects. Sir Geoffrey Hawkins, born in 1895 and married to a daughter of the 7th Duke of Buccleuch, had served with distinction in both World Wars; he retained his office until 1964.

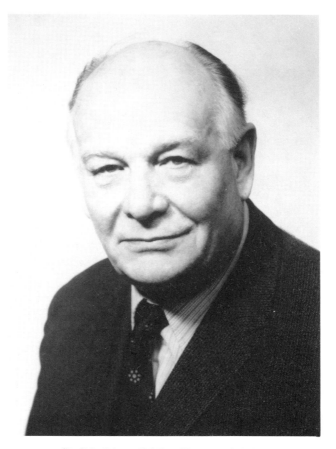

Sir Gyles Isham, 12th Bt., Chairman 1956–73.

Lieutenant-Colonel R. L. Findlay of Naseby Woolleys, Rugby, became Chairman of the Farm and Grounds Sub-Committee, in succession to Sir Gyles; he resigned in 1960 on leaving the county, succeeding to a baronetcy in 1962. His successor as Chairman was Lieutenant-Colonel R. A. Collins.

The contribution made by the 7th Earl Spencer was outstanding. Elected a Governor in 1920 as Viscount Althorp, he succeeded his father in 1922. In 1943, he joined the Management Committee and the Furnishing and Decoration Sub-Committee, revealing the thoroughness with which he applied himself to the many responsibilities he undertook. He became a member of the Expenditure Sub-Committee in 1948. On becoming, like his father, Lord-Lieutenant and therefore the Hospital's Perpetual President in 1952, he continued as a Trustee both of the Hospital and of the

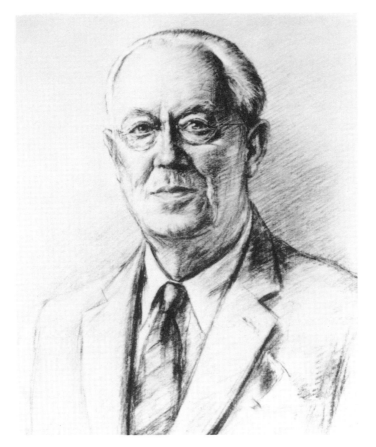

The 7th Earl Spencer, TD, President 1952–67.

Superannuation Fund, duties which he had first undertaken in 1947. He took a close interest in all aspects of the Hospital's work, but it was to the investment fund and the superannuation scheme that he particularly directed his attention. He attended regularly both the Management Committee and the Finance Sub-Committee meetings: only after the Trust Deeds for the new Superannuation Scheme had been satisfactorily completed did he resign his trusteeship in 1961. His two fellow Trustees were Mr, later Sir John Hobson, MP, who in 1960 agreed to serve on the Law and Parliamentary Committee of the Association of Independent Hospitals of which St Andrew's was a member, and H. C. M. Stockdale. A fourth Trustee during 1950–4 was W. A. R., later, Sir William Collins, Chairman and Managing Director of William Collins, the publishers, who made several generous donations of books to the Hospital's library.

Mr Stockdale announced at a meeting of the Finance Sub-Committee in February 1958 that he had seen a representative of Personnel Administration Ltd., management consultants, who were prepared to carry out a preliminary survey into reducing expenses, as wage increases over the previous two years had added £18,000 per annum to the cost of running the Hospital. In May, the consultants reported that they could cut running costs by £15,000 per annum without lowering the Hospital's standards, for which their fee would be £2,500 for approximately four months' work. This was accepted, although the Superintendent declared that he refused to co-operate so far as the medical staff was concerned; they were therefore excluded from the investigation.

The consultants' first report in March 1959 was primarily concerned with office procedures, the equipment used and the re-organisation of the administraton. The most controversial recommendation was that the Medical Superintendent should be relieved of the administration, much of it of minor importance, with which he was too much occupied, and that this should become the responsibility of an Administrative Officer. This proposal was resisted strongly by Tennent. If this new officer was to be on the same level as himself, he was prepared to resign; he had in 1938 turned down the appointment of an administrative officer, arguing that it would lead to dual control and therefore to much friction. The consultants, however, pointed out that this recommendation represented standard modern hospital organisation. It was eventually decided that an Administrative Officer should be appointed with clearly defined duties, that he should be guided by the general directions of the Medical Superintendent, who was to remain in overall charge, and that he was to be directly responsible to the Management Committee for administrative matters. The Committee was anxious to retain Tennent's services and this arrangement was accepted by him.

Three further reports were discussed that summer. They covered cost control techniques and staffing, office routines and the need for more publicity about St Andrew's; teaching hospitals and all provincial psychiatrists and general practitioners needed to be circularised with literature about the hospital. Sir Gyles, in his 1959 report, said that the recommendations so far approved should enable the Hospital to effect savings of some £8,200 per annum, and that the changes so far made had reduced running expenses by about £6,000 per annum. He also announced the appointment of Lieutenant-Colonel J. W. M. Hipkin as Administrative Officer. Hipkin had relieved the Medical Superintendent of all non-medical administrative work and was responsible, subject to the general direction of the Superintendent, for the condition and state of repair of the hospital buildings, works and equipment. His first report appeared in the 1960 Annual Report.

One recommendation which was not accepted, at least for the time being, was that Bryn-y-Neuadd should be closed down. This rest home and estate with its tenanted farm continued to be used throughout Tennent's superintendency. Both he and the Management Committee were convinced of the beneficial effect of holidays there, especially on patients long-resident in St Andrew's. In 1959 Mr Geoffrey Nickson of Conway, and in 1961 Lieutenant-Colonel H. G. Carter of Beaumaris, Anglesey, joined the Management Committee with a watching brief over the home.

In 1959 there was a major step forward in the nation's attitude towards the mentally ill and the administration of the services provided. In a debate in February 1954 Mr, now Sir Kenneth Robinson, then Labour Member of Parliament for St Pancras North and later Minister of Health, 1964–8, declared in the House of Commons:

> That this house, while recognising the advances made in recent years in the treatment and care of mental patients, expresses its concern at the serious overcrowding of mental hospitals and mental deficiency hospitals, and at the acute shortage of nursing and junior medical staff in the Mental Health Service, and calls upon H. M. Government and the hospital authorities to make adequate provision for the modernization and development of this essential service . . . There are shortcomings, many shortcomings, but they are not the responsibility of any particular government; they are the responsibility of numerous successive governments, and of the local authorities as well, and are perhaps due even more to public apathy and ignorance.

A Royal Commission on Mental Illness and Mental Deficiency was set up under the chairmanship of Lord Percy. The Mental Health Act, 1959, was a long one, containing 146 clauses and 8 separate schedules, but it repealed 15 whole Acts and 37 Acts in part. The then Minister of Health, Mr Derek Walker-Smith, now Lord Broxbourne, explained to the House:

> They [the then existing laws] are certainly complex, difficult, and in many respects out of date. Consequently, in replacing the mosaic . . . of law and procedure produced by our fathers and forefathers with a single contemporary design, we are making a clean sweep. But this holocaust of the laws made by our predecessors does not carry any condemnation of their actions. They, particularly in the nineteenth and early twentieth

century, laboured for progress in their day as we do in ours. [He added]: One of the main principles we are seeking to pursue is the re-orientation of the mental health services away from institutional care towards care in the community.

In his report for 1960, Dr Tennent briefly explained the major innovations of the Act. The changes:

enable patients suffering from mental illness to obtain treatment in the same way as people suffering from physical illness, without formality. It is envisaged that by far the majority will be admitted on this basis. Provision has been made also for those patients who, in their own interests or for the protection of others, must be compulsorily admitted and detained in hospital. Where such is necessary, safeguards for wrongful detention have been provided even though the Magistrate has no part now in ordering the detention.

Both an admission and a treatment order had now to be made on the recommendation of two medical practitioners, while an emergency order, which was to last for three days only, had in future to be made by a Mental Welfare Officer or a relation of the patient and backed by one medical recommendation.

All forms of mental illness or disability, have been included in the single designation 'mental disorders'. Provision for compulsory detention recognises four groups of mentally disordered patients

1. Mentally ill
2. Severely subnormal
3. Subnormal
4. Psychopathic

The facilities of appeal against detention which have been provided with the establishment of Review Tribunals are welcomed . . . We hope that such provision will allay the anxieties of those whose stay in hospital may be prolonged particularly as if, on enquiry, the Tribunal are satisfied with the evidence, they have the power to discharge the patient. The New Act has been warmly welcomed by all of us.

The 1959 Act dissolved the Board of Control and transferred its functions of inspection and review of individual cases to Mental Health Tribunals, one to be established for each Regional Hospital Board. This ended a period of growing friction between the Board and the Hospital in the fifties. The causes of this friction are not clear from the records available but the Committee recorded that it was disturbed by the general attitude of the Commissioners at the end of their autumn 1957 visit and by the unhappy atmosphere they left behind them. The visit of a senior Commissioner was requested. It was also decided not, in future, to include the Commissioners' reports in the Annual Reports.

Chapter Twelve

RECENT DEVELOPMENTS (1962–1988)

O n Sunday, 28 January 1962, Dr Thomas Tennent died suddenly while holidaying in Switzerland. His death came only months before he had planned to retire after twenty-four years devoted service to St Andrew's. Sadly, he did not live to see his plan for a separate occupational therapy and leisure activities centre come to fruition. He had made many innovations in the treatment of patients and had helped keep St Andrew's in the forefront of psychiatric hospitals. Apart from his development of occupational therapy and recreational activities, he actively encouraged research within the Hospital. It was he who had persuaded the Governors that the pathology laboratory, in addition to carrying out routine investigations, should undertake fundamental research into the neuropathology of mental disorders and who engaged Dr McLardy.

On Dr Tennent's death, his deputy Dr D. J. O'Connell was appointed Medical Superintendent and Dr J. E. McLaughlan became his deputy. One of Dr O'Connell's first functions was to propose the vote of thanks to HRH the Duchess of Gloucester for opening the new occupational/recreational unit which was called Gloucester House. In the meanwhile, Priory Cottage, a large Victorian house which had become vacant on Dr Tennent's death, became the School of Occupational Therapy.

In the same year, the Governors decided to set aside £10,000 to carry out much-needed routine repairs and redecoration previously limited by post-war restrictions. This proved the start of a great programme of

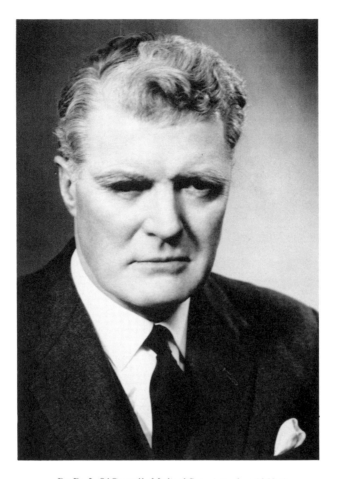

Dr D. J. O'Connell, Medical Superintendent 1962–6.

improvements which was designed to provide the best possible facilities for staff and patients.

For some years, the Governors had been concerned by the relatively high costs of maintaining Bryn-y-Neuadd, particularly as it was now only fully occupied for about four months in the year. In 1963 they decided to accept an offer from the Welsh Hospital Board who were anxious to secure a home in North Wales for the treatment of mentally impaired patients. It was hoped that most of the permanent staff there would be employed by the new owner but, in the event, only two were kept on.

In his report to the Committee for 1964, Dr O'Connell drew attention to the continuing change in the Hospital's population in that many more patients of advanced age were being admitted. He pointed out that much of

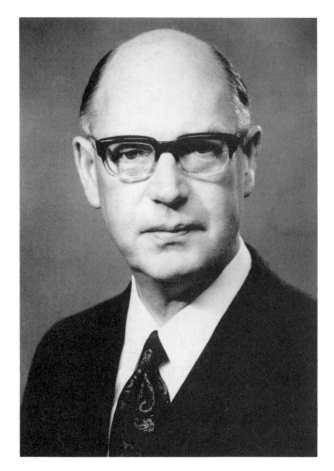

Dr James Harper, Medical Director 1966–75.

the available accommodation was not particularly suitable for nursing this type of patient and he suggested that consideration be given to providing a modern geriatric unit. This was to be actively pursued by Dr O'Connell's successor.

Dr O'Connell retired in April 1966 after thirty-nine years of loyal service to St Andrew's. The Committee held a number of meetings to decide on the appointment of his successor, assisted in their deliberations by Dr D. L. Davies, Dean of the Institute of Psychiatry. Seven candidates were interviewed and Dr James Harper, Medical Superintendent of Crichton Royal Hospital, Dumfries, was appointed, taking up his duties on 1 May 1966.

In his first report to the Committee, Dr Harper reviewed some of the major changes in the practice of psychiatry since the early 1950s. He pointed out that the number of patients in mental hospitals throughout the country had been falling in spite of continued high admission rates and that this was equally true for St Andrew's. This was because most patients required relatively short stays in hospital and very few young patients went on to become chronic hospitalised invalids. The fall in numbers of long-stay in-patients would have been even more dramatic had it not been for the increase in the admissions of elderly patients with dementing illness.

Dr Harper pointed out that there was a growing demand for private medical treatment, but that people's expectations of the standards of accommodation and of privacy were increasing. He presented a paper to the Governors outlining the developments which he felt were necessary if the Hospital was to retain its position of eminence. His suggestions were accepted by the Committee and they recommended that the following projects be undertaken:

That a new building for the Nurse Training School should be provided by converting some existing buildings.
That Wantage House be substantially upgraded.
That a modern psycho-geriatric unit be developed within the main hospital.
That consideration be given to the building of a new admission unit.

The Governors approached Mr K. J. Allsop, ARIBA of Messrs Gotch, Saunders and Surridge, as architect to the Hospital for all these works. To provide the necessary capital, the Committee looked to the sale of the land occupied by the farm at Moulton Park, some of which had already been sold off at satisfactory prices during the fifties, and the monies used to help pay for the building of Gloucester House. In 1965, the county boundaries were changed, whereby some 214 acres of Moulton Park farm land now came under Northampton Borough and thus fell within the bounds of the plans for development. Uncertainty over the land's eventual future made it difficult to farm effectively; its sale on the open market was impossible because planning permission would not be forthcoming until the new Town Development Corporation was established.

By 1969 seventy-six acres of land had been sold to the Northampton Corporation. The money, in accordance with the regulations of the Charity Commissioners, formed part of the Permanent Endowment Fund. This meant it could not be used to pay for repairs, but only for new buildings. In 1970, all the remaining land was sold to the Development Corporation. The original purpose of the farm had been to supply produce to the

Hospital, to provide some accommodation for suitable patients and possibly to be the site of the Hospital if circumstances made the Billing Road site untenable. The money from the sale of the farm was partly invested in property in the Lune Valley, while the remainder was used to pay for the new buildings, including the new admission unit.

Dr Harper in his Annual Report for 1967 had pointed out that Wantage House, though in its day a very advanced concept, had several defects. With the great increase in the number of short-stay admissions, it was no longer large enough. Secondly, by modern standards, it was rather spartan and required considerable modernisation. The only way to carry out the work would be to close half the unit at a time and this, he felt, would interfere disastrously with the work of the whole Hospital. He expressed the opinion that a new admission unit was an urgent necessity. The opening of such a building would enable the necessary changes to be carried out in Wantage House and the two buildings would then be complementary to each other. Patients with minor nervous afflictions would be admitted to the new unit, while those with more severe illnesses requiring greater observation and nursing care would continue to be admitted to Wantage House.

The Planning Sub-Committee, accompanied by the architect Mr Allsop, visited a number of hospitals and nursing homes to study the most recent developments and to form an idea of the standard of accommodation which private patients might expect.

While plans for the new unit were being drawn up, a number of other projects in the list of proposals were pursued. The new School of Nursing was opened on 7 November 1967 by Dr J. O. F. Davies, Secretary of the Central Committee on Post-Graduate Medical Education, Royal College of Physicians. The third floor of the hospital building was brought into service by installing three lifts. The ward area was extensively and attractively modernised. This extra accommodation enabled the Hospital to accept fifty-three patients from Barnwood House in Gloucester which had closed down.

It was decided that the South Wing of the main hospital building should be adapted to form a comprehensive psycho-geriatric unit for both sexes. It was also agreed that the villas in and around the hospital grounds which provided accommodation for long-standing schizophrenic patients, although fulfilling a definite need, had a limited life span and should eventually be replaced with flats or bedsitting rooms.

In September 1970, work was started on the new admission unit. There was an initial set back, as the original contractor went into voluntary liquidation, but a new contract was negotiated with Messrs Simcock and

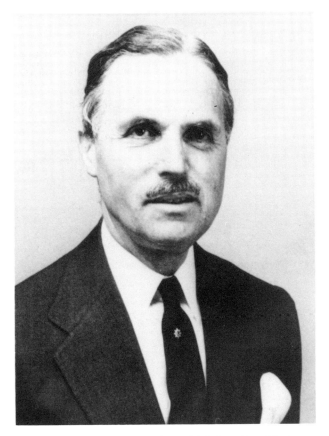

Lt-Col. John Chandos-Pole, CVO, OBE, President 1967–84.

Usher Ltd. Work was resumed in April 1971, and completed in time for the formal opening ceremony on 3 October 1972. This new building was named Isham House in appreciation of the work as Chairman since 1956 of Sir Gyles Isham, who had announced that he would be retiring from this post in 1973 and would be succeeded by Viscount Kemsley. Sir Gyles died in January 1976 after a short illness, having served as a Governor for thirty-one years and as Chairman for seventeen – a length of time exceeded only once in the Hospital's history.

Isham House was formally declared open by Lieutenant-Colonel John Chandos-Pole, President of the Hospital, in brilliant sunshine before an invited audience of 300. The principal guests were Lord Aberdare, Minister of State, Department of Health and Social Security, and the Mayor and Mayoress of Northampton, Alderman K. R. and Mrs Pearson.

This new building was planned, both in design and furnishings, to resemble a conventional hospital as little as possible. There were forty-six single bedrooms, of which thirty-six on the first floor had en-suite bathrooms. Each bedroom was equipped with a telephone and colour television. Public rooms included a commonroom opening on to a spacious terrace facing south across the Nene Valley. The clinical areas included individual consulting rooms and a treatment and recovery room. Some minor modifications have since been made internally, but the basic design has proved extremely successful. Most of the changes have been dictated by a need to provide more consulting rooms as the numbers of medical and paramedical staff have increased.

While Isham House was under construction, another additional building was planned and work started. This was the patients' social centre which joined on to Gloucester House to provide shopping and canteen facilities for patients and their visitors together with a hairdresser's salon and

The opening of Isham House, 3 October 1972. Left to right: Mr George Heritage, Dr James Harper, Sir Gyles Isham, Bt., Lord Kemsley.

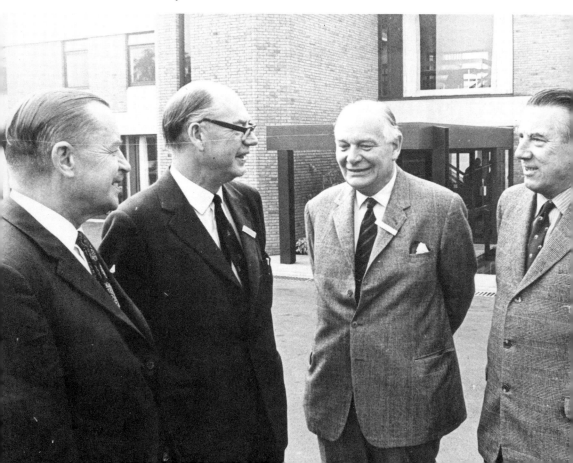

Beauty Centre. This facility was made possible by a generous gift from Mr G. R. F. Tompkins and was opened on the 3 July 1973 by the Duchess of Grafton.

These new buildings meant that the Hospital now had an admission campus including the admission units, Wantage House and Isham House, and a social, occupational and recreational centre formed by Gloucester House and the Tompkins Centre. Thus, it was well placed to face a future in which the continuing need for the main hospital building was somewhat uncertain. However, while this new construction work was in progress, extensive improvements and repairs had been carried out in the old building as well. By the end of 1973, all the patient accommodation in the North Wing had been upgraded and work had started to convert the South Wing into a modern psycho-geriatric unit.

Sadly, Sir Frederick V. L. Robinson, Bt., who had been a Governor since 1920 and Chairman from 1949 to 1956, when he became a Vice-President, died in 1975. His service to the hospital thus covered a period of fifty-five years. Dr James Harper also retired in 1975. On his arrival at St Andrew's, he had clearly seen the need for the Hospital to adjust to the changing demands in psychiatric treatment and had been responsible for the programme of building and reconstruction which left the Hospital well-equipped to meet the challenges of the time.

Dr Harper was succeeded by Dr Gavin Tennent, son of Dr Thomas Tennent, the former Medical Superintendent. Before his appointment, Dr Tennent had been Medical Superintendent at St Brendan's Hospital in Bermuda. He had previously held the post of Director of Research to the Special Hospitals, and had a particular interest in both forensic and adolescent psychiatry. Having grown up in Priory Cottage, he brought with him an extensive awareness of the history and traditions of St Andrew's but clearly recognised that to survive the Hospital had to provide new and different services.

He pointed out in his report to the Governors in January 1975 that:

St Andrew's has to face two different but related problems. First the alteration in the pattern of in-patient care and secondly the diversification of psychiatric interest in treatment programmes. The general pattern of care has moved from a model based on hospitals (and in-patient populations) to the treatment of the patient in the community.

St Andrew's was originally developed for the care and treatment of people living in Northamptonshire and there would seem to be a potential for the hospital to adopt a more community-orientated approach. There is almost certainly scope for the expansion of out-patient services, the development of various types of hospital accommodation and the provision of day care facilities for both the mentally ill and the psycho-geriatric patient.

Within the Hospital itself there is scope for the provision of more specialised treatment programmes both for the medium-stay patient, who requires rehabilitation and resocialisation, and for the short-stay patient for whom specialist care is required such as in an adolescent treatment.

These developments were rapidly initiated and St Andrew's embarked on the most radical change in both patient population and treatment philosophy in its history.

The time was favourable in many ways to this course of action. The major building works had been completed and the wards within the main Hospital could now be used as mixed sex wards with fairly limited structural alterations. The psycho-geriatric unit (named The Harper Unit in honour of Dr James Harper) was able to take the majority of very elderly or physically frail patients from other wards. The extra beds provided by Isham House allowed half of Wantage House to be used as temporary accommodation for patients, as other wards were altered or their function changed. However, the most vital factor was the particular talents of people holding senior staff posts and the co-operation they received from the Management Committee under the chairmanship of Lord Kemsley.

The Chief Administrative Officer at that time was Mr George Heritage He had joined the staff in 1928, some ten months after the opening of Wantage House, and had worked his way up the administrative ladder to become Secretary in 1948 and Administrative Officer and Secretary when the two posts were amalgamated on the retirement of Lieutenant-Colonel Hipkin in 1965. Heritage possessed an unrivalled knowledge of the Hospital and its workings and held the view that the purpose of administration was to facilitate the running of the Hospital – not to be an end in itself. His enthusiasm and energy remained unabated and, when he retired in 1979, his outstanding service to the Hospital over a period of fifty-one years was appropriately recognised by his being made a Governor. He is the only member of staff ever to have been honoured in this way. His place was taken by Mr David Harries, previously Head of Administrative Services with Kettering Health Authority.

The Director of Nursing was Mr David Smith, who had joined the hospital in 1974. Mr Smith had considerable experience in psychiatric nursing and was also much involved in the work of professional nursing

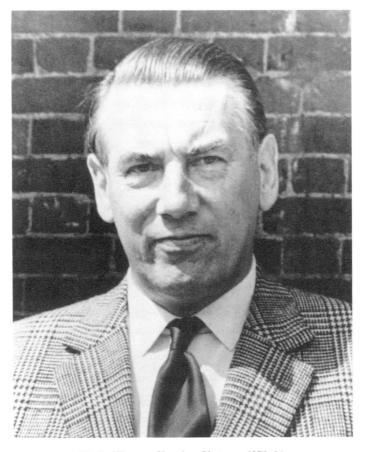

The 2nd Viscount Kemsley, Chairman 1973–84.

bodies. His range of contacts within nursing both in Great Britain and overseas was enormously helpful in finding places for staff to be seconded for special experience to help in developing specialised treatment units within the Hospital.

Finally, a key new appointment was made in October 1975 when Mr Anthony Bedford was appointed as Senior Psychologist. The post was originally set up in collaboration with Pfizers Pharmaceutical Ltd in order to carry out a joint research programme. Part of his time had been available for clinical work and he had demonstrated how valuable a contribution psychologists could make to the work of the Hospital. From

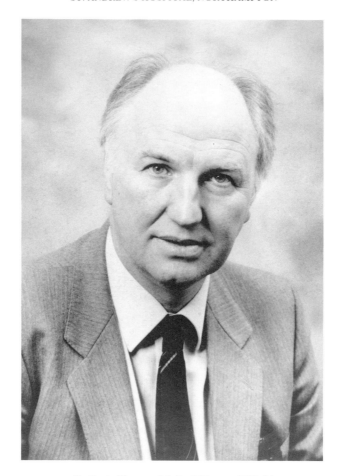

Dr Gavin Tennent, Medical Director 1975–84.

one psychologist in 1975, the department had grown by 1988 to five consultant psychologists supported by seven technicians.

Dr Tennent, from his involvement with forensic and adolescent psychiatry, had become aware of the lack of facilities within the NHS for adolescents with moderate to severe behaviour disorders. Such young people were often initially referred to the Child Guidance Service but, on attaining school-leaving age, were no longer regarded as appropriate for this facility. They then became the responsibility of the Social Services who could provide accommodation and care, but relatively little in terms of specific treatment. Most departments of adult psychiatry rightly took the view that, if such young people needed in-patient management, they were quite inappropriately placed in adult psychiatric wards. Inevitably, a substantial proportion of these youngsters came into conflict with the law and ended up in the penal system. While some responded to the 'short sharp shock' approach, a substantial number did not and then formed the young recidivist population.

Dr Tennent believed that it might be possible to help such young people by utilizing a behaviour management approach, with treatment extending over a period of a year to eighteen months. The Governors agreed that a small unit should be established on a trial basis and in January 1977 a ward was opened. It was called the John Clare Unit to commemorate the Hospital's most famous patient. The unit was run on a 'token economy system' designed to reinforce patients' positive behaviour and to discourage the negative aspects which lead to their rejection by ordinary society. In addition to the basic ward programme, most patients also had individual programmes allowing for immediate reinforcement of appropriate behaviour.

The ward programme was carried out by a multi–disciplinary team of doctors, nurses, psychologists, occupational therapists, social workers and ancillary staff. The need for clear communication between all members of the treatment team was recognised and there were frequent and regular meetings of all grades of staff with an emphasis on honest and frank expression of opinions.

The ethical dilemma inherent in any system designed to modify a person's behaviour, when that individual may be relatively unmotivated to change, was fully recognised by all those involved in the programme. It was decided that such methods were justifiable, given that a series of safeguards were incorporated and that these were themselves the subject of constant and continuing scrutiny and review.

The demand for the service of the unit rapidly increased and within a year of opening, there was a waiting list for admission. Certain lessons had been learnt even at this early stage. A suprisingly high percentage of patients were found to have some kind of psychiatric disorder in addition to their obvious behaviour problems. These disorders included schizophrenia, manic depressive illness and severe neurotic conditions. Most striking of all, however, were the high numbers who exhibited symptoms suggestive of underlying brain damage as revealed by detailed psychological testing and electroencephalographic studies. This finding led to the use of more purely medical forms of treatment than had initially been expected.

A second aspect which rapidly became apparent was that those patients who were less intellectually bright did less well than their fellows. This in part was due to the pace of the programme being too fast, and in part to their tendency to be exploited by their brighter colleagues. It was therefore decided to open a second unit for young people with both mild mental impairment and severe behaviour disorders. Both groups had a need for statutory education, and many had a need for special remedial education. A teaching department was therefore established.

In August 1977 a second unit was opened, named after Admiral Sir Geoffrey Hawkins, which was designed to take up to nineteen patients. In the same year, it was decided to develop a third unit along behavioural lines to take patients with a combination of severe mental illness and marked behaviour disorders. These patients present a major management problem both in the community and in ordinary 'open' psychiatric wards, because of their unwillingness to participate in treatment and their tendency to behave in an unpredictable and sometimes violent fashion. With the move towards open-door facilities both in traditional mental hospitals and in the newer general hospital psychiatric units, such patients have become increasingly unacceptable and have tended to drift into the penal system. The proposed solution has been the establishment of regional secure units within the health service. However, these have been slow to become established and, in some cases, have declined to take patients needing relatively long periods of in-patient care. This third unit, opened in the latter part of 1978, was called the Hereward Wake Unit to commemorate the long link between the Hospital and the Wake family.

While these developments were taking place in the main hospital building, the function of the admission units was also changing and developing. Throughout its history, St Andrew's has provided care and treatment for people with alcohol problems. However, there was no specific treatment programme for such patients and in 1976 it was decided to develop a special unit for this purpose. The patients would continue to be admitted to Isham House, but they would come under the care of one consultant who would have a specific team of therapists carrying out a treatment approach which emphasised the behavioural and educational aspects of the drinking problem. The course was planned to last 4–6 weeks and aimed to teach the patient alternative coping skills. The main methods used were intensive training in social skills, relaxation techniques, small group discussions and cognitive training. Follow-up of patients was recognised as being vitally important and, to help patients who found getting to Northampton difficult, follow-up sessions were arranged in Harley Street.

In parallel to the development of units with an essentially behavioural approach to treatment, a group psychotherapy unit was established in October 1977. Here treatment consisted of daily small group psychotherapy sessions, supplemented by a structured programme of relaxation therapy, recreational activities, projective art sessions and psychodrama. The programme was designed to last for a period of three months.

In 1977 Dr Peter Eames joined the consultant staff. He had served in the RAF as a neuropsychiatrist and had a special interest in the interface between psychiatry and neurology. One of his first tasks at St Andrew's was the establishment of a department of physiological measurement. The major task of this department was to carry out electroencephalography (EEG) but it was also equipped to do electromyography. Before the opening of this facility in May 1977, all patients who required EEG studies had been referred to St Crispin Hospital, Northampton. In the first six months, over two hundred recordings were performed. The finding that a substantial number of the young people in the behavioural wards had abnormal EEGs led to it becoming an almost routine examination in newly admitted patients. A later development was the use of ambulatory machines which allowed recordings to be taken while the patient went about his normal day's activities. By recording any abnormal behaviour during this time, it was possible to demonstrate whether there was any corollation between behaviour and the presence of any disorder in electrical brain rhythm.

Shortly after his arrival, Dr Eames also became responsible for the development of a unit which at the time was unique in the United Kingdom. He had long been interested in the rehabilitation of young brain-damaged people, a group for whom provision within the health service was far from satisfactory. He was aware that among people sustaining severe head injuries (usually as a result of road traffic accidents) there was a subgroup who, in addition to their physical and intellectual handicaps, developed severe behaviour disorders. Their unacceptable behaviour often led to them being excluded from ordinary rehabilitation units and sometimes resulted in their being treated in the so called 'back wards' of psychiatric hospitals. Dr Eames proposed that a small unit be established to try and treat this type of patient along behavioural lines.

It was realised that such a unit would require a high staff-to-patient ratio and that numbers could only build up slowly. Patients would be likely to have physical handicaps in addition to their psychological difficulties, so physiotherapy and speech therapy would need to be provided. The unit was opened in 1975, using the East Wing of Wantage House which had been suitably adapted. The unit was named after Lord Kemsley and rapidly became a focus of interest for all involved in the rehabilitation of the brain injured. Staff from the unit have lectured extensively both in Great Britain and overseas, while large numbers of people from a wide variety of professions have visited it.

The patients coming into the adolescent behavioural wards were mainly admitted either under sections of the Mental Health Act or under Court Orders relating to Child Care Legislation. In both, there was need for a considerable amount of social work and it was no longer possible for the one social worker employed by the Hospital to cope with the case load. In February 1979, Mrs Mary Lees was appointed Principal Social Worker with the task of developing a department of social work to meet the changing needs of the Hospital.

Another aspect of the Hospital's involvement with the community was the increasing use of voluntary helpers to supplement the work of the professional staff. While the Hospital throughout its history had made use of the good services of local people, their help had always been organised on a spare-time basis. A full-time Voluntary Organiser was appointed, who rapidly developed links with local schools and other youth organisations and encouraged children and young people to spend time helping in the Hospital as part of their community studies.

This development did not usurp the role of the Friends of the Hospital. The Friends saw their task mainly in the area of fund raising. Over the years their help had been of the greatest value in purchasing a wide range of items which has greatly contributed to the patients' comfort and entertainment.

Throughout the 1970s the demand for the Hospital's services continued to grow. The numbers of short-stay admissions went on rising, while a totally new population of medium-stay patients was being admitted to the main hospital wards. The length of time spent in hospital by the short-stay patients also diminished so that the actual work load of the staff became greater. In order to meet these demands, the number of staff employed in the medical and paramedical categories increased.

Apart from pressure on staff, the rising number of short-stay patients began to impose strain on the available accommodation. Although the original intention had been to run Isham House and Wantage House largely on parallel lines, there was a good deal of 'consumer resistance' to being admitted to Wantage, once Isham House was fully functional. Despite extensive modernisation, Wantage House's basic structure precluded the provision of *en suite* bathroom facilities, while the public rooms were small and rather gloomy. Consideration was given to the building of a second admission unit very similar in design to Isham House.

Meanwhile, two other developments were in hand: the establishment of a sheltered workshop and the building of a surgical/medical unit. It had been agreed that the old laundry building near the Bedford Road would be made available to Workbridge Enterprises, a charitable organisation, for use as a sheltered workshop on the understanding that a number of places would be available for suitable patients from St Andrew's. The hospital accordingly gave a donation of £40,000 to help with the reconstruction of the building, which was leased for a period of twenty-one years, the first two years rent-free.

In 1975, proposals were considered for the development of a new medical/surgical hospital in Northampton and Mr Christopher Davidge, a grandson of Christopher Smyth, the Hospital's Chairman from 1896 to 1932, was appointed Chairman of the Steering Committee for this project. It was agreed that, if the financing difficulties could be resolved, St Andrew's would make a site available and assist in the running and management of the hospital.

The Three Shires Hospital, as this surgical unit was now called, was to be built on the site of the grass tennis courts. The Charity Commissioners agreed to a scheme whereby St Andrew's donated £100,000 in return for three beds being available for patients from St Andrew's. The construction was finished slightly ahead of schedule in February 1982, and formally opened by HRH the Duchess of Gloucester on 18 May of that year.

During 1980, the Committee continued to examine the possibility of building a second new admission unit. It had to satisfy itself that there was a genuine need for such a unit and that it could not be achieved merely by adapting or extending existing accommodation. The architects showed that building a new unit was the better option. The site decided on was the south-west corner of the sports field, and Messrs Gotch, Saunders and Surridge were appointed architects.

In January 1981, the Committee approved the layout of the unit and at the time it was decided to meet half the costs from the Permanent Endowment Fund, the rest being met out of income. Tenders were received and the contract went to Linford (Midland) of Cannock. Work started in early August 1981.

The building of this new admission unit, to be called Spencer House to mark the long association between Lord Spencer's family and the Hospital, was at first beset with problems. Some unexpected ground fissures necessitated remedial work, and the extremely severe winter weather caused further delays. However, lost time was made up and the building was handed over to the Hospital on the 25 March 1983, just one month behind schedule.

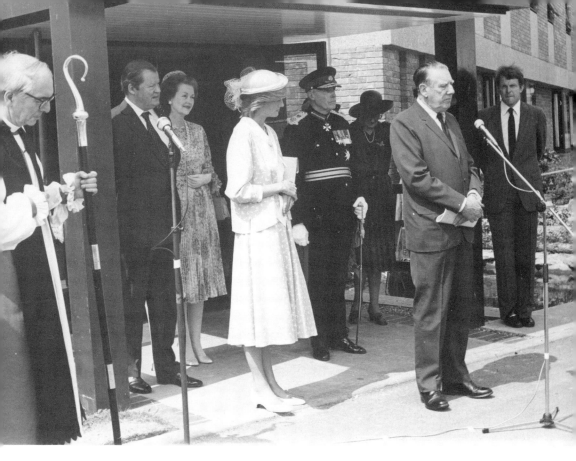

HRH the Princess of Wales being welcomed by Lord Kemsley at the opening of Spencer House, 12 July 1983.

The official opening of Spencer House, including the unveiling of a memorial plaque, took place on a warm and sunny 12 July and was performed appropriately by Lord Spencer's daughter, HRH the Princess of Wales, who arrived by helicopter to the great excitement of the assembled staff and patients. Before the opening ceremony, the royal party visited the psycho-geriatric wards where Her Royal Highness spent much time talking to the patients to their evident delight. Some 1,500 people lined the route from the main Hospital and were rewarded by Her Royal Highness stopping to speak to many of them.

The opening of this new unit occurred at a time when some marked changes were taking place in the provision of private psychiatric treatment in Great Britain. There had been a considerable expansion of private in-patient facilities, particularly in the the London area, mostly by profit-making American companies. This development meant, not only that there was increased competition for patients, but also for experienced staff. One advantage that these new units had was that they were sited in

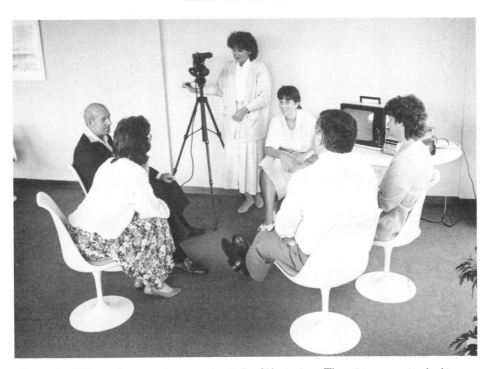

Occupational Therapy has come a long way since its 'craft' beginnings. Therapists are now involved in many forms of treatment.   ABOVE: *Social skills group.*   BELOW: *Orientation therapy.*

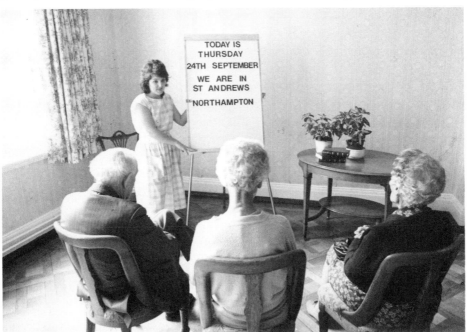

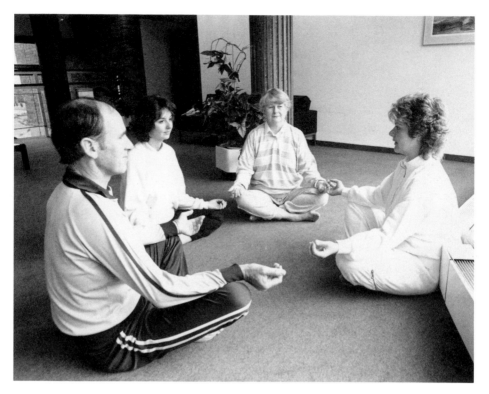

Relaxation class.

large centres of population and could thus provide in-patient treatment nearer the patient's own home. It seemed likely that St Andrew's would suffer a fall off in short-term admissions from the London and Birmingham areas.

Fortuitously, in February 1983, the Governors were approached by the Directors of Bowden House Clinic in Harrow-on-the-Hill. The clinic was experiencing financial difficulties and had been approached by an American company with a view to being taken over. The Directors however contacted St Andrew's as they felt that it would be more appropriate to be associated with a British charitable trust. After examining the legal and financial implications, the Governors decided to take over the running of the clinic, which took place on 23 June 1983. Dr David Curson, who had been in charge of the alcohol treatment unit at St Andrew's, assumed the day-to-day medical responsibility for Bowden House. It was appreciated that a considerable capital sum would need to be injected to bring the buidings up to the appropriate standard and to undertake desirable expansion, but it was also realised that the clinic was ideally situated for further development to meet the need for in-patient facilities in the Greater London area. In retrospect, 1983 can be seen as a year in which the Governors of St Andrew's decided upon a policy of expansion and development at a period when, for the first time in its history, the Hospital was facing serious, mainly American, competition.

This decision was influenced by the report of a Sub-Committee which had been established to carry out a study of the options open to the Hospital for its long-term development. The members of the Sub-Committee were Sir John Robinson, 11th Bt., grandson of Sir Frederick V. L. Robinson, Mr Arthur Jones, Conservative M.P. 1962–79, and Mr Simon Forster. Sir John, whose family had long been associated with St Andrew's, had been Deputy Chairman of the Management Committee since 1982. Their report was considered at a meeting of the Policy and Planning Sub-Committee on 18 March 1984. Though the report had been completed by December 1983, it was agreed that the Governors should have time to consider it in detail and be able to submit their own written assessments before discussing it.

The report began by recognising that the Hospital had to compete in an

Physical treatment plays an important part in therapy. Modern drugs enable many psychiatric disorders to be treated rapidly and effectively.

The pharmacy.

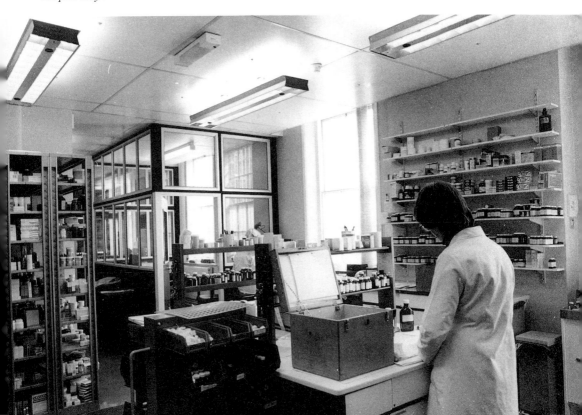

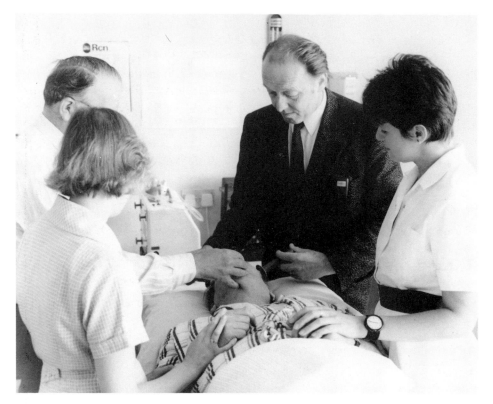

Some very distressed patients, who do not respond to drug treatment, may require electrical treatment.

increasingly commercial environment, while continuing to exercise its charitable role. It was also felt that its annual charitable contribution of some £500,000 was not sufficiently publicised.

There was considerable discussion as to the extent to which St Andrew's should change from a mainly Northampton-based charity to a more national enterprise with satellite units in different parts of the country. The conclusion was that such units might be developed as and when the opportunity arose but that to pursue an expansionist policy actively might place too great a strain on the resources of the Hospital both in management and financial terms.

Dr Tennent felt strongly that there was a need to develop such units. The behavioural wards were finding it difficult to discharge patients because of the lack of suitable facilities in the areas from which they had been admitted. He was not in favour of establishing a hostel in the Northampton area, as this would create a pool of former patients for whom the Hospital would have continuing responsibility and who would also make demands on the local social services. He also recognised that some of the young people being referred to the behavioural units did not require the level of security provided and might be better managed in a more open setting.

Some time previously, the senior medical and psychological staff had formed a limited company to develop private out-patient services in London and to offer management advice to other independent psychiatric units. Dr Tennent proposed that a new company be established to set up an adolescent unit independent of St Andrew's. A suitable site was found in Dorset and in due course a unit, originally called Spyways, was opened.

In the Sub-Committee's report, concern had been expressed that the development of separate units in this way and the involvement of medical staff in contractual arrangements with other organisations could lead to a conflict of interests. As time passed, these concerns became more marked. Early in 1985, after much discussion with the Governors, Dr Tennent decided to tender his resignation as Medical Director so that he could be more actively involved in the establishment of independent units.

In the period following Dr Tennent's resignation, a number of senior medical staff and psychologists also left the hospital to take up new posts. In the short term, this created problems of consultant cover in the behavioural wards but new staff were rapidly recruited and the work of the units was able to continue without too much disruption.

Shortly before these events, Lord Kemsley, having reached the statutory age, retired from the chairmanship. Sir John Robinson was elected in his place with Mr Arthur Jones as Vice-Chairman. The Committee under its new leadership was faced with the need to make urgent decisions about the future of the behavioural units. When the Sub-Committee considering the development of the Hospital had been taking evidence, a number of people had expressed concern that the development of the behavioural units might have a detrimental effect on the image of the Hospital which could lead to a falling off in admissions to the short-stay wards. The Committee felt that this view had not been substantiated but recommended that the proportion of beds allocated to the behavioural units should remain approximately the same.

As half Wantage House was not currently in use, it presented an opportunity for a major reconstruction of the wards occupied by the behavioural units, because patients could be moved there while building work was undertaken. The aim was to improve the facilities in each of these wards for the treatment and rehabilitation of a reduced number of patients.

The first major change was to move the John Clare Unit from the third floor down to the second, and to move Nesbitt Lodge Ward, which was an

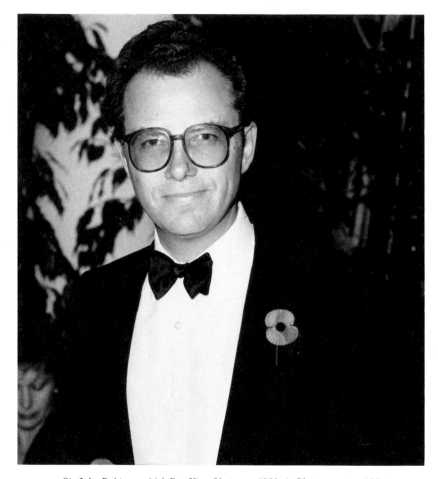

Sir John Robinson, 11th Bt., Vice-Chairman 1983–4, Chairman since 1984.

open rehabilitation ward, up to the third floor. Structural alterations were carried out so that the new Nesbitt Ward had two self-contained flatlets which gave patients the opportunity to practice the skills required to survive independently in the community before they were discharged. The ward was organised so that patients could progress from the very structured and supportive environment of the other units to the more demanding situations they would face outside hospital. The inevitable problems which arose could now be dealt with by staff who were familiar with the patients and who had the full resources of the behavioural units at their disposal.

Having completed the changes on the John Clare Unit and Nesbitt Lodge Ward, major alterations were started in the Hereward Wake Ward.

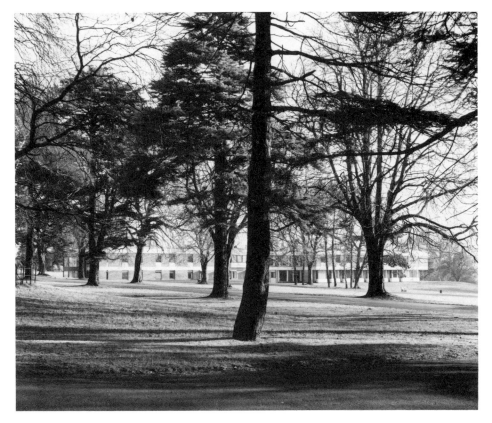

Isham House.

This unit dealt with the most severely mentally disturbed patients in the Hospital, many of whom were referred to St Andrew's because the hospitals in their own locality could not cope. The ward had always presented major structural problems and, in order to improve substantially the working environment, major alterations were put in hand. The bed number was reduced from thirty-one to twenty which allowed for the development of greatly improved day rooms and dining facilities. All this work was accomplished in a remarkably short time and was virtually completed by August 1985.

Now that the patients had been moved back to their own wards, the future use of the East Wing of Wantage House, now vacant again, could be tackled. This was one of the many tasks facing Dr John Henderson when he took up the post of Medical Director in that August. Dr Henderson came to the Hospital from the World Health Organisation, where he had been

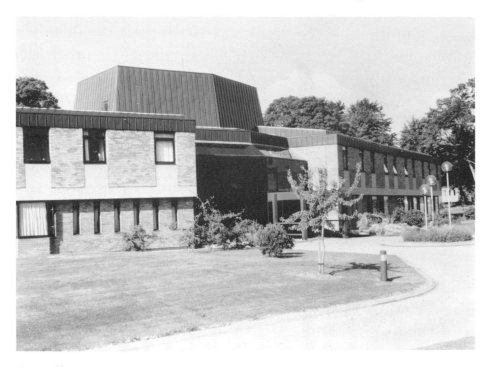

Spencer House.

Regional Officer for Europe with responsibility for establishing and developing mental health programmes. Prior to joining the World Health Organisation, he had been Principal Medical Officer to the Scottish Home and Health Department from 1972 to 1976 and before that Physician Superintendent at Bangour Village Hospital in West Lothian. Thus he brought to his new post a wealth of experience in medical administration.

Shortly after he took up his post, the Governors arranged a study weekend to re-evaluate the aims and purpose of the Hospital because many Governors had expressed the wish to have an opportunity to discuss topics in greater depth than was possible at monthly committee meetings. In this way a number of matters could be considered free from the usual pressures of urgent committee business. This weekend took place at Ettington Hall in November 1985 when Governors and senior hospital staff spent many hours in a free-ranging examination of a number of important subjects, some of them based on brief discussion papers submitted beforehand.

As a result of these exchanges, a number of changes in the management structure and function were proposed and subsequently considered by both

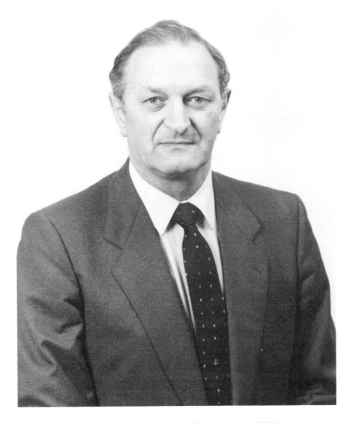

Dr John Henderson, Medical Director since 1985.

the Management Committee and the Bi-annual Court of Governors. It was agreed that, for a trial period, a number of existing Sub-Committees should be disbanded; Management Committee meetings should be reduced from monthly to quarterly, and a newly formed Finance and General Purpose Committee should meet monthly. The intention of these changes was to streamline the decision-making process to enable the hospital to respond more rapidly to changing circumstances. After a trial period, it was decided to revert to a monthly meeting of the Management Committee which was to be limited to nineteen Governors.

A major problem in effective management during the early 1980s was the relative slowness with which data could be produced and evaluated. Computers had been introduced into the work of the Hospital on a somewhat *ad hoc* basis and by 1985 there were systems in twelve different areas dealing with everything from clinical activities, such as attention

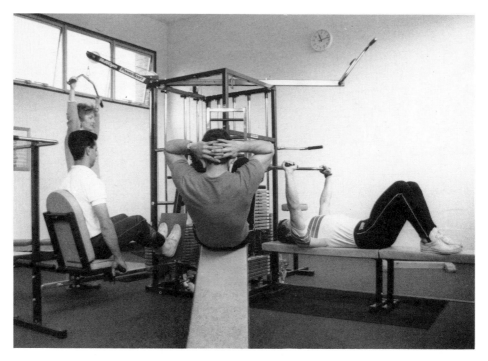

Physical recreation is an important facet of treatment. A multi gym provides a range of graduated exercise. The swimming pool was extensively rebuilt in 1988. ABOVE: *The multi gym.* ABOVE RIGHT: *The swimming pool, 1962.* BELOW RIGHT: *The swimming pool, 1988.*

retraining, to data searches in the medical library. In March 1985 the Management Committee approved the appointment of a Computer Technician and set up a Computer Sub-Committee. The Sub-Committee recommended that priority be given to the computerisation of the treasury accounting system which in turn would link to medical records and admissions. Provision of word-processing facilities was also recommended.

From 1985 onwards, the work of renovation and rebuilding continued unabated. The development of the behavioural units with the introduction into the Hospital of many young people had led to a far greater utilization of the sport and recreational facilities of the Hospital. The small gymnasium in the main Hospital was inadequate for their needs and in 1979 a new gymnasium was built on to Gloucester House. At the same time an additional squash court was added and, later, a sauna and jaccuzzi incorporated into the swimming-pool area.

It was recognised that the pool itself was reaching the end of its useful life and that a major rebuild would be necessary. The increasing use made of

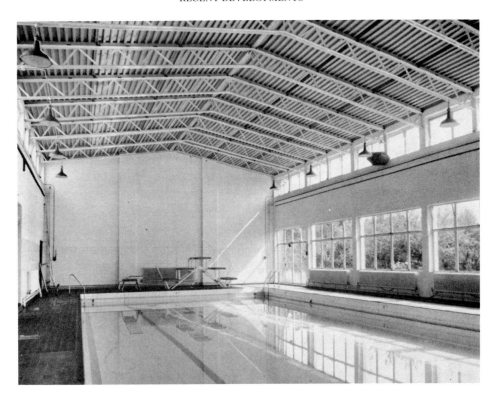

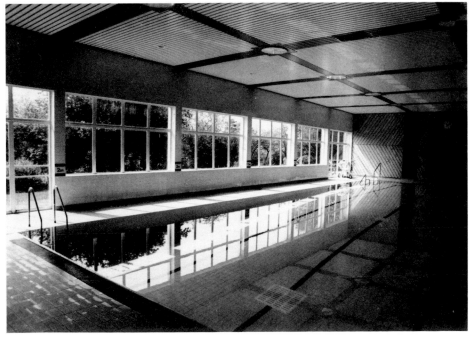

the pool by patients with physical handicaps, associated with brain damage, meant that the original step-down design was no longer appropriate; it was thought that a level-deck design would provide greater convenience and safety. The Management Committee commissioned a study of the possible alternatives that could be achieved within a certain budget. This study suggested that the pool could be improved with a more frequent water change-over, a new filtration plan for improved hygiene and a suspended ceiling to better condensation conditions. Work on the conversion was started in March and completed by September 1987. The new pool, much more attractive than the original rather spartan structure, proved very popular with both staff and patients. The improved sporting and recreational facilities were used not only by the young people on the behavioural units but also formed an integral part of the treatment programmes both for short-stay patients and for the physically fitter patients in the long-stay and elderly infirm wards as well.

The major undertaking during this period was to provide a new wing at Bowden House with twenty extra beds in a new building equivalent in standard of design to Isham and Spencer House. Patients would then be moved from the existing building into the new wing while extensive modernisation was carried out. Work began on the new building in the autumn of 1986 but took longer to complete than had been predicted, which made for difficult working conditions and the first patients were only admitted to the wing in January 1989.

In 1985 the Governors decided that the 150th Anniversary of both the founding and the opening of the Hospital should be celebrated by a variety of events starting in 1986 and continuing to the end of 1988. The first external event was an exhibition of the history of the Hospital which was staged for a month at the Abington Abbey Museum – appropriately in view of its previous connection with Dr Thomas Prichard, St Andrew's first Superintendent. The exhibition was a considerable success and attracted some ten thousand visitors.

The Hospital acted as host to a number of national and international conferences during the two-year period. In June 1987 the Intractable Pain Society held its spring meeting there; the topic, *Psychological Methods of Pain Control*, reflecting St Andrew's interest in behavioural techniques. In October 1987, the Kemsley Unit was the subject of a seminar for the Head Injury Social Work Group, and later in the same month a conference was organised by the nursing staff on the subject of *Nursing Skills in Specialist Units*. Nursing staff also organised two very successful conferences, the first on the management of aggression, and the second organised jointly with the Royal College of Nursing Mental Handicap Society.

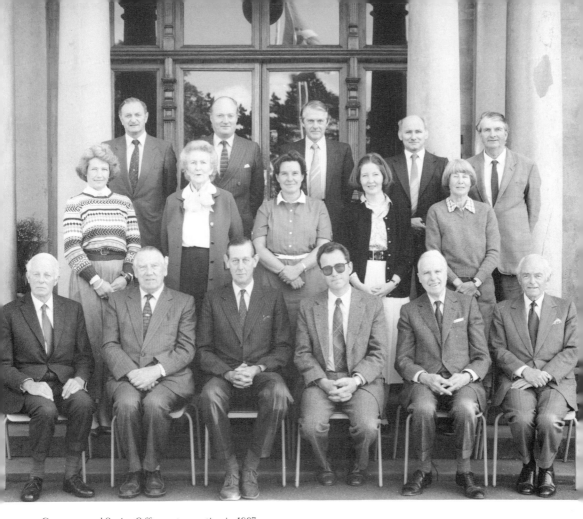

Governors and Senior Officers at a meeting in 1987.
Front row, left to right: Major Sir Hereward Wake (Vice-President); Lord Kemsley (Vice-President);
Mr J. L. Lowther (President); Sir John Robinson (Chairman); Lieutenant-Colonel John Chandos-Pole
(Vice-President); Mr Arthur Jones (Vice-Chairman).
Middle row, left to right: Mrs A. B. X. Fenwick; Mrs J. Morgan; Lady Juliet Townsend; Lady Braye;
Mrs H. C. Henderson.
Back row, left to right: Dr J. H. Henderson (Medical Director); Mr S. S. Forster; Mr D. R. Harries
(Admin. Officer); Mr J. P. McIntegart (Director of Nursing); Major J. M. Fearfield.

On Sunday, 19 June 1988, a special service was held in the hospital chapel by the Lord Bishop of Peterborough, the Rt. Rev. William Westwood. The final celebrations took place on the evenings of 4 and 6 November. On the Friday a firework display for patients, staff and families was staged in the hospital grounds. On the following Sunday, a Gala Concert was performed at the Derngate Theatre before an invited audience, attended by

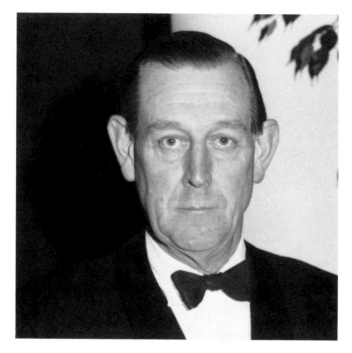

John Lowther, Esq., CBE, President since 1984.

the hospital's President Mr John Lowther, Lord Lieutenant of Northamptonshire, and the Mayor of Northampton, Councillor Ronald Liddington. The concert was given by the Northampton Youth Orchestra who accompanied two soloists, both of whom had previously won the Young Musician of the Year Award. The choice of orchestra and soloists was significant in that it symbolised the confidence with which St Andrew's views its own future and the challenges of the 21st Century.

ADDENDA

Presidents

1838–41	The 10th Earl of Westmorland, KG
1842–66	The 2nd Marquess of Exeter, KG
1866–72	The 3rd Lord Southampton
1872–1908	The 5th Earl Spencer, KG, PC
1908–22	The 6th Earl Spencer, KG, GCVO, PC
1922–51	The 5th Marquess of Exeter, KG, CMG, TD
1952–67	The 7th Earl Spencer, TD
1967–84	Lieutenant-Colonel John Chandos-Pole, CVO, OBE
1984–	J. L. Lowther, Esq., CBE

Chairmen of the Management Committee, 1838–1856
Chairmen during these years were elected at each Committee meeting. The following gentlemen
served in this capacity at one or more meetings: name and title are those finally held:

The 5th Duke of Grafton
The 2nd Marquess of Northampton
The 3rd Earl Spencer
The 4th Earl Spencer, KG
The 3rd Lord Southampton
The Hon Philip S Pierrepont
The Rt Hon R Vernon Smith, MP
The Rev Sir George Robinson, 7th Bt
Edward Bouverie Esq
The Very Rev Dr George Butler
Langham Christie Esq
Cary C Elwes Esq

The Rev R Geldert
Charles Hill Esq
The Rev J P Lightfoot
John Mercer Esq
Samuel Percival Esq
John Reddall Esq
Henry B Sawbridge Esq
Thomas Sharp Esq
William Smyth Esq
The Rev William Wales
Allan A Young Esq

Chairmen and Vice-Chairmen of the Management Committee from 1856 onwards.

1856–65	Rev. Sir George S. Robinson, 7th Bt.	William Smyth, Esq.
1865–70	William Smyth, Esq.	The Very Rev. Lord Alwyne Compton
1870–9	The 6th Duke of Grafton	The Very Rev. Lord Alwyne Compton
1879–82	The 6th Duke of Grafton	The Rev. Maze W. Gregory
1882–93	The 4th Marquess of Northampton, KG	The Rev. Maze W. Gregory
1893–7	The 4th Marquess of Northampton, KG	Christopher Smyth, Esq.
1897–1917	Christopher Smyth, Esq.	Lieutenant-Colonel J. Rawlins
1917–20	Christoper Smyth, Esq.	Rev. H. H. Crawley
1920–32	Christopher Smyth, Esq.	Sir Charles V. Gunning 7th Bt., CB, CMG
1932–8	Sir Charles V. Gunning 7th Bt., CB, CMG	Major A. H. Thurburn
1938	The Rt. Hon. Sir George Stanley, GCSI, GCIE, CMG	Sir Kenneth Murchison
1938–49	Sir Kenneth Murchison	The 6th Lord Braye
1949–51	Sir Frederick V. L. Robinson, 10th Bt., MC	The 6th Lord Braye
1951–6	Sir Frederick V. L. Robinson, 10th Bt., MC	Rear-Admiral Sir Wellwood Maxwell, KBE, CMG
1956–64	Sir Gyles Isham, 12th Bt.	Admiral Sir Geoffrey Hawkins, KBE, CB, MVO, DSC
1964–73	Sir Gyles Isham, 12th Bt.	Lieutenant-Colonel A. V. C. Robarts
1973–80	The Viscount Kemsley	Lieutenant-Colonel A. V. C. Robarts
1980–83	The Viscount Kemsley	Derek Lawson, Esq.
1983–84	The Viscount Kemsley	Sir John Robinson, 11th Bt.,
1984–	Sir John Robinson 11th Bt.	Arthur Jones Esq.

Members of the Management Committee from 1856 onwards.

The name, title and decorations listed are those finally held.
(* indicates life Vice-President)

The 5th Duke of Grafton	1856–63	
The 6th Duke of Grafton	1856–82	
The 3rd Lord Southampton	1856–63	*
The Rev. Sir George S. Robinson, 7th Bt.	1856–73	*
Edward Bouverie, Esq.	1856–7	
The Rev. Canon Henry J. Barton	1856–72	
Charles Britten, Esq.	1856–8	
The Rev. William Butlin	1856–78	
William Collins, Esq.	1856–71	
The Rev. Henry Crawley	1856–8	
James Mash, Esq.	1856–84	
John Nethercoat, Esq.	1856–67	
George Osborn, Esq.	1856–66	
William Smyth, Esq.	1856–72	*
The Rev. Chancellor William Wales	1856–88	
William Williams, Esq.	1856–62	
Cary Charles Elwes, Esq.	1856–8	
Henry Terry, Esq.	1856–71	
General E. W. Bouverie	1857–70	
The Rt. Rev. The Lord Alwyne Compton, Bishop of Ely	1858–80	*
The Rev. George Robbins	1858–71	
The 5th Earl Spencer, KG, PC	1859–67	*
H. O. Nethercote, Esq.	1860–85	
W. H. I. Mackworth Dolben, Esq.	1862–72	
The Rt. Hon. G. Ward Hunt, Esq., MP	1863–78	
William Grant, Esq.	1865–8	
The Hon. F. W. C. Villiers	1867–91	
Sir Rainald Knightley, Bt.	1867–91	
J. H. Webster, M. D.	1867–74	
H. M. Stockdale, Esq.	1868–71	*
The Rev. G. S. Howard Vyse	1868–93	*
Rev. Christopher Smyth	1869–94	*
The 7th Duke of Grafton, KG, CB	1870–9	
John Beasley, Esq.	1870–2	
Colonel S. G. Stopford Sackville	1871–1900*	
Rev. Maze W. Gregory	1870–1905*	
J. M. C. Fairclough, Esq.	1871–9	

J. H. B. Whitworth, Esq.	1871–8	
R. Lee Bevan, Esq.	1871–89	*
G. L. Watson, Esq.	1872–4	*
The Rev. J. P. Lightfoot	1874–88	
Dr W. A. Barr	1875–92	
The Rev. J. W. Field	1877–83	
G. L. Watson, Esq.	1877–91	
The 4th Marquess of Northampton, KG	1879–97	
Christopher Smyth, Esq.	1879-1932*	
The Rev. Sir Frederick L. Robinson, 9th Bt.	1879–91	
Sir George W. Gunning, 5th Bt.	1880–1903	
E. P. Monckton, Esq.	1883–1900*	
The Rev. Randolph Skipworth	1884–96	
Edward Grant, Esq.	1885–1909	
Lieutenant-Colonel John Rawlins	1885–1917*	
C. W. H. Sotheby, Esq.	1885–7	
Admiral Sir Drury Wake, KCIE, CB, RN	1887–91	
The Rev. H. H. Crawley	1890–1920	
The Rev. L. H. Loyd	1891–1905	
The Lord Knightley	1891–1932*	
Spencer Pratt, Esq.	1891–1901	
Lieutenant-Colonel F. E. Sotheby	1891–1907	
The Rev. A. A. Longhurst	1892–4	
F. H. Thornton, Esq.	1892–1904	
Herbert Sartoris, Esq.	1893–1900	
The 5th Lord Erskine	1894–1906	
Major Price Blackwood	1894–1902	
Lieutenant-Colonel John Henry Lowndes	1894–1906	
Henry Lloyd, Esq.	1896–1901	
The Rev. F. N. Thicknesse	1896–1906	
Henry Wickham, Esq.	1899–1905	
R. D. Carey, Esq.	1900–29	
Thomas F. Hazlehurst, Esq.	1900–16	*
C. Falconer MacDonald, Esq.	1900–20	
Colonel J. V. Nugent	1900–5	
H. M. Stockdale, (jnr.), Esq.	1903–31	*
B. Wentworth Vernon, Esq.	1903–5	
Major Alexander Bell	1904–9	
The Hon. E. A. FitzRoy	1905–15	
Sir Hereward Wake, 12th Bt.	1905–15	
A. H. Sartoris, Esq.	1905–35	

Sir Vere Isham, 11th Bt.	1906–18	
Sir Charles V. Gunning, 7th Bt., CB, CMG	1906–50	*
Colonel J. Hill, CB	1907–17	
Major Leslie Renton	1910–37	*
Colonel Henry Wickham	1912–22	*
The 7th Lord Vaux of Harrowden	1913–33	*
R. B. Loder, Esq.	1914–30	*
Gervase Elwes, Esq.	1916–19	
The 6th Lord Erskine	1919–45	
Major A. H. Thurburn	1920–38	*
Sir Frederick V. L. Robinson, 10th Bt., MC	1920–56	*
The 1st Lord Hesketh	1921–37	*
The 4th Lord Annaly, MC	1923–52	
Major-General Sir Hereward Wake, 13th Bt., CB, CMG, DSO	1923–48	
Lieut.-Colonel H. G. Sotheby, DSO, MVO	1924–54	
Major C. J. C. Maunsell	1925–48	
The Lord Brooke of Oakley	1928–44	
Lieutenant-Colonel Geoffrey Elwes	1929–32	
Stephen Schilizzi, Esq., OBE	1929–47	
Miss Mary Bouverie, OBE	1929–41	
Colonel N. V. Stopford Sackville, OBE	1930–48	
Sir Kenneth Murchison	1932–52	*
Colonel T. A. Thornton CVO	1932–77	*
W. M. Plevins, Esq.	1933–40	
Captain G. E. Bellville	1934–67	*
F. Vincent Gompertz, Esq., CIE	1933–54	
The Rt. Hon. Sir George Stanley, GCSI, GCIE, GMG	1936–8	
Rear-Admiral Sir Wellwood Maxwell, KBE, CMG	1937–65	*
Mrs Wentworth Watson	1937–52	
The 6th Lord Braye	1937–52	*
Mrs. St. John Mildmay	1937–50	
Brigadier-General M. F. Gage, DSO	1938–50	
Major J. Cross	1939–55	
R. W. F. Cartwright, Esq.	1940–3	
Mrs Scott Robson	1941–4	
A. E. S. Guinness, Esq.	1942–8	
Lieutenant-Colonel P. Y. Atkinson, MC	1942–51	
The 7th Earl Spencer, TD	1943–67	
Captain P. H. Wykeham, MC	1944–57	
Major J. C. Grant-Ives	1947–57	

H. C. M. Stockdale, Esq.	1947–81	*
Major Sir Reginald Macdonald-Buchanan, KCVO, MBE, MC	1949–66	
Major Sir Hereward Wake, 14th Bt., MC	1949–85	*
The Viscountess Dilhorne	1950–63	
Sir Gyles Isham, 12th Bt.	1952–76	*
Lieutenant-Colonel R. A. Collins, DSO	1953–71	
Lieutenant Colonel Sir R. L. Findlay, 3rd Bt.	1954–9	
The 8th Earl Spencer, LVO	1955–8	
Admiral Sir Geoffrey Hawkins, KBE, CB, MVO, DSC	1956–80	*
Lieutenant-Colonel A. V. C. Robarts	1956–82	
Lieutenant-Colonel John Chandos-Pole, CVO, OBE	1957–	*
Lieutenant-Colonel D. D. P. Smyly, DSO	1957–66	
Mrs T. A. Thornton	1957–64	
Major R. Chaplin	1958–68	
Major J. K. Maxwell, MC	1960–78	
G. W. Nickson, Esq.	1960–5	
Lieutenant-Colonel P. W. Dollar	1963–84	*
Derek Lawson, Esq.	1963–84	
Mrs H. V. Phelps	1964–8	
Colonel Ivo Reid, OBE	1964–	
S. F. Bennett, Esq.	1966–78	
The 2nd Viscount Kemsley	1966–	
Mrs J. Morgan	1967–	
Major P. de. L. Cazenove, TD	1968–75	
Major J. M. Fearfield	1968–	
Mrs H. C. Henderson	1968–	
Michael Robinson, Esq., OBE	1968–70	
Mrs R. N. Richmond-Watson	1970–	
Christopher Davidge, Esq., OBE	1971–	
J. L. Lowther, Esq., CBE	1971–	
The Viscountess Ward of Witley	1972–8	
A. J. Macdonald-Buchanan, Esq.	1972–80	
Major David Watts-Russell	1973–9	
Lionel Stopford Sackville	1974–	
R. T. Gibbs, Esq.	1974–	
J. S. Schilizzi, Esq.	1974–85	*
Mrs A. B. X. Fenwick	1976–	
The 7th Marquess of Northampton	1977–85	
The Lady Braye	1978–	
H. deL. Cazenove, Esq.	1978–	

Governors, 1988
(Not members of the Management Committee)

Robert Fellowes, Esq.

A. N. Foster, Esq.

A. G. Heritage, Esq.

Captain J. Macdonald-Buchanan, MC

The Lord McGowan

W. D. Morton, Esq, CBE

The Marquess of Northampton

Peterborough, The Rt. Rev. Wm.
  Westwood, Bishop of

Mrs Peter Player

S. J. Richmond-Watson, Esq.

Professor Sir Martin Roth

Colonel Lord George Scott

The Earl Spencer, LVO

Sir James Spooner

Mrs J. M. Tice

Medical Superintendents

Dr T. O. Prichard 1838–45

Dr P. R. Nesbitt 1845–60

Dr E. Wing 1860–5

Dr J. Bayley 1865–1912

Dr D. Rambaut 1913–37

Dr T. Tennent 1937–62

Dr D. J. O'Connell 1962–6

Dr J. Harper 1966–75

Dr G. Tennent 1975–1984

Dr J. H. Henderson 1985–

INDEX